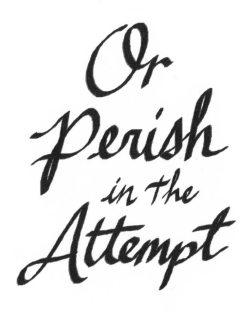

Or Perish in the Attempt

Wilderness Medicine

 *in the*

Lewis & Clark Expedition

By David J. Pe

Foreword by Moira Ambrose • Illustrations by R.P. "Bob" Morgan

ISBN: 1-56037-226-5 hardbound
1-56037-225-7 softbound
Library of Congress Control Number:
2002102970
© 2002 Farcountry Press

For more information on our books write:
Farcountry Press, P.O. Box 5630, Helena,
MT 59604; or call: (800) 821-3874; or visit
www.farcountrypress.com
Created, produced, and designed in the
United States. Printed in Canada.

For Marti

My wife, best friend,

and a clear voice in the wilderness

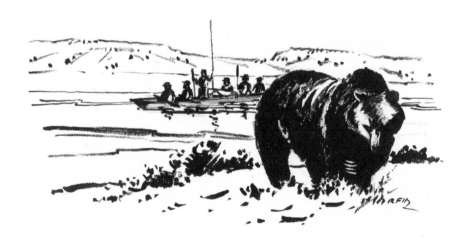

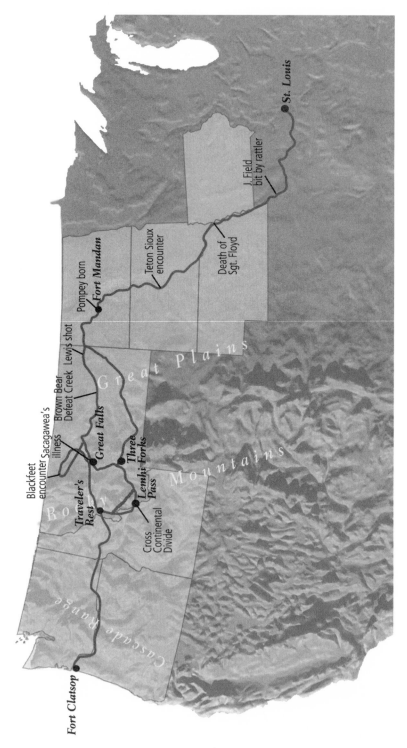

St. Louis

J. Field
bit by rattler

Death of
Sgt. Floyd

Teton Sioux
encounter

Fort Mandan
Pompey born

Lewis shot
Defeat Creek
Brown Bear

Sacagawea's
illness

Blackfeet
encounter

Great Falls

Three
Forks

Lemhi
Pass

Cross
Continental
Divide

Traveler's
Rest

Great Plains

Rocky Mountains

Cascade Range

Fort Clatsop

4

CONTENTS

Acknowledgments

Sometime during the several hundred hours I spent researching material in preparation for a lecture I presented to the annual University of California San Diego Wilderness Medicine Conference in the summer of 2000, my wife Marti encouraged me to write a book about the topic of my lecture: "The Lewis and Clark Expedition: Wilderness Medicine in Early America." I quickly came up with a couple of reasons why I would not do that. Not then...not ever!

During a canoe trip on the Missouri River in May 2000, through the White Cliffs area, my friend David Hendrick, after hearing me babble for hours about the expedition and medicine, asked me why I didn't write a book about it. I told him the same couple of reasons I had told my wife, but this time with less conviction. By the end of the trip, my resistance was replaced with enthusiasm. I came home full of ideas and started writing about my two favorite aspects of the trip: the wilderness experience of the Corps of Discovery and the medicine of the era. In your hands rests the product.

Special thanks to all the following people and special apologies to the many more who in some way helped me accomplish this labor of love:

my maternal grandparents, Frank and Anna Beniger, who left Europe in the early 20th century and came to Montana on their own voyage of discovery and gave me so many wonderful childhood memories;

Mom and Dad, Ann and Leonard Peck, for their love, encouragement, support, and patience, and for allowing me to run around the hills and wade through the creeks of Santa Barbara, and then taking me to Montana to do the same;

Justin, my son whose antelope hunt and poem about Montana are still talked about around campfires in the "Big Sky Country";

my Montana aunts: Funsie Hysell and her husband, Floyd, of East Helena, who took me camping and gave me the opportunity to become addicted to those good times by a babbling creek and crackling camp-fire, and their daughter Kim Waltee and her husband Mark for all the fun times we've shared; Elsie Magennis and her husband Ernie for all they have given to me during my life; Dolly Hanshaw and her late husband, Bob, for supplying me with so many good memories; and my uncle Frank Beniger, who sat with me by Prickly Pear Creek and showed me how to pan gold;

Keith and Becky Bortnem and Keith's dad, Al Bortnem, all of Great Falls, for their friendship all these years since medical school, all our great outdoor adventures on the Missouri and in the Little Belt Mountains, and for all those nights I've spent on their living room sofa;

my brother Leonard, holder of twenty-one patents in infrared technology during his thirty years with Hughes Aircraft, for his help with ballistics, physics, and general research, and my brother Randy, who was always willing to answer a physics question on the phone even though he was too busy designing and building his high-tech machines. They are the smart ones in the family;

my friends David Hendrick and his wife Stephanie Nigh, who always liked what I wrote and offered endless encouragement during the early days of this manuscript;

Moira Ambrose for graciously reading my original manuscript and offering valuable suggestions and encouragement, and her husband Steve for writing *Undaunted Courage* and all his other books that have enriched my life;

my editor, Barbara Fifer, for her good humor, professionalism, literary insights, and Lewis and Clark scholarship;

Deirdre Price, Ph.D., for her valuable advice with editing.

all my former students of biology at McClintock High School, Tempe, Arizona;

Gary E. Moulton for his fabulous edition of *The Journals of the Lewis & Clark Expedition*;

Mr. Bard Salcido, M.A., my fabulous college American history professor, Santa Barbara, California;

all my friends at Sharp Rees-Stealy Medical Group, Inc., San Diego, California;

and the following people, who graciously gave advice, feedback, or help on various aspects of the text:

Brian Acord, M.D., Sharp Rees-Stealy Medical Group, San Diego, Department of Obstetrics and Gynecology;

Keith Aune, Ph.D., Montana Department of Fish, Wildlife and Parks Wildlife Research Lab, Bozeman;

Keith Bortnem, D.O., Great Falls Orthopedic Associates, Montana;

Jeff Broadbent, Ph.D., Assistant Professor of Food Microbiology (and my former student in high school biology), Utah State University, Logan;

Robert S. Cox, Manuscripts Librarian, American Philosophical Society, Philadelphia, Pennsylvania;

Todd Damrow, Ph.D., M.P.H., Montana Department of Public Health, Helena;

Gordon Defendorf, Montana Historical Society, Helena;

Bena Fisher, M.D., Department of Neurology, Sharp Rees-Stealy Medical Group, San Diego, California;

Bill Foreyt, Ph.D., Professor of Veterinary Parasitology, Washington State University, Pullman;

Fred Fung, M.D., Medical Toxicology, Sharp Rees-Stealy Medical Group, San Diego, California;

Lee Grunden, Ph.D., Professor Emeritus of Pharmacology, Western University of Health Sciences, Pomona, California;

Betty Hall, Lewis & Clark Trail Heritage Foundation, Great Falls, Montana;

Ken Marr, Ph.D., Adjunct Assistant Prof. of Botany, University of Montana, Missoula, Montana;

Leland Rickman, M.D., Division of Infectious Diseases, University of California at San Diego.

Tom Schwan, Ph.D., Medical Entomology, Rocky Mountain Labs, Hamilton, Montana;

Jeremy Skinner, Librarian, Lewis & Clark National Historic Trail Interpretive Center, Great Falls, Montana;

Ellen Steinsapir, M.D., Department of Urgent Care, Sharp Rees-Stealy Medical Group, San Diego, California;

David Worley, Ph.D., Professor Emeritus of Veterinary Parasitology, Montana State University, Bozeman;

Garo Yerevanian, M.D., Department of General Surgery, Sharp Rees-Stealy Medical Group, San Diego, California;

Foreword

Toward the end of August 1975, our family stopped to visit Aunt Lois Ambrose at her house in Bloomington, Illinois, on our way home to New Orleans for the school year. Before parting, Aunt Lois gave my husband, Stephen Ambrose, a history professor at the University of New Orleans, the Biddle Edition of the Journals of Lewis and Clark. Once home he commenced reading them. That autumn, whether gathered in the shady garden or around the dinner table, he began to tell us what the Corps of Discovery was up to. He'd bring a volume from the Thwaites Edition to read aloud to us. He adopted the pronunciation of these 18th century Virginians who'd kept their journals in the early 19th century. We began to know them. Their favorite expressions, "We Proceeded On," "Muskeetors verry trublesom," "Rained the forepart of the day," entered our speech. Our conversations included the Captains and York. Sacajawea, Pompey, Charbonneau—why, we had friends in New Orleans with that name! Drewyer, Colter, Shannon took up places in our imaginations. They had made this most excellent journey together, across the unknown Louisiana Purchase and beyond. Oh, what a story!

At the peak of family goodwill that Christmas morning Steve asked us all to consider what we should do to celebrate the Bicentennial of the United States. Our faces turned toward his, eyes wide, hearts thumping. Who would say it first? Who would be the one to call out, "We Proceeded On" or "Ocian in view—O the Joy"? Stephenie would be sixteen in April, Barry fourteen in March, Andrew twelve, Grace just ten, and Hugh eight. They were tried and true campers from the beginning of our blended family, and they were unanimous. They enlisted their great friend Mickey Fluitt, nineteen years old, artist and college student whose enthusiasm matched their own.

He painted "Lewis and Clark Expedition" across the front of the pickup truck so it could be read in rear view mirrors. The "Corps of Discovery '76" decorated the VW bus. Cassettes of the Beatles, Earl Scruggs, the Moody Blues, Bob Dylan, and Joan Baez, bags of M&Ms and raisins, quarters, magic tricks, crayons, paper, pens, books went in with the camping gear and the food staples, red beans, brown rice, chicory coffee, and granola. Two canoes went on top of the pickup. Grace brought her bike lashed on the back. The dog, Bib, took his place. We proceeded on, timed to leave Wood River, Illinois on May 14 just like the captains.

Steve consulted his maps and the Journals to put our evening camps in the locations described by the captains. Though the Missouri River was much changed, we paddled Independence Creek and visited Sgt. Floyd's bluff. The farther west we went the closer we got to their path. When we reached Montana we ventured off the trail to replenish our store of books and treats at the University of Montana Copper Commons.

There we found *Only One Man Died*, a medical history of the Corps of Discovery written by "Frenchy" Chuinard, M.D. It proved to be an eye-opening read for us. From then on we included that aspect in our acquaintance with the sites as Stephen continued to read aloud to us what the Journals told of each one. We hiked to the sulphur spring where Lewis had gone to prepare the vile drink to help Sacajawea in her illness. We marvelled at the endurance and good luck of the Corps—no bones broken, no wound that didn't heal. We reached their camp Fort Clatsop on the Pacific Ocean—O the Joy—we made it home safe and sound. Stephenie made her plans for the University of Montana. We all expected to return to the scenes of visionary enchantment. We did.

Years later with the publication of *Undaunted Courage*, a young physician made our acquaintance. His love of the trail, the captains, the Corps matched Stephen's and mine. His knowledge of medicine and his experience as a practicing physician brought a new depth of interest to our discussions of this achievement in U.S. history. We got to know one another. He was building a log cabin in Montana. The log cabin going up for us wasn't far from his site. We met his wife, and Dr. David and Dr. Marti Peck entered our lives.

At dinner at their cabin one evening in 1999, Dave brought up a medical history of the Corps illustrated with his own excellent photographs of important sites. He'd made charcoal portraits of the main characters in U.S. medicine in that period. He'd prepared it to present to his peers at an annual wilderness medicine convention. That evening Dave showed us a few of the photographs and talked about the high points of the narrative. In his opinion, the Corps, with regard to their medical supplies and practice were definitely, "up the creek without a paddle," as Dave first thought of calling this book.

By the fall of 2000, Dr. Peck had completed his manuscript. He sent it to me to read. I was captured by the vigorous description he wrote for each of the medical episodes in the Journals of Lewis and Clark. The solid ground of my understanding I'd felt so confident upon opened up before me full of bacteria, venoms, viruses, exhaustion, wild animals, and the greatest example of general good luck in the history of U.S. exploration. Dr. Peck gives us a detailed colorful canvas of the state of U.S. medicine at the turn of the 19th century by introducing us to the physicians of the day and the medical men who taught them. This book holds up our national epic to the light of modern medical knowledge to the wonder, delight, and gratitude of the reader. Read it for the thrill. Enjoy!

Moira Ambrose
Helena, Montana
August 2001

Introduction

I had the great fortune to be raised by a family with ties to Montana. Although I grew up in Santa Barbara, California, roaming on the beach and sliding on old cardboard boxes down hillsides of dry wild oats, I spent many days of youthful bliss with my mother's family in western Montana doing the outdoor activities that many kids just dream about. Fishing with my grandfather on blue-ribbon trout streams, camping in the western Montana mountains, panning for gold or just sitting by the side of a clear mountain creek, provided me with enough daydreams for the rest of my life.

As I have moved into my adult years, new Montana experiences have been added. Introducing my son Justin to the same fascinations that captivated me as a young person, building a log cabin, more hunting and fishing trips, trail riding with friends in the deep woods, and an intense interest in the history of the area, have added to the quality of my life in ways I can never fully express in words. Part of my early exposure to Montana also included a superficial knowledge of the Lewis and Clark Expedition.

Through the years, many books have been written about numerous aspects of this epic trip and great American adventure. Then I received a copy of Stephen Ambrose's fascinating account of the expedition, *Undaunted Courage: Meriwether Lewis, Thomas Jefferson and the Opening of the American West*, as a birthday present from my wife. It provided the critical mass that sparked my deep interest in the expedition and led to this book.

Or Perish in the Attempt is a book about medicine and science as practiced and conceived in the early 19th century, and the numerous wilderness adventures and hardships that threatened this small band in the hostile environment of unexplored America of 1804-1806. Quotes from expedition journals have been reproduced with the captains' original and very creative spelling, as presented in the edition so excellently edited by Gary E. Moulton and published by University of Nebraska Press.

The field of wilderness medicine encompasses a wide variety of health issues, such as hypothermia, heat-related illnesses, animal envenomations and attacks, high-altitude sickness, and food- and water-related issues. The Lewis and Clark Expedition was truly the epitome of the wilderness medicine experience. They encountered a multitude of medical problems during their twenty-eight-month stay in the wild.

As a physician, I enjoyed peering back into the world of science that gave birth to the medicine of the expedition. The stairway of progress is often built on individual steps of error and faulty assumptions. Scientific and medical advances are the result of the incorrect ideas of yesteryear which, when disproved, led to new experimentation and discovery. The medical beliefs of the early 1800s were a morass of incorrect assumptions, based on faulty ideas concerning the nature of the human body and disease. The medical practice that resulted was equally inadequate, which makes the great success of the Corps of Discovery an even more remarkable feat. (If readers want to more fully appreciate the medicine of Lewis and Clark, they will enjoy reading Appendix One before reading Chapter 3. This material briefly covers the evolution of western medical thought from antiquity to the time of Lewis and Clark.)

I often think—while repairing a wound or examining a patient with severe abdominal pain—what a tremendous weight it must have been for Lewis and Clark to handle these same problems with none of the knowledge, training or experience I have acquired over the last seventeen years. They had no laboratory to check their patient's blood count or computerized scanners to look into an abdomen. The hands the captains laid on the bodies of their patients were not those of trained physicians. They didn't possess even the rudimentary medical training that an 1803 physician had. They had what amounted to a few weeks of first aid training and some practical medical knowledge obtained during their army careers. Their challenge was staggering—their luck was phenomenal!

As an outdoorsman, some of the most thrilling moments of my life have been while sitting atop the Bitterroot Mountains with gale force winds blowing me around, looking in every direction as the captains did, and seeing...more mountains; canoeing through the White Cliffs of the Missouri River past the enchanted rock formations and sleeping under the stars—the same stars that York, Sacagawea and John Ordway gazed at as they drifted off to sleep; looking upward while boating through the Gates of the Mountains, that five-mile, rock-lined spectacle on the Missouri River near Helena, Montana.

I have ultimately written this book so that the physician/teacher/historian/scientist within me can gain a greater understanding and, thereby, a greater appreciation for this fascinating topic. As a lover of the outdoors and the adventure it offers, I can walk the trails with my friends of two hundred years ago and allow myself to relive the expedition in my own small way. I will never experience being a member of the Corps of Discovery, in part, because I was born 175 years too late. But in my sometimes overly romantic imagination, I see myself with those hearty men somewhere in the Rocky Mountains, carrying my own 1803 Harpers Ferry rifle, stalking an elk with George Drouillard or playing my banjo along with Pierre Cruzatte and his fiddle around the campfire, somewhere along the banks of the great Missouri or in the thick evergreen forests of Oregon.

But should the truth be known, I could not have made that trip. In my physical prime, which was years ago, I would not have finished a week with these tough men; rowing and towing their boats up the Missouri, climbing thousands of feet up a steep Bitterroot slope in eight inches of snow, running for their lives from an enraged grizzly bear, or sitting around a campfire, pulling inch-long cactus spines from the soles of their feet. As close as I'll get is to travel and visit some of the areas that these heroes visited and to imagine their adventures through eight thousand miles of early American wilderness.

I invite you along, and hope that you discover some of the same magical admiration I feel for the men of the Corps of Discovery. The wilderness adventures and incredible hardships they experienced are the epic of the American wilderness story. The wilderness medicine that they practiced was at various times both surprisingly wise and incredibly ignorant. Although the Corps of Discovery certainly ranks as one of the greatest explorations of all time, the group was, at least in a medical sense, profoundly unprepared.

If you are ready, pack your gear, sense of curiosity, and imagination, and let's get started!

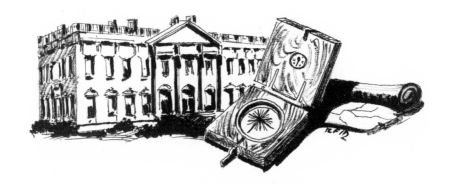

🌿 1 🌿

POLITICS AND PASSION

The Exploration of the American Wilderness

I can't say I was ever lost, but I was bewildered once for three days.
—*Daniel Boone*

A love for the wilderness and outdoor adventure are born into the heart and mind of nearly every American, or, at the least, learned early in life. It is nurtured and grows in some more than in others, but it is difficult to grow up in the United States without a strong love of the vast open expanses with which we North Americans are blessed. Coupled with our love of the wilderness comes a fascination with the people who blazed the trails into the wild. That sense of awe and admiration for these pathfinders is cultivated and personified by American icons of the wilderness, men such as Jim Bridger, Kit Carson, Joe Walker, John Muir, Richard Byrd, and the most famous of all, Meriwether Lewis and William Clark.

Even if one has never visited the wilderness, nearly any city dweller in America that you might stop on the street could tell you something about the Grand Canyon, Old Faithful Geyser, the Everglades, or the Grand Tetons.

Some experience wilderness and its adventure in rather normal ways: camping, photography, backpacking, fishing, hunting, or skiing. Others are more radical in their tastes and perform death-defying (-seeking?) feats by kayaking off 100-foot waterfalls, ice diving, or participating in extreme treks. The majority are content to relax in a lounge chair with a soda or beer and a bag of chips, watching travel and adventure programs on the tube. Any way we do it, Americans love the outdoors and we love the idea of exploration, challenge, and adventure.

Inherent in these activities is the factor of competition. It's us against Mother Nature. We marvel at the Iditarod sled race and at the tenacity of men and women, as we watch their teams of dogs pull them over narrow snowy trails for a thousand miles, through wintry Alaskan forests, even through the dead of night. We wonder at the physical stamina of athletes competing for three weeks in the Tour de France bicycle race. We stand in awe of the surfer who has the courage to catch a thirty-foot wave, and we wait to see whether he successfully rides it or gets swallowed by several tons of water. We love to experience, either first hand or vicariously, the challenge and thrill of a dangerous and risky physical adventure.

This is why we Americans love Lewis and Clark and their band of hardy explorers. In their story the fullness of the wilderness and its daunting physical demands are fused indelibly together, wrapped in a setting of an adventurous era, staged in lands of stunning beauty, and made relevant by our collective American experience. Those of us living in the 21st century are able to visit many areas in the American west that are virtually unchanged from the time when Lewis and Clark explored them. We can walk on the trails that once showed their moccasin prints, read their journals, camp at their campsites, and experience their thoughts, frustrations, fears, and excitement.

North America in the early 1800s was a land ripe for exploration. The majority of the 5.5 million Americans who were living at the beginning of the 19th century lived within fifty miles of the eastern seaboard.[1] Our eastern coast had been under Euro-American settlement for nearly a century and a half, and urban centers in the east were buzzing with activity. The major cities of Boston, New York, and Philadelphia were growing steadily, offering the era's city comforts and conveniences.

But optimistic and inspired immigrants who came to the United States in search of political freedom and a piece of the economic action, and those restless Americans who did not want to live as domesticated city-folk, provided a constant tide pushing against the North American wilderness. These people required land on which to build cabins, grow crops, and raise families and livestock. Those who were inclined not even to follow the farming life set out to virgin territory, to explore new lands or obtain furs, and to be a part of the progressing boundary of the frontier. West of the Appalachians were vast areas of virgin forests, land waiting to be cleared and settled, areas where a man and his family could live unencumbered by city life or even escape all contact with civilized living.

Fifty years prior to our independence from England in 1776, various ethnic groups, including German and Scots Irish immigrants, had pushed the line of the frontier westward into the Shenandoah Valley of Virginia and Carolinas and up the Mohawk River in New York. By the time of the American Revolution, the frontier had been moved to Kentucky and Tennessee and the upper Ohio River Valley.[2] In the early 1800s, heading west meant opportunity and freedom as well as possible riches, many dangers, backbreaking hardships, and certain adventure.

The fire of westward expansion was also being fueled by large land owners in the South who needed fresh land to grow their crops of tobacco and cotton. Farther north, in the Ohio Valley, vast forests were cleared for farms producing corn and other crops. Whether for money or personal independence, people needed land, and thus the edge of civilization steadily progressed farther west towards the Mississippi River.

But, in early 1803, the United States ended at the Mississippi River. England, Spain, France, and Russia all had interests in securing portions of North America. In the words of historian Robert Leckie, "the French had sought fur, the Spanish gold and the English land."[3] Although distant nations had dreams of holding land in North America,

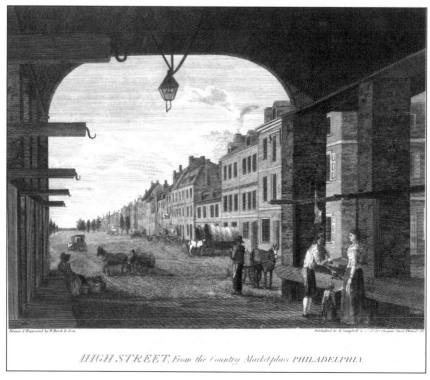

A Philadelphia market about the time Lewis was there. LIBRARY OF CONGRESS, LC-USZ62-3239

thousands of miles of Atlantic and Pacific oceans made the dreams hard to fulfill. Support for civilian populations and military troops in a land so far away was difficult at best.

France claimed the wilderness lands immediately west of the Mississippi, and beyond that the Missouri River drainage. The British and Russians also had their eyes on the continent's expansive open lands and its financially attractive fur trade. The surface of the wealth available through trapping beaver had only been scratched. British influence by way of the fur trade was pushing southward from Canada and was being felt in the upper Missouri River area (in what today is North and South Dakota) through commerce with the Indian tribes. The British fur companies operating in the area provided Indians with guns and goods in exchange for beaver pelts that brought a handsome profit when shipped to London. Control of the continent and its great wealth was in hot dispute. If the young United States of America wanted to expand, something would have to change.

Well, change it did. In 1803, Napoleon Bonaparte of France decided that his hold on France's land in North America was weakening. In order to keep the vast territory of Louisiana, numerous troops would have to occupy the area and be supplied by ships sailing from France. Ultimately, French citizens would need to settle here. With his frequent sorties against the British, Napoleon did not want to risk losing Louisiana to England, should his military fortunes go sour, as they did at the hands of rebel slaves in Haiti in 1801. Napoleon sent French troops to Haiti, led by his brother General LeClerc, to subdue the insurrection. More than 27,000 Frenchmen, including his brother, were wiped out by an epidemic of yellow fever.[4] To make the best of a bad situation, the French emperor offered to sell France's entire North American land holdings, nearly 827,000 square miles, to the United States for $15 million, about $18.14 per square mile. In the third year of his first term, President Thomas Jefferson thought this French pastry too tempting to resist and jumped at the offer. The U.S. Senate ratified the deal on October 20 of 1803. On the morning of October 21, the United States had nearly doubled in size. Much of the vast wilderness west of the Mississippi was now part of America.

The land included in the Louisiana Purchase was virtually unknown to white Americans. Many believed it to be a wasteland filled with sagebrush and ground squirrels. Except for the port of New Orleans and a few settlements on the Mississippi, it seemed an area of plains, forests, and wild animals. Some of the people there were believed to be, according to historian Gary E. Moulton, "numerous, powerful and warlike nations of savages, of gigantic stature, fierce, treacherous and cruel: and particularly hostile to white men."[5] The area was mysterious and uncharted. No white man had set foot farther west in Upper Louisiana than a cluster of Indian villages on the Missouri in what today is North Dakota.

In addition to the 17th and 18th centuries being a time of exploration, they were also a time of great mental awakening in a society that wanted answers to many questions. Science was beginning to unlock many secrets about the nature of the world. Physics had made remarkable progress through the genius of Copernicus, Kepler, Galileo, and

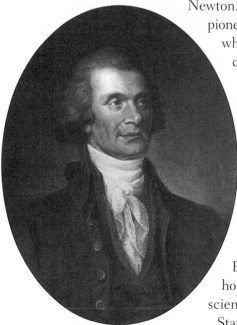

Thomas Jefferson, from a U.S. Capitol mural. LIBRARY OF CONGRESS, LC-D416-9856

Newton. Great Britain's Robert Boyle did pioneering work in the study of gases, while others were exploring the chemical world of strange solutions called acids and bases. Seeking answers through a rational approach to nature led the world into a period called the Enlightenment. America fell in with this European movement, and although early America did not provide a great volume of groundbreaking scientific work, we did have our Benjamin Franklin, David Rittenhouse, and other notable men of science. Fortunately for the United States, we also had a political leader who reveled in these disciplines.

President Thomas Jefferson was one of the most inquisitive and forward-looking individuals of his time. He was a member of the prestigious American Philosophical Society of Philadelphia, whose rolls read as a "Who's Who" of the American scientific community of the early 1800s. Jefferson had intense interests in botany, zoology, ethnology, and geography, and collected information about the western wilderness. Since the 1770s, he had wanted to have the area explored, document its flora and fauna, learn about its inhabitants, and find a feasible river route to the Pacific, the elusive Northwest Passage. In addition, he believed the sometimes belligerent Indians could be pacified. A trading relationship with them would benefit American business interests, but the British were accelerating their trade and trapping activities in the Missouri River Valley and farther west into the mysterious Rocky Mountains. For the Anglophobic Jefferson, an exploration of the area would have to occur quickly. If Jefferson's goals could be accomplished, British and Spanish influence would be minimized in the shadow cast by the Americans.

Several failed attempts had been made to explore the area during the later 1700s. Now that the Louisiana territory belonged to the United States, it was vital to investigate this region, gain scientific information about the land, solidify our possession of it and, in general, get to know our new backyard. Jefferson proposed to Congress to send a group up the Missouri River to its headwaters and over the range of mountains, then onward to locate the Columbia River and follow it to the Pacific. (American sailors under Robert Gray had located the Columbia's estuary in 1792, and named the river that flowed west into it.)

Considerations about the proposed trip required great wisdom in choosing the route, size of the exploration team, its goals, needed supplies, and plans for contingencies including probable contact with belligerent natives. A key decision President Jefferson faced was: Who would command this exploration? The leader would need numerous talents and abilities.

For starters, the commander must be able to make scientific observations and accurately record what he witnessed. The area would need to be mapped, so the leader would have to be able to calculate latitude and longitude. He would then have to draw accurate maps of the areas through which he travelled. He would have to describe in a scientific manner any biological discoveries. The leader would have to know a great deal about the flora and fauna in the eastern United States so that he would be able to identify which plants and animals were new to science in the western region. His mind would have to be inquisitive and his eye remarkably observant. An ability to inspire confidence in his men would tax his leadership talents.

He would have to be knowledgeable about mineralogy and geology. He needed diplomatic abilities for meeting Indian tribes and French and British nationals along the Missouri. All would have to be effectively, firmly, but respectfully dealt with, and informed that they were now operating within United States territory. The leader would also be responsible for the physical welfare of the men who accompanied him on the trip.

This was to be a military operation, a reconnaissance "in force"—Jefferson hoped for a peaceful foray, but there was no guarantee of that. Enough uncertainties were involved to make even the most confident leader a bit uneasy. The distance of the proposed trip was unknown, and it would have to be covered by boat, foot, and horseback. The talent and toughness required of such a leader, and the commitment required to complete all these tasks, coupled with the strength and endurance required for the daily grind of the exhausting work eliminated all but the hardiest and most intelligent. And, of course, getting to the Pacific was just half the battle; they would have to come back. Accomplishing the first half of the trip would be fruitless if they could not return with their new-found information. Who in the world could ever qualify for all that would be required?

President Jefferson already had someone in mind, and the person lived in his house.

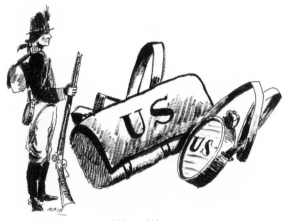

MERIWETHER LEWIS AND WILLIAM CLARK

The Right Stuff of 1803

A Friend may well be reckoned the masterpiece of Nature.
—Ralph Waldo Emerson

The leader of the exploration of North America would be none other than a boy from Jefferson's neighborhood. A young man who grew up in the woods, who became a United States Army officer, and then came to live in the President's mansion, at the request of the President himself. This man was the President's personal secretary, Captain Meriwether Lewis, a twenty-eight-year-old fellow Virginian whom Jefferson described as having a "firmness of constitution & character, prudence, habits adapted to the woods, & a familiarity with the Indian manners & character, requisite for this undertaking."[1]

August 18, 1774, Lewis's birth date, was probably a sultry day in Albemarle County, Virginia Colony. Within walking distance of the

Lewis home was Monticello, the estate of the thirty-one-year-old Thomas Jefferson, the learned, wealthy, and influential citizen already involved in the movement to break its American colonies away from Great Britain. Four-year-old sister Jane probably awaited baby Meriwether's coming with anticipation. The proud parents were William Lewis and his wife and first cousin, Lucy Meriwether Lewis. William's family had been in America since 1635, and owned large tracts of land in Virginia. A third Lewis child, Rueben, was added to the clan in 1777.

Meriwether was born into relative comfort, but his position did not result in having uncalloused hands. As a young boy, Meriwether loved the outdoors and roamed the Virginia woods, becoming as comfortable in the outdoors as he was inside his home. When he was only eight years old, he frequently went out in the dead of night with his dogs to hunt and trap raccoons and possums in the forest. Season and weather conditions mattered little to the young Lewis as this outdoor boy even plowed through frozen streams in pursuit of his quarry. Writing in later years, a family friend noted that the boy had "the highest degree of self-possession in danger."[2]

Part of Lewis's early outdoor education came by way of his mother. Lucy was a self-sufficient frontier woman as well as a noted herbal doctor of the area. Although lacking a formal medical education, she created many of her own remedies and utilized them to treat her family and others who sought her care. Undoubtedly, young Meriwether learned first-hand about herbal medications and their use from his mother, treatments that were the backbone of medicine in the early 1800s.

That Lucy Lewis knew a good deal about doctoring and herbs was not enough to save her husband from an early death in 1779, however. After falling off his horse into a rain-swollen stream in November while returning to the Revolutionary battlefield from a leave at home, William Lewis took sick with a fever and cough. With nine-year-old Jane, four-year-old Meriwether and two-year-old Reuben likely keeping vigil by the fireside, their father's condition deteriorated quickly in spite of probable application to his chest of the best and freshest herbal poultices available in Albemarle County. Within days he was dead, probably the victim of the "chief of the four horseman of death"—pneumonia.

Already possessing a good deal of outdoor knowledge, and a rudimentary medical-botanical background, Lewis started to develop his leadership skills as a young man of twenty. Looking for more excitement than life as a farm manager offered, the youth enlisted in the Virginia militia, which was called out by President Washington in 1794 to put down the "Whiskey Rebellion." The revolt in western Pennsylvania was sparked and fueled by frontiersmen's refusal to pay federal taxes levied on their whiskey. Serving first as a private, Lewis seemed well suited to military life, and he was promoted later that year to officer ranks, becoming an ensign. In 1795, Ensign Lewis joined the regular army.

Within miles of Lewis's birthplace, on the day he was born, a young boy was probably running around his Virginia home, tormenting his siblings or aiding with the family chores. That four-year-old lad was William Clark.

The genes that express themselves in a man's mental and physical toughness certainly existed in the Clark family. Few could boast of having an older brother as revered in the annals of adventurers as George Rogers Clark. William was born of Scottish background on a farm in Caroline County, Virginia in 1770. The Clark family knew Thomas Jefferson as they had previously resided in a log cabin near present Charlottesville and Jefferson's home of Monticello.[3] The Clark family was quite a flock, with six sons and four daughters, with William being the ninth of the ten children. Military service to the United States was highly esteemed in the Clark family; the older brothers all fought in the Revolution, and four of the six Clark boys, including William, would become high ranking officers.[4]

During some of the darker days of the American Revolution in 1778, days when the outcome of the war for independence leaned in favor of the British, great bloodshed took place in the Ohio River valley. Americans who lived on this frontier were few and isolated. The British took advantage of this by supplying and encouraging hostile Indian tribes to strike at American settlements. The Indian attacks were vicious and merciless, killing and scalping American settlers of all ages, male and female.

Someone was needed to silence the British and their Indian allies. The Virginian who answered this call was General George Rogers Clark, of Virginia. General Clark and his militia of 127 men endured horrific hardships and marched for seventeen days through icy forests and swamps to capture a British fort at Vincennes, Illinois Territory. Other military actions, in 1780, against the Shawnee Tribe in the Ohio Valley, have indelibly written George Rogers Clark's name in American Revolutionary hall of fame.[5] All this occurred while this man's younger brother, eight-year-old, red-haired, explorer-in-training William, was at home in Virginia, playing soldier.

In 1784, three years after the revolution's final shot, the Clark family pulled up their Virginia roots. Fourteen-year-old William and his family moved down the Ohio River to Louisville, Kentucky, settling near one of the forts that George had built during his campaign against the British in 1778. On this edge of civilization, in a splendid wilderness with all its fascinations and dangers, William Clark grew to manhood. He loved the outdoor life and hearing George's stories about his adventures, and the hardships during that frozen winter of 1778-1779.

At nineteen, William joined the militia and was soon promoted to the rank of captain. In 1791, he transferred to the regular U.S. Army as an ensign, and became a lieutenant in March of 1792, under the command of "Mad" Anthony Wayne, the rash but splendid fighting general of the American Revolution. Until 1796, when he resigned his Army commission and returned to Kentucky, Lt. Clark distinguished himself as an able commander and a brave soldier. During one episode, commanding seventy men and a packtrain of seven hundred horses, Lt. Clark drove off a larger force of attacking Indians, winning tributes from General Wayne. Enjoying Wayne's great confidence, young Clark was also sent on several sensitive and demanding trips into Spanish territory along the Mississippi River in present-day Missouri and Tennessee, gaining intelligence on Spanish military fortifications and activities. During one of his missions, he met with Spanish officers who occupied a small area of U.S. territory near today's Memphis, informing them, in no unclear terms, that the United States government did not want them there. The Spanish were impressed with this confident young soldier, calling him an "enterprising youth of extraordinary activity." Enjoying the respect of friend and foe, the "extroverted, even-tempered, and gregarious" Lt. Clark was not simply relying on his famous family name, but was making a name for himself.[6]

Most of us can probably look back on our personal histories and pinpoint certain moments when we either made an important decision that turned our lives in a beneficial direction or met an acquaintance who ultimately proved to have a great influence on the course of our lives. The fall of 1795 would prove to be such a time in the lives of both Meriwether Lewis and William Clark. The United States Army provided a meeting ground for the young men who would go on to become icons of American exploration.

America in the late 18th century was hardly a picture of fidelity and harmony. Contentious politics were the rule as the young nation debated various viewpoints on how to run the newly-invented form of government. Most discussion centered on the conflicting philosophies of the Republican and Federalist parties. Jefferson, who had served as Vice President in the John Adams administration, was the leader of the Republican party and champion of its ideals. Jefferson disagreed on almost every issue with the Federalists, headed by President Adams and his Secretary of the Treasury, Alexander Hamilton. Republicans supported a weaker national government, emphasizing the rights of states to govern themselves. The Federalists wanted a strong central government at the expense of states' rights.

The majority of U.S. Army officers in the late 1790s were Federalists, including a young Lt. Eliott who happened to be serving in the same unit as Ens. Lewis. Lewis, on one September evening in 1795, managed to get himself into some very hot water. Under the influence of alcohol, he insulted and slapped Lt. Eliott, apparently after forcing his way inside Eliott's quarters. To make matters worse, he allegedly challenged Eliott to a duel. The twenty-one-year-old Lewis had mixed his emotions, fueled by the energy of youth, with some whiskey, and the result was explosive. A court-martial was initiated, charges were brought and a trial held, but Lewis was found not guilty.[7]

To separate his feuding young officers, General Wayne transferred Lewis to a new unit: the Chosen Rifle company of elite riflemen-sharpshooters, commanded by another young former Virginian, now-Captain William Clark. Through the winter of 1795-1796, then spring and early summer, Lewis and Clark likely had daily contact, talking politics and sharing their life stories. Having spent their boyhood years outdoors in the same neighborhood must have forged a strong bond between them.

In July of 1796, only six months after their meeting, William Clark resigned his army commission and returned to Kentucky. He had taken ill, and his famous brother had fallen on hard times. George was drinking excessively, financially broke, and emotionally drained. These problems called William home. His brother needed his help.

But the admiration between the two young army officers would not be forgotten.

By 1800, Lewis, showing great dependability and leadership, was promoted to captain. His army duties as a paymaster allowed him to travel far and wide on horseback, becoming ever more adept at living outdoors, and gaining confidence in his ability to meet any challenge put in his way. By his twenty-sixth year, Meriwether Lewis was an experienced military leader as well as a tough, knowledgeable, and able outdoorsman. In addition to his star's rising in the army, his old neighbor just happened to be running for the Presidency of the United States.

The Presidential election of 1800 was one of the most contentious in American history. The Electoral College's initial balloting was indecisive, with numerous deals being cut in smoke-filled rooms. In the end, on February 17, 1801, and after thirty-six ballots in the House of Representatives, Thomas Jefferson was elected over the Federalist-sponsored candidate, Aaron Burr. One week later, President-elect Jefferson sat down and dipped his quill into its well of black ink and started writing to a boy who used to live in his neighborhood in Virginia. That young man was now serving as a captain in the army of the United States.

One can only imagine what Captain Lewis was doing during the morning that the letter arrived. Perhaps he just finished some of his paymaster paperwork. Or perhaps he had been outside the fort's log walls, discussing the recent election. An army supply train of horses plodded past the gates of the fort. The soldiers looked forward to these arrivals and the news from the outside world that accompanied them. Letters from parents, brothers and sisters, or sweethearts were highlights in spartan military life. The horses were unloaded and soon mail call was underway. The men crowded closer to try to hear their names called. Captain Lewis perhaps hoped he would get a letter from his mother or brother telling him about his progress in school, or perhaps from one of the pretty young ladies of Virginia he knew. The name "Captain Lewis," is shouted, a letter is extended from an outstretched arm. In the letter, Lewis read:

Dear Sir   *Washington Feb. 23, 1801*

The appointment to the Presidency of the U.S. has rendered it necessary for me to have a private secretary, and in selecting one I have thought it important to respect not only his capacity to aid in the private concerns of the household, but also to contribute to the mass of information which it is interesting for the administration to acquire. Your knolege of the Western country, of the army and of all it's interest & relations has rendered it desireable for public as well as private purposes that you should be engaged in that office... [8]

Undoubtedly, young Lewis's eyes opened a bit wider as he scanned this remarkable invitation to join the highest level of American government. He was being asked to come to the nation's capital and live in the President's House. Who could turn down such an offer? The salary was $500 per year, and the President added the spectacular assurance that "you would be one of my family." Only an utter fool could refuse such an offer, and that fool would certainly not be Meriwether Lewis.

His return letter of March 10 joyfully accepted the invitation. His baggage was soon gathered into bundles and secured on three Army pack horses that trudged their way east on the muddy road to Philadelphia and then another hundred miles through the budding broad-leafed forests to the new capital.

Meanwhile, Jefferson had moved to Washington, D.C., to set up his administration and organize his staff. With a minimum of pomp and circumstance, wearing the clothes of an ordinary citizen and shunning the public extravagance that his two predecessors practiced at their inaugurations, Jefferson went to work. He appointed cabinet members with the names of Madison, Gallatin, Smith, and Dearborn—names that grace some of Montana's splendid rivers today.

By April 1, 1801, Lewis had moved into the partially completed presidential mansion on Pennsylvania Avenue and assumed his duties as private secretary to President Jefferson and his honorary role of "one of my family." This was certainly not army life on the frontier. There were balls, state dinners with foreign diplomats, and long fireside conversations with the President about his many interests, including western exploration. Meriwether Lewis was living a life of privilege and opportunity, and his personal star was destined to rise yet higher.

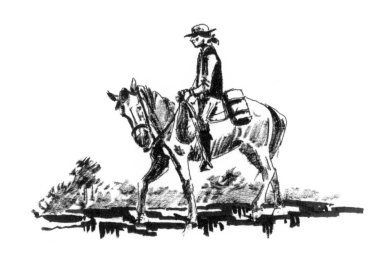

⚛ 3 ⚛

JUST DOING THE BEST WE CAN

Development of American Medicine: 1620-1803

Hemorrhages seldom occur where bleeding has been sufficiently copious.
—*Benjamin Rush*

At this point in our journey, we will depart from the current trail into another section of the historical forest and hike along the narrow, winding, and precarious trail that was early American medicine. What was happening in American medicine would directly influence the medical practice of Lewis and Clark and thus contribute to the success or failure of their mission. Without an understanding of the practice of medicine during the late 18th and early 19th centuries in America, the medicine of Lewis and Clark is bizarre and baffling. With an understanding, the medicine is simply bizarre.

In some ways it is a difficult task for those of us who live in the 21st century to understand the world of two centuries ago and the medical thought of early American physicians. The concepts of germs, contagious diseases, and parasites are at least vaguely familiar to nearly everyone in the modern world. Other forms of disease such as cancers, diabetes, or coronary heart disease are understood in a rudimentary manner by a majority of the general public. Most people have the idea that a cancer grows and ultimately kills, that high blood pressure is not a good thing, and that a high fat diet should be avoided. Nearly everyone knows that it is a good idea to wash your hands after you visit the toilet, and that it is not a good idea to let someone who has a cold or the flu cough in your face.

During most of history, including the time of Lewis and Clark, infectious illnesses in various forms took a staggering number of people into early graves, often with a helpful push from their learned physicians. The viral diseases of smallpox, measles, influenza, and yellow fever mercilessly swept millions of Americans, young and old alike into the great beyond. Bacterial infectious diseases such as diphtheria, tuberculosis and syphilis were other scythes used by the Grim Reaper. Malaria infected millions. The tiny parasite that causes the illness was as yet undiscovered, and the disease was believed to be caused by inhaling air found around swamps. Infectious diseases made living to old age an unlikely proposition, and made the death of a young mother or father, child or infant, a tragically common occurrence. Aside from their own immune systems, people in early America were nearly defenseless against these maladies.

The diseases of aging—such as congestive heart failure, osteoarthritis and stroke—were not as prevalent then. Many Americans alive in 1801 died of infections before they had an opportunity to grow old and suffer from these problems. If our ancestors did live long enough to have their bodies fail from age, treatments for these problems were just as inadequate as those used to fight infection. The medical profession understood virtually nothing about the true nature of disease. There was a great deal of ignorance and it was spread around in a very liberal fashion.

On the day in 1801 when Meriwether Lewis rode into Washington, unloaded his gear and took up his new duties as the President's personal secretary, American physicians were treating thousands of sick patients across the country, in city boarding houses and frontier cabins.

Just Doing the Best We Can

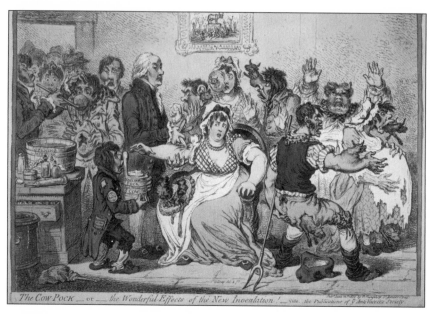

A British cartoon from 1802 portrays Edward Jenner inoculating for smallpox—and the results. LIBRARY OF CONGRESS. LC-USZC4-3147

The patients came with wounds, tumors, breathing difficulties, and fever. Mysterious 19th century names such as apoplexy, imposthume, tissick, timpany, dropsy, and consumption were penned on the medical records of the day. In terms of efficacy, the treatments for these illnesses ranged from mildly helpful to worthless, with many going further down the continuum into the dangerous category.

A visit to your local physician could provide you with a treatment plan that included Bateman's Pectoral Drops of dilute alcohol, opium, red sanders, camphor and anise oil. Bateman's acted as a diaphoretic (sweat inducing) and diuretic (urine producing), thought to rid the body of morbific, or diseased, matter. If you were feeling a bit fatigued, various tonics such as Bitter Infusion, consisting of gentian, orange peel, coriander seeds, and dilute alcohol, would likely spark you up a bit and get you back to your old self. Another popular health tonic was a mixture of dilute sulfuric acid. Skin injuries or irritations could be treated with Goulard's Extract, a cooling wash made of lead salts. Your bowels could be made to move with any number of potent cathartics, in theory removing disease-producing elements lurking in your intestines. Blistering was a process accomplished by the application of ground up beetles to the patient's skin, a process thought to stimulate congested internal organs.

With such varied and ineffective treatments available, it is no wonder that much of the public lacked faith in the medical profession. A poem circulated in Philadelphia outlined the advantages to having two physicians, and summed up the cynicism many Americans felt towards the medical profession during that era:

> One prompt Phisician like a sculler plies,
>   And all his Art, and skill applies;
> But two Phisicians, like a pair of Oars,
>   Convey you soonest to the Stygian Shores.[1]

The physician of the early 19th century was like a hunter with a rubber knife going out in search of a grizzly bear. He very well may be able to find one, but once he did, he would not be able to do anything about it.

Along with faulty assumptions about disease, there was very little formal training available in America for a student of medicine, a situation that probably benefitted the public. In Virginia, only one out of

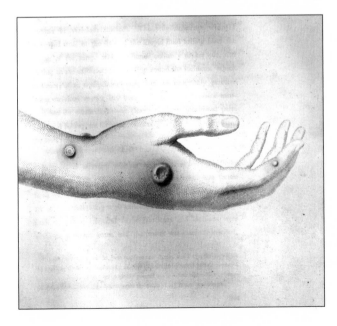

The milkmaid's hand with cowpox blisters from which Jenner developed the smallpox vaccination.
LIBRARY OF CONGRESS.
LC-USZ62-95255

Just Doing the Best We Can

every nine practicing physicians had a medical degree in the early 1800s and, until 1765, there had been no formal academic medical programs in the nation. The vast majority of American physicians had on-the-job-training, serving apprenticeships of five to seven years with experienced physicians. A young man who desired a medical education would petition an established physician, make his interests known, and if the practitioner wanted to take on the ambitious young student, the apprentice would pay the physician for the privilege to come live in his house, do chores, clean the stable, file prescriptions, and gain medical experience by observing and helping his mentor.[2] Practical experience was the route that most young colonials took to become recognized physicians and place M.D.s after their names.

It must be emphasized, though, that lack of formal medical education also had some advantages. The informally trained, apprenticed American physicians received a strong clinical emphasis that stressed patient contact and empirical observation of their treatments. The result was, as historian Daniel Boorstin states, "immediate transfer of wisdom of the practitioner to the student," that often resulted in "the American doctor being a more successful healer in his daily rounds."[3] The lack of formal training spurred American physicians to open-minded experimentation that resulted in improvements in their clinical practices. Lucy Meriwether Lewis was a classic example of this informally trained frontier physician who experimented with herbal treatments (also known as "simples") and their medicinal use.

The terms "botanist" and "physician" were nearly synonymous in the 18th and early 19th centuries, and many physicians came to their practices through a study of botany, and vice versa. Dr. Benjamin Smith Barton, professor of medicine at the University of Pennsylvania and an advisor to Meriwether Lewis, wrote the first comprehensive American work on botany.[4] Common herbs used by European physicians were, of course, often unavailable to American physicians. This biogeographical reality forced Americans to rustle the bushes and find their own efficacious medicinal plants.

Another example of early American medical practice that would influence medicine during the time of the Lewis and Clark Expedition was that of protecting a patient from a deadly infectious disease by introducing some of the "catagion" from a patient who had survived the illness. Such was the procedure employed against the deadly smallpox. Discovered by Turkish physicians and carried to Britain then to colonial America, it was literally and figuratively on the cutting edge of science and medicine at the time.

The Puritan minister Cotton Mather (1663-1728) had used the innovative procedure of inoculation to protect the citizens of Boston during a smallpox epidemic during the early 18th century. Inoculation consisted of taking a bit of infectious material obtained from a blister of a victim of smallpox and placing it into a superficial wound made on the recipient. A small percentage of recipients contracted the severe form of the disease and died, but this new procedure was shown beyond doubt to decrease the incidence of the deadly illness. No one understood why or how it occurred, but the results were undeniable. Great numbers of people were saved from an early grave, and a large trail sign was placed on the previously uncharted path of understanding infectious disease and its treatment.[5]

By 1798, inoculation was replaced by a newer and better procedure—vaccination. This process was developed by the English physician Edward Jenner, who used material from blisters of victims of a milder form of the disease that primarily affected cattle. (Latin *vacca*, for cow, hence vaccination.) Jenner didn't know it at the time, but the cowpox virus is similar to the smallpox virus. The viruses are sufficiently similar to provide the vaccinated human immunity to the more virulent smallpox.[6]

While most practicing physicians from the time of the founding of our country to the early 1800s received their entire medical training through apprenticeship, many affluent and ambitious young Americans who really wanted prestige in the medical world traveled to Europe, often to the University of Edinburgh. Once there, the person would usually study for two years to fulfill the requirements for an M.D. degree. It was here, overlooking the green hills of Scotland, where the academic portion of medical training was provided to young American minds filled with mush. These physicians-in-training came to sit and learn about the latest theories of disease and the human body, supplied by two of the most exalted teachers of the day, Dr. William Cullen and his protege, Dr. John Brown.

Great progress during the 16th and 17th centuries in the fields of chemistry and physics and, to a lesser degree, in biology provided numerous discoveries that influenced physicians to develop theories of disease based on isolated scientific discoveries. Thus the latest exciting discovery in any branch of science might lead some physician down the path of creating a new medical doctrine.

Cullen developed a theory that life existed in a state of nervous excitement produced by environmental stimuli. He believed that disease was a result of what he termed a "spasm of the nervous system." His theory was based on a recent discovery that a muscle would contract if the nerve supplying it was stimulated.

John Brown developed an extension of this theory and an entire framework of medical practice that had a huge following in the colonies and early days of the United States. Brown believed that all disease was the result of too little, or too much nervous stimulation. He categorized diseases into these two groups, and his treatments consisted of trying to counteract the nervous system's excess or deficiency. If Brown's patients suffered from what he determined to be insufficient excitation, he would "stimulate" the patient—with alcohol being his drug of choice. If the patient's nervous system required a bit of "destimulation," Brown's answer was his favorite sedative: opium.

Diseases were also thought to be caused by poisons, or "morbific matter," found in the body. In addition to alcohol and opium, any number of medications existed to help rid a patient of these elements, chiefly through purging their intestines with cathartics, inducing them to vomit with emetics, or causing them to sweat or urinate.

Such was the case for the physician whose methods and practice had a great influence on American medicine during the years of 1776 to 1810. Without question, his status in the American medical world was at the top. He was one of the most illustrious, highly regarded, but controversial personalities of his day. He is also a main player in our story of the Lewis and Clark Expedition. He was Dr. Benjamin Rush (1745-1813).

Rush was born on a farm twelve miles northeast of Philadelphia, in the small village of Byberry, Pennsylvania, on Christmas Eve 1745. The Rush family tree had been planted in the colony for sixty-two years, having been uprooted from England in 1683. Young Benjamin's childhood had been marked with tragedy, like so many others in those days, by the loss of his father when he was only six years of age. Fortunately

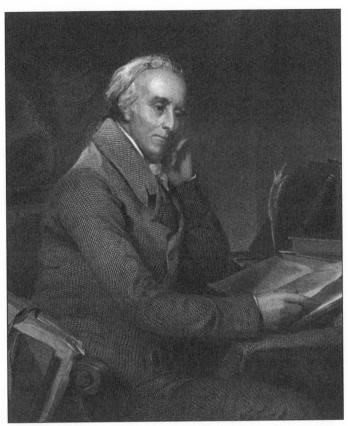

Benjamin Rush.

for Benjamin, while he was still a young boy his mother's guidance led him to pursue an early education at Nottingham, Maryland.[7]

The school and its master had earned a great reputation for its work with bright young colonials. Benjamin's rise to prominence was under the watchful eye of his headmaster, the Reverend Dr. Finley. For five years young Ben learned Greek and Latin, English, mathematics, and other classical subjects. It was said that Dr. Finley "trained his pupils for both worlds" and it was here in Nottingham Academy that Rush's life of study, devotion, and practice of his Christian faith was set in motion.

By the age of thirteen, Rush had finished his preparatory classes and entered the college of Princeton in nearby New Jersey. Before he reached his fifteenth birthday he had completed all the requirements for his Bachelor's degree and graduated in 1760.

Deciding to follow the path to a career in medicine, he returned to Philadelphia in 1761 and joined the renowned Dr. John Redman, serving a five-year apprenticeship. Dr. Redman was a great fan of intestinal purgings, accomplished with oral doses of Glauber's salts (sodium sulfate). Rush's apprenticeship included duties as nurse, coachman, and prescription clerk. He was the good doctor's assistant in minor surgeries and learned his medical skills through experience. Rush's great intellect was displayed when he translated *Aphorisms of Hippocrates* from Greek into English during these years.

A great advantage of Rush's training in Philadelphia was the opportunity to be around some of the very best medical teaching available in the colonies. He had the good fortune to come within the sphere of influence of two other notable physicians, William Shippen and John Morgan, also alumni of Dr. Finley.[8] Young Rush was one of ten favored students to attend the first formal anatomy lectures held in the colonies, under Dr. Shippen. While sitting in the amphitheater at the new University of Pennsylvania, next door to Independence Hall in Philadelphia, Rush watched the master anatomist dissect muscles, nerves and organs, enlightening the eager students on the intricacies of the human body.

John Morgan, the great innovator in American medical education, taught the young Rush *materia medica*, the study of medications— including the numerous herbal remedies that had been discovered in the colonies. Rush learned about their preparation, dosing, indications, and side effects.

The rigors of Rush's medical apprenticeship as well as his abbreviated formal education must have been remarkable, as during the five years he lived with and worked under Dr. Redman, Rush missed fewer than two weeks of work. In 1766, Benjamin Rush had finished his apprenticeship period and thus the practical side of his medical training ended. Next would come the dogmatic and theoretical influence of European medicine, an influence that would make Rush one of the leaders of American academic medicine.

Twenty-one years of age and full of ambition, the practical doctor now set off to Scotland and the University of Edinburgh. Here he would come under the influence of the theories of William Cullen and John Brown.

For two years in Scotland, he burned the midnight oil, studying Cullen's theories of "nervous excitation" and the effect on bodily solids as the cause of disease, and Brown's corollary that disease was caused by "variations in nervous excitability." Rush took in the teachings of his mentors and his medical thought became an interesting mixture of American practicality and European dogma, with a healthy dose of nonsense thrown in by both groups. It was a strange brew of ideas.

Toward the end of his residence in Edinburgh, Rush completed a research project pertaining to the digestive process. The question he was attempting to answer was whether or not fermentation played any role in digestion. His methods were novel, and included eating a dinner and inducing himself to vomit. He noted that the vomit was acidic. So he took a dose of alkaline salt to neutralize any acid that might be in his stomach and then dined on some beef, peas, bread, and beer. Three hours later he induced himself to vomit again and noted once more that the contents of his stomach were acidic. Then he ate chicken, cabbage, unleavened bread and water, and again waited three hours and forced himself to vomit. The burning question must have been: Will the vomit be changed? Again, the contents were acidic. From this set of observations accomplished with two grains of tartar emetic and a small amount of self sacrifice, Rush concluded, "an inference can be drawn, that the aliment in the human stomach, in the course of three hours after deglutition, underwent the acetetous fermentation."[9] In June of 1768, only twenty-two years old and after seven years of studying medicine as apprentice and scholar and authoring a simple physiological research project, Rush was awarded his M.D. degree by the medical faculty at the University of Edinburgh.

The Philadelphia that Dr. Rush returned to in 1769 was awaiting him with open arms. He was now a lettered professional, well spoken, well versed, with a noted aptitude for polished conversation and convincing rhetoric. Both his professional and personal fortunes were taking off. He was appointed Professor of Chemistry at the Medical College of Philadelphia, and together with his old tutors Drs. Shippen and Morgan, he helped mold young Americans into learned physicians. Through the coming three decades Dr. Rush would help educate thousands of physicians.

When Rush returned to Philadelphia from Europe, he found Ameri-

Just Doing the Best We Can

can society in a profound uproar. Political interest and controversy were at a feverish pitch, with the colonists becoming ever more irritated with their mother country across the Atlantic. Being at the center of Philadelphia society, Rush rubbed shoulders with such revolutionaries and prominent American thinkers as Benjamin Franklin, George Washington, Thomas Jefferson, and John Adams. As the next several years saw increasing tensions between the Americans and the British, the young doctor's political tendencies became decidedly revolutionary. He was elected to the Second Continental Congress and, on a hot July day in 1776, risked his life and professional future by penning his signature on a document declaring that he would no longer consider England his mother country and that he and the rest of the colonies were now and hence forth in active rebellion. During the war years that followed that first *American* July Fourth, Rush served his country as a physician general, publishing his observations about diseases of the army and the state of army hospitals. Every practicing physician and patriot in America became acquainted with the name of Benjamin Rush.

In 1790, a full twenty years into his medical career, Rush took his place in medical history and became a theorist, developing his own ideas about the nature of disease. Up until this point, he had been a great admirer of the theories of Cullen and Brown, his old Edinburgh professors. But he also slowly became disenchanted with some of their concepts. Benjamin Rush now provided the medical world with his own—a doctrine that would profoundly influence American medicine for decades to come.

Rush theorized that disease was the result of a hyperactive state of the blood vessels, that he termed "hypertension." He believed that all fevers were a result of an irritation within the blood vessels, or as he put it, "the higher grades of fever depend upon morbid and excessive action in the blood-vessels." (Rather than being a symptom of a disease, "fever" was believed to be a specific disease entity—and there were numerous types of fevers.) Of course, if irritation causing a disease is taking place within the blood vessels, something must be its source. Rush's conclusion was that, "The blood is the most powerful irritant which acts upon them."

Bloodletting had been practiced for centuries, but Benjamin Rush enlightened the world to the "irritating" nature of blood and provided what he considered theoretical justification for the practice. Bloodletting would rid the body of this "morbid and excessive" action of blood on the vessels.

Rush began to bleed his patients for nearly every ailment. He would assess the degree of "hypertension" by interpreting the patient's pulse, both its rate and strength. Then, using a sharp blade called a lancet, he made an incision in a vein usually in the patient's arm or hand, and allowed the patient's blood to flow into a pan. The bleeding was continued until Rush decided that the proper amount of blood had been removed for the condition being treated. This could amount from a few ounces or up to eighty ounces of blood per day, or until four-fifths of a patient's blood was removed.[10] His proof of the effectiveness of his bloodletting therapy was that a good bleeding would relax a tense patient! He also made the profound observation that "hemorrhages seldom occur where bleeding has been sufficiently copious." Surgeons...are you listening?

Rush's approach to medical treatment was not to sit idly by and allow nature to take its course. He told his students, "we can have no reliance on nature, gentlemen. We must turn her out of doors in our practice, and substitute for her efficient art."

In July of 1793, perhaps while Rush was making his rounds in the University of Pennsylvania hospital, a boatload of white immigrants sailed up the Delaware River to Penn's Landing, several blocks from Rush's residence at 3rd Street and Walnut. These folks were fleeing racial strife in Haiti, where some slaves had been staging a bloody rebellion against whites. The seemingly routine arrival would lead to a devastating disaster for the unsuspecting residents of Philadelphia and further notoriety for Benjamin Rush.

Within days, Philadelphians started getting sick—very sick.[11] First came terrible chills, fever, and headache. Arms, legs, backs, and chests ached with severe and debilitating pain. The victim would often begin to feel better for a few hours, maybe even a few days. With the decreased symptoms, the illness seemed to have passed and recovery seemed assured. But as quickly as a cat pounces on its prey, the black vomit came, sometimes mixed with bright red blood. Within hours the unfortunate man, woman or child could not hold anything down. Within days, eyes and skin turned yellow. Urine output dwindled, with sub-

Just Doing the Best We Can

sequent dehydration. As the deadly sequence continued, the patient became lethargic, and delirium, shock, and coma set in. The pathetic victim wasted away and died.

Between July and November of 1793 this scenario was repeated more than four thousand times in the homes and boarding houses of Philadelphia. Young children, who a few days earlier were happily playing with their toys, became lifeless corpses. Young women recently married left their new husbands widowers. Horse-drawn hearses clopped through the streets day and night. In an attempt to protect themselves some citizens hid inside their homes. Many packed up a few belongings and left the city as quickly as possible. Normal life within the City of Brotherly Love came to a deadly and terrifying standstill.

This was the yellow fever, also known as the "Great Sickness" or the "Bilious Plague." Its cause was completely unknown to Benjamin Rush and the two other doctors who remained in Philadelphia. An effective treatment was equally unknown, but this state of ignorance did not cause the medical community to surrender. Numerous therapeutic approaches resulted with some fascinating treatments. Some of the favored ones included placing an open container of vinegar in a room or alongside a hot iron. Smoking cigars seemed to help ward off the disease and many inhabitants from children to the elderly walked around town with cigars sticking out of their mouths. Odiferous camphor either applied to the skin or worn in a bag around the neck seemed efficacious as well. Some chewed garlic cloves. But even the hopeful users of these methods often came down with the deadly symptoms.

During this plague, Dr. Rush worked himself to exhaustion. At times he saw up to 120 patients a day, attempting to relieve suffering without regard to the patient's financial standing. He was even called on to treat the British minister's family. He frequently had to ignore the pleadings of help from people on the street as he rode by in his carriage on his way to help his patients. He ate his meals while dozens of patients waited in his house for treatment. Others outside Philadelphia petitioned him to avoid the fever by leaving the city, but his stellar character would not allow him this self-serving escape. After one friend suggested a quick exit, he wrote, "I was resolved to stick with my principles, my practice, and my patients, to the last extremity."[12]

What Rush possessed in compassion and diligence on behalf of the victims of the yellow fever plague of 1793, he lacked in effective treatment. For nausea and vomiting Rush encouraged his patients to "drink plentifully gruel, or barley water, or chicken water." He encouraged producing blisters to the "sides, neck or head" by application of ground up Spanish beetles to the skin, to draw fluid to the skin's surface from irritated and congested internal organs. Another adjunctive therapy was to wrap the patient's legs with flannel soaked in vinegar and water. "When the pulse is full and tense," Rush directed that windows were to be opened to let in cool air. Floors of the sickroom were to be sprinkled with vinegar.

Rush, as previously mentioned, bled many of his patients, often repeatedly, often more than once daily. To his already famous therapy of bloodletting, he added purging of the bowels. The combination of these treatments was very appropriately termed a "depleting" therapy. His favorite purging agent was calomel, a mercury salt (mercurous chloride). Calomel is a profound intestinal irritant which Rush administered in whopping doses of ten to fifteen grains per day.[13] When the calomel was combined with the magnum-powered herbal cathartic, jalap, obtained from the root of a Mexican vine (*Exogonium jalapa*), this dynamic duo produced a potent intestinal irritation and spirited bowel movement containing large quantities of bile.[14]

He credited the healing power of calomel, calling it "the Sampson [*sic*] of the Materia Medica." His opponents countered with public ridicule and some clever sarcasm, stating they agreed with Rush's assertion of it being "a Sampson," not because of its efficacy, but because "it has slain its thousands." The British diplomat's family was treated with Rush's big three therapies with apparent success. Although thoroughly "depleted," at least they survived. Rush was delighted and wrote of his success to his wife Julia, "Four persons in the British minister's family will swell the triumphs of mercury, jalap and blood-letting."[15]

Even though Rush was ridiculed by his detractors and sarcastically referred to as "the bloodletter," his fame and influence on American medicine was unquestionably great as well as controversial. His own humility and devaluation of his medical practices were manifest in a letter he wrote in his closing years. He wrote, "Of the poor services I have rendered to any of my fellow creatures I shall say nothing. They

Just Doing the Best We Can

were full of imperfections and have no merit in the sight of God. I pray to have the sin that was mixed with them, forgiven."[16]

Some physicians and historians have revered his medical contributions such as improving treatment of the mentally ill. In honor of his work in the field, the American Psychiatric Association designated Rush as the "Father of American Psychiatry." His early support of inoculation for the American army undoubtedly saved thousands of Continental soldiers from the ravages of smallpox. His untiring efforts on behalf of the stricken population of Philadelphia in 1793 as well as his thirty-two years of medical teaching at what became the University of Pennsylvania certainly qualify him as a man of great caring and compassion, and for his time, a noted physician and patriot. His aggressive stand against slavery led to the founding of the first Anti-Slavery Society in Philadelphia. He was an ardent supporter of Dickinson College and improved educational opportunities for American women.

Other medical historians have been profoundly critical of Benjamin Rush's medicine, with one writing, "Benjamin Rush had more influence upon American medicine and was more potent in the propagation and long perpetuation of medical error than any man of his day. To him, more than to any other man in America, was due the great vogue of vomits, purgings, especially of bleeding, salivation and blistering, which blackened the record of medicine and afflicted the sick almost to the time of the Civil War."[17]

The controversy surrounding the man continues to the present day among medical historians. Perhaps the ultimate irony is that Rush could be so progressive and correct with many of his non-medical ideas as well as being a visionary in his support of just social causes and yet be so completely incorrect in his theory of disease and thus his practice of medicine.

On a late-spring day, in May of 1803, a young man from Washington rode into downtown Philadelphia from Lancaster. He had come to meet with and learn from several of the leading American scientists of the day. Letters of introduction to these men of science from the President had preceded this young traveler by two months. Dr. Andrew Ellicott, of Lancaster, had just spent three weeks instructing him on the use of the sextant, artificial horizon, and chronometer in fixing longitude (for the purpose of map making). Dr. Caspar Wistar, a leading American physician/naturalist and Professor of Anatomy at the University of Pennsylvania would add to the young man's knowledge of fossils and medicine. Professor Robert Patterson would refine his training in figuring longitude. Dr. Benjamin Smith Barton, botanist, physician, and a leading naturalist, would bolster the student's knowledge of description and taxonomy.

The traveler from the nation's capital also came to meet with one of Philadelphia's most famous citizens: Dr. Rush. This young man, who had little practical medical training and even less theoretical medical knowledge, directed his horse down the cobblestone streets lined with brick houses, to the front of a Philadelphia home on the corner of Walnut and 3rd, just three blocks from Independence Hall. The sign on the front of the house read, "Benjamin Rush, M.D." The dusty and tired traveler swung off the horse and tied the reins of his mount to one of the many hitching posts that lined the street. He walked up the stairs approaching the front door with a large dose of awe, as if he were entering some sort of temple. The young man gently knocked on the door and awaited a response from inside. He was there to be instructed about the practice of medicine and other related topics. This young man would soon be responsible for the health of a few dozen men under his command in remote territory. Being assigned such a monumental responsibility, it is truly ironic that he would serve the shortest medical apprenticeship in American history—about two weeks. His training would be intense and important. His responsibility was daunting. His medical professor would be Benjamin Rush. His name was Meriwether Lewis.

Just Doing the Best We Can

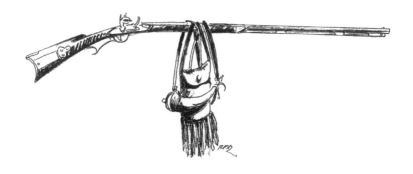

☙ 4 ☙

INTO THE STARTING BLOCKS

The Expedition Prepares

Great oaks from little acorns grow.
—Proverb

Plans for the expedition were already in full stride by the time Meriwether Lewis rode into Philadelphia for his whirlwind series of lectures and practicums with the stars of American science and medicine in 1803. A full two years had passed since Lewis had left active army duty and traveled to Washington to assume his duties as the President's personal secretary. It was his good fortune during this time to have had access to all the resources of the American government, including powerful and knowledgeable men and access to the best available maps of the western country. In addition, he had the full attention of President Jefferson.

By early June, Meriwether Lewis's short medical internship was completed and Benjamin Rush reported to President Jefferson on his progress.

Dear Sir,   *Philadelphia, June 11th, 1803*
I have endeavored to fulfil your wishes by furnishing Mr. Lewis with
some inquiries relative to the natural history of the Indians. The
enclosed letter contains a few short directions for the preservation of
his health, as well as the health of the persons under his command
His mission is truly interesting. I shall wait with great solicitude for its
issue. Mr. Lewis appears admirably qualified for it. May its advantages
prove no less honorable to your administration than to the interests of
science....From, dear sir, your very respectfully and sincerely,
                                                        Benjn: Rush[1]

With advice from Dr. Rush, Lewis hit the streets of Philadelphia securing the supply of medicines that he would likely require during the long stay in the wilderness. These were purchased with taxpayer money from the apothecary shop of Gillaspy and Strong at 103 South Second and 243 High Street in Philadelphia. The list included such herbal cathartics as powdered jalap and rhubarb. Other cathartic salts such as sodium sulfate, known as "Glauber's salts," and magnesia were purchased in the unlikely event that the jalap couldn't do the job. Various emetics (which produce vomiting) such as ipecacuan, and the antimony-potassium compound called tartar emetic were added to the medicine chest. Nutmeg, clove and cinnamon were purchased to flavor foul-tasting medicines as well as lessening the intestinal griping of some of the cathartics. Topical analgesics (pain relievers) such as gum camphor, tragacanth, and calamine ointment would help with skin problems.

Pain and other nervous system problems such as "excessive nervous stimulation" could be handled by Captain Lewis with a half pound of the best Turkish opium as well as laudanum, an alcoholic tincture containing about 10 percent opium. And certainly not of least importance to the men of the expedition would be the thirty gallons of medicinal wine and a supply of whiskey.

The biggest quantity of any medication purchased was the fifteen pounds of powdered Peruvian bark, which was one of the few really beneficial items Lewis purchased. The "barks" were obtained from a

Benjamin Rush's Rules of Health

Dr. Rush to Capt. Lewis for preserving his health.   June 11.1803.

1. When you feel the least indisposition, do no attempt to overcome it by labour or marching. *Rest* in a horizontal posture. Also fasting and diluting drinks for a day or two will generally prevent an attack of fever. To these preventatives of disease may be added a gentle sweat obtained by warm drinks, or gently opening the bowels by means of one, two, or more of the purging pills.

2. Unusual costiveness is often a sign of approaching disease. When you feel it take one or more of the purging pills.

3. Want of appetite is likewise a sign of approaching indisposition. It should be obviated by the same remedy.

4. In difficult & laborious enterprises & marches, *eating sparingly* will enable you to bear them with less fatigue & less danger to your health.

5. Flannel should be worn constantly next to the skin, especially in wet weather.

6. The less spirit you use the better. After being *wetted* or *much* fatigued, or *long* exposed to the night air, it should be taken in an *undiluted* state. 3 tablespoonfuls taken in this way will be more useful in preventing sickness, than half a pint mixed with water.

7. Molasses or sugar & water with a few drops of the acid of vitriol will make a pleasant and wholsome drink with your meals.

8. After having had your feet much chilled, it will be useful to wash them with a little spirit.

9. Washing the feet every morning in *cold* water, will conduce very much to fortify them against the action of cold.

10. After long marches, or much fatigue from any cause, you will be more refreshed by *lying down* in a horizontal posture for two hours, than by resting a much longer time in any other position of the body.

11. Shoes made without heels, by affording *equal* action to all the muscles of the legs, will enable you to march with less fatigue, than shoes made in the ordinary way.

tree that grew in Peru and were taken back to Europe by missionaries, which earned it another name, the "Jesuit bark." Peruvian bark was first used extensively by the famous 17th century English physician Thomas Sydenham on various diseases manifested by fever. It was also a popular tonic or cure-all. It answered for a treatment of snakebites and just about anything else the practitioner could think of.

Lewis packed fifty dozen of the calomel-and-jalap "Bilious Pills of Dr. Rush," also known as "Thunderclappers." The extent to which medical thinking of the day believed that a disease was either caused by or contributed to by poisons in the intestines can be easily appreciated by this quantity.

Two medications that would prove to be in short supply by the end of the trip were six ounces of "Sacchar. Saturn. Opt.," Latin for sugar of lead (lead acetate), and four ounces of "Vitriol Alb.," Latin for white vitriol (zinc sulfate). Towards the end of the trip, the lead acetate at thirty-seven cents, and the zinc sulfate at twelve cents, would prove to be the best bargains in the medicine chest. During the return, Lewis would wish for much more of each of these "eyewash" ingredients.

President Jefferson was interested in using the latest advances in medicine to help ensure the success of the expedition and to help protect what he called the "noble savages" along the Missouri. Jefferson instructed Captain Lewis to take along a supply of the "kinepox," the lymphatic substance obtained from blisters of the patients who had been vaccinated with the cowpox virus. This blister fluid could be collected and sent in protective glass tubes. Jefferson had received some of this lymphatic material from Dr. Waterhouse of Boston as well as Dr. Edward Jenner of England and had used the substance to successfully vaccinate between seventy and eighty of his family members.[2] Jefferson exhorted Lewis to inform the Indians of its benefit and use it to protect them from smallpox.

Lewis was well aware of the impending scourge of mosquitoes that awaited him and the Corps while spending their days on the river. Lewis wisely purchased "Muscato Curtains" and "8 ps Cat Gut for Mosquito Curtins," as well as some 19th century DEET[3] in the form of tallow and hog's lard, which the men could smear on their exposed skin.

In addition to his medicines, Lewis also purchased some basic surgical tools, as well as three "Clyster Pipes," or enema syringes. Enemas could be used if the Thunderclappers failed to treat what Dr. Rush called "unusual costiveness" or constipation—a sure sign, at least to Dr. Rush, of approaching sickness.[4]

Lewis's knowledge from the army of soldiers' frequently contracting venereal disease led him to purchase medicines to utilize when this problem arose. The four pewter penile syringes would be used to treat gonorrhea by injecting a solution up the penile urethra. This solution could have been made from the listed medication "balsam copaiba," an oily, resinous substance containing benzoic or cinnamic acid, obtained from a South American tree. Mercury compounds such as calomel (mercurous chloride, an inorganic mercury salt), used to treat syphilis and act as a cathartic and diuretic, and mercury ointment to be used as a topical (applied to the patient's skin) syphilis treatment, were on the list. I can just see the men lining up with anticipation as the enema and pewter penile syringes were being loaded!

A tourniquet for $3.50 (it must have been embroidered or laced with gold), patent lint (a cloth material used to pack wounds), dental instruments, three "best lancets" to get rid of some of that irritating blood, in addition to various canisters, bottles, and two wooden medicine chests rounded out the shopping list. Total cost of the medical supplies was $90.60.

One of the chief aims of the exploration would be to encourage friendly commerce with the Indian tribes along the Missouri and to bring them into the American trading sphere and within government influence. Lewis purchased a vast assortment of merchandise to be utilized as both presents and trade items with the tribes. Pounds of red, blue, and white beads, earrings, 500 brooches, 4,600 needles and 2,800 fish hooks, ribbons, scissors, thimbles, cloth, and some cast iron corn mills were among the items obtained in Philadelphia. The list of supplies goes on—steels for making fire, pots, blankets, stockings, shoes, shirts, tape, ink powder, tomahawks, knapsacks, fishing lines and hooks, would all be of great value as trade items. Another item that would prove to be a most sought after item by the men of the expedition and the Indians alike—130 rolls of "pigtail" tobacco. All of these supplies, which cost the taxpayers $2,324, were loaded onto an Army wagon and transported westward. A fifty-five-foot keelboat, under construction in Pittsburgh, awaited the goods and their voyage down the

Ohio River, then up the Mississippi and finally up the Missouri.

The distant Pacific Ocean was only one goal of the voyage of discovery. The unknown country the group passed through would need to be mapped. Surveying tools such as a level, plotting instruments, two-pole chain, compasses, magnet, sextant, and chronometer were procured.

Some Indian tribes on the already explored lower Missouri were known to be aggressive with traders coming up their river. Many traders had been robbed of their goods and forced at gun- and arrow-point to backtrack down the Missouri River to St. Louis. Since the Corps of Discovery would ascend this dangerous portion of the river, they would have to be a powerful outfit. Armament would be provided in part by fifteen .54-caliber flintlock rifles produced at the national armory at Harpers Ferry, Virginia. These single-shot blackpowder rifles had the approximate stopping power of a modern-day .357 magnum—deadly to most game animals or humans within about 150 yards. Slings were added to make carrying the weapons easier. Flintlocks are worthless without flints, powder, and ball. The list included 500 rifle flints, fifty pounds of "best powder," bullet molds, and 420 pounds of "sheet lead" to be shaped into canisters holding the powder, and later melted over campfires and poured into bullet molds.

Thus, in early June, with much of the ground-laying work completed and many supplies gathered, Lewis began his horseback ride to Washington for some last-minute conferences with the President and his cabinet.

Had Lewis sensed during his tutorials in Philadelphia that there was just too much for one officer to do? Or was it a desire for the companionship of another officer with whom he could share the burdens of command? Whatever the motivation, at some time after his return to Washington, during one of his conversations with Jefferson, Meriwether Lewis spoke to the President of his desire to add another officer to the Corps of Discovery. Jefferson liked the idea and agreed.

With the President's approval and the Secretary of War's monetary allowance to add "one Lieutenant," Lewis sat down on June 19, and penned a letter to his old friend and Army commander, the now-retired Captain William Clark, who was living on the Ohio River in Clarksville, Indiana Territory: "From the long and uninterrupted friendship and confidence which has subsisted between us I feel no hesitation in making to you the following communication."[5]

Into the Starting Blocks

The letter invited Clark to join the Corps of Discovery as a captain. If Clark accepted, Lewis instructed him to begin to recruit men suitable to the hardships that they would encounter, men who were toughened outdoorsmen and soldiers, avoiding those whom Lewis termed "soft-palmed gentlemen, dazzled by dreams of high adventure." Clark was to wait for Lewis's arrival via the Ohio at Clarksville, across from Louisville, Kentucky. Lewis sent the letter westward and departed Washington for Pittsburgh on July 5, 1803.

Details of the trip were taking shape quite nicely. The Secretary of War, Henry Dearborn, began sending letters in early July to Army officers along the route, instructing them to furnish Captain Lewis with cash to be used for "recruiting service" and as payroll for members of the expedition. Dearborn told commanders of Fort Massac on the Ohio and Fort Kaskaskia on the Mississippi to furnish Captain Lewis with the men needed to help with passage of the supply-laden keelboat. Dearborn added, "If any non-commissioned officer or private in your Company should be disposed to join Capt. Lewis, whose characters for sobriety, integrity and other necessary qualifications render them suitable for such service, you will detach them accordingly."[6]

Meriwether Lewis's letter reached his old friend by the middle of July, while Lewis was spending days in head-banging frustration over delays in the keelboat's construction in Pittsburgh. Clark enthusiastically replied on July 18: "The Contents…I recived with much pleasure. The enterprise &c is Such as I have long anticipated and am much pleased with,"[7] adding in a letter of July 24, "My friend I join you with hand & Heart and anticipate advantages which will certainly derive from the accomplishment of so vast, Hazidous and fatiguing enterprize."[8]

The stage was now set and the players were ready. The mysterious and unexplored American west was a vast wilderness that some thought inhabited by living examples of megalonyx (extinct giant ground sloth) and possibly other Ice Age animals.[9] Some believed that active volcanoes were strewn across the western landscape and that the land was inhabited by vicious giant natives who disliked white men. All this wild and unknown territory would soon be before Meriwether Lewis and William Clark.

Even though the boats that would carry him up the Missouri contained thousands of pounds of the latest trade goods and supplies, the lessons from Dr. Rush and his colleagues could not provide Lewis with medical skills equivalent to his naturalist and leadership abilities. Lewis's practice would consist of the use of a few herbal and chemical medications, some of his mother's medical-herb knowledge and some practical medical skills acquired during his army career. In addition, Dr. Rush had added a pinch of European medical theory flavored with the influence of Cullen's beliefs in "nervous excitement" and Brown's love of opium and alcohol. Rush also threw a generous dose of bloodletting into the explorer's medical bag of tricks. Lewis's superficial knowledge and skill would have to suffice in caring for the health of his men and himself.

Illnesses and injuries awaited around every turn of the trail and bend of the river, medical problems of which Lewis and Benjamin Rush had no understanding of at all. The trip would have been a challenge to any modern physician accompanying the Corps of Discovery, even possessing a 21st century bank of knowledge. There would be no laboratories for blood counts or various body chemistry studies. No CT or MRI scanners. No radiology services. No knowledge of bacteria or the basic medical sciences. No surgical suites with bright lights. No autoclaves to sterilize instruments—and not many instruments to sterilize. For Lewis and Clark there would only be a little bit of practical knowledge, some theoretical nonsense, and a small supply of mostly worthless medications.

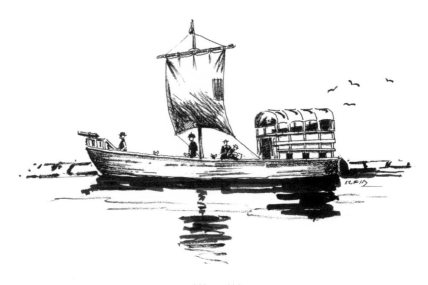

⚓ 5 ⚓

"MISQUTRS" ON THE OHIO

The Trip Gets Underway

From small beginnings come great things.
—Proverb

Meriwether Lewis's departure from Pittsburgh had been delayed for weeks by boat builders who were perhaps treating themselves for "insufficient nervous stimulation," and were, as Lewis described, "incorrigible drunkards" who continually frustrated his attempts to leave. The fifty-five-foot keelboat was weeks overdue, and on some days the master builder didn't ever show up for work. Lewis passed the weeks in frustration, trying to encourage and/or intimidate the builder to complete the job.

While passing the days, Lewis started building the expedition team with the purchase of one of its first members. This particular explorer-in-training had a decidedly non-military attitude and slobbered a good deal of the time. But he had the right amount of enthusiasm as well as a good warm fur coat. Seaman, a black Newfoundland dog, would provide numerous adventures of his own during the expedition, from being kidnapped to catching squirrels for dinner. He would also be a lifesaver to the men with his barking alarm, warning of approaching dangers.

Finally on August 31, with most of the supplies tucked tightly inside the keelboat's hull and more on their way by wagon to Wheeling, then in Virginia, Lewis set sail on a rapidly falling late-summer river. Captain Lewis and the eleven men assigned to aid his transit floated and sometimes towed the keelboat through the shallow waters. Only a few miles downstream, at Beaver, Pennsylvania, Lewis purchased the first pirogue, already needing to lighten the keelboat's load. Between bouts of scraping its wooden hull on the streambed rocks yard by yard and mile by mile, the big boat floated southwestward among the beautiful broadleaf forests lining the banks of the Ohio. What a relief to finally be under way and approaching the reunion with William Clark.

While Lewis and his rivermen slowly made progress toward Clarksville, Indiana Territory, Captain Clark was busy interviewing the men who would make up the nucleus of the small exploratory army. Numerous men expressed interest in joining the effort but some lacked the needed skills and outdoor proficiency, while others were simply "gentlemen's sons" who had never done a hard day's work in their lives. Lewis and Clark would chose their men from essentially three groups: Ohio valley frontiersmen, U.S. Army enlisted men, and French settlers of Illinois and Missouri.

One of the first men "chosen" to accompany the Corps of Discovery was Captain Clark's slave York, euphemistically referred to as "servant." But to be chosen for a task carries the implication that you have applied for the position, and it is highly doubtful that York had much say about his presence on the upcoming trip. York had been selected as a youth to be William Clark's body servant. Clark was probably just a few years older than York, and the two youths grew up together hunting, fishing, horseback riding, and probably getting into various brands of childish mischief.[1] This man would prove to be a valuable member of the group. The positive effect he would have on the North American Indian nations the group would encounter as well as his personal contributions to the Corps' success were profound.

"Misqutrs" on the Ohio

The remainder of the men Clark chose were young men who had grown up in the untamed woods of Kentucky. They possessed many of the same outdoor skills of their commanders and in addition had talents of carpentry, blacksmithing, hunting, sign language, and linguistics.

Two of the three sergeants selected for the Corps of Discovery were first cousins. Charles Floyd, one of the youngest of the entire group, about twenty-one years of age, was probably from a farm near present St. Matthews.[2] Young Floyd was sworn into the Army of the United States on August 1, 1803, as a member of the Corps of Discovery. His cousin Nathaniel Pryor, recruited on October 20, had been born in Virginia in 1772 and moved with his family to Kentucky at age ten. In 1798, Nathaniel married Patty Patten, who may have died in childbirth, as he was apparently not married in 1803 at the expedition's outset.[3]

Two members of the team were brothers Reubin and Joseph Field. Clark apparently recruited the brothers at their family farm in southwestern Jefferson County, Kentucky. Individualism and unfamiliarity with military regulations, along with a fondness for whiskey, got Reubin into some trouble during the first winter camp across the Mississippi from St. Louis. Both brothers fell into the routine of military discipline, though, and were praised in 1806 by Captain Lewis as "Two of the most active and enterprising young men who accompanied us" who "acquitted themselves with much honor."[4]

Private John Shields was likely born in Harrisonburg, Virginia, in 1769, one of a family of eleven children. The Shields family moved onto the frontier of the Smoky Mountains' Tennessee foothills. Here he became an apprentice blacksmith under the watchful eye of his brother-in-law. In 1790, he married in Kentucky. In 1803, at thirty-four years of age, the oldest member of the team and apparently still married, he joined the expedition. His skill and ingenuity would be boons to the team and contribute significantly to its success.[5]

Shortly after Captain Lewis had left Pittsburgh he met a man he thought had the makings of a great team member. The fame of this man has transcended two centuries, along with that of Lewis and Clark. His name was John Colter. He was born in 1775 in Virginia, and by 1803 lived near Maysville, Kentucky. Twenty-nine years of age and standing five feet, ten inches tall, with blue eyes, shy disposition and a quick mind, Colter would go down in history as one of America's greatest mountain men and the white discoverer of future Yellowstone National Park's wonders.[6]

Lewis also picked the youngest member of the team. At eighteen, George Shannon would prove to have a real talent at losing himself or his equipment in the wilderness. He started out a poor hunter, but necessity improved his skill.

Scots Irish William Bratton had been twelve when his family moved to the frontier of Kentucky. He was described as being more than six feet in height, square of build, reserved, and of strictest morals.[7] Bratton had skills as a gunsmith and blacksmith, and he would provide an interesting medical problem during the trip.

One of the thousands of Pennsylvanians who moved to the Kentucky territory was George Gibson from Mercer County near Pittsburgh. Gibson was to prove a talented hunter, horseman, interpreter and fiddle player—and to suffer one of the most severe injuries among the men.[8]

More men would be added to the growing Corps of Discovery of North America, as it made its way down the Ohio to the Mississippi and up to winter camp across the river from St. Louis. Some later accepted into the Corps volunteered from Forts Massac and Kaskasia in present-day Illinois: John Newman, the French-Omaha Francois Labiche (who enlisted officially the following May), Patrick Gass, John Ordway, John Boley, and John Collins.[9]

At Fort Massac would be civilian George Drouillard, hired as an interpreter and Lower Missouri guide. He turned out to be a most valuable hand throughout the trek.[10]

By the spring of 1804, the corps would also include Silas Goodrich and Hugh McNeal, Robert Frazer, and future mutineer Moses Reed, along with John B. Thompson, William Werner, and John Robertson. Formally enlisting in May 1804, Pierre Cruzatte was a one-eyed boatman who had traveled the Missouri River all the way to the Mandan-Hidatsa villages. Of French-Omaha birth, Cruzatte specialized in piloting, or guiding, boats up the treacherous Missouri. He was also a talented fiddler who played beside many a campfire while the men sang, danced, and blew off steam after a hard day's work.[11]

On September 8, at a stop in Wheeling, Virginia, Lewis nearly added a physician to the group. While Lewis sat on the keelboat that was docked there, he joyously stuffed himself with juicy watermelons. In between bites, he talked with some local men, and a young physician wandered down to the boat and joined in the discussion. The young doctor was William Ewing Patterson. He was the son of the math professor in Philadelphia who had tutored Lewis four months earlier. Discussions about the upcoming trip, mixed with bites of watermelon and the prospect of exploring the unknown west, appealed to the young doctor. Lewis wrote that Patterson "expressed a great desire to go with me." Probably pleased at being relieved of his medical duties, Lewis told him to be ready to go the next day. Dr. Patterson "instantly set about it" and went home to prepare his personal supplies and medicines. The following afternoon, the hour scheduled for departure came and went without the appearance of Ewing Patterson. Lewis wrote, "Dr could not get ready I waited untill thre this evening and then set out." Did Dr. Patterson change his mind? Did he have second thoughts about going into such a treacherous wilderness? Perhaps he went home to celebrate and drank too much. The young man was said to be an alcoholic, and later rumors had it that he had gone west in an attempt to kick the habit.[12]

Although some have written that the presence of a physician would have been a great advantage to the team, I believe the practical skills that most physicians had in 1803 were not much better than those that Meriwether Lewis possessed, and Lewis was not burdened with as much erroneous theory. As an amateur, Lewis was probably more conservative in his treatments than a trained physician, whose unfounded confidence in his medical abilities would likely have made him more aggressive. It was probably the start of Lewis's and the Corps' great luck that Dr. Patterson did not make it to the keelboat that late summer afternoon, leaving the captains to their own enormous common sense.

Besides, medical problems that individual Corps members suffered would affect the entire Corps' effort. Sick individuals at home are unfortunate. Sick traveling companions become a hindrance and possibly are dangerous to the entire team. They did not need an alcoholic physician along to add to their troubles.

Without Dr. Patterson but with the addition of a second pirogue, Lewis left Wheeling. Along the way he encountered two women living along the river, emigrants from Pennsylvania. Lewis noted in his journal that the ladies suffered from goiter, an abnormal enlargement of the thyroid gland situated in the neck. They "had contracted the disorder since there residence on the Ohio."

Goiter can occur due to a variety of causes. If the ladies were related, the goiters could have been caused by hereditary underproduction of thyroid hormone, which led in a series of pathological steps to the gland's enlargement. Their diet could have been deficient in iodine, an element necessary in the production of thyroid hormone. They also could have been eating a tremendous amount of certain foods that can cause this problem. Turnips, cabbage, and other members of the plant family *Cruciferae* (mustard family) contain a chemical (glucosinolate) that, when broken down in the body, produces a another chemical (goitrin) that blocks the body's normal process of incorporating iodine into the thyroid hormone, thus effectively blocking its production. When the gland underproduces thyroid hormone, a goiter can develop.

Although the women's move to "the Ohio" would not have caused their goiters, this area did support a disease that would affect the expedition during its three summers on the trail. Here the fabric of the Lewis and Clark story, and the fate of the Corps of Discovery, becomes inextricably woven with threads of the biological phenomenon of parasitism. That is, the biological principle that some organisms cannot live on their own. These organisms are sometimes, as in the case of viruses, too small to be seen with the human eye, and in other cases, parasitic intestinal worms as long as thirty feet. Parasites are either unable to obtain their own food supply or replicate themselves, and do so at the expense—and even death—of their host organism. Although the offending parasites were usually very small, the threat they posed to the Corps of Discovery was immense.

A serious parasitic problem with which the people living in early America had to contend was an illness they called "intermittent fever," or "ague." It was also known by other names: "autumnal," "bilious," "remittent," "congestive," "miasmatic," "marsh," "malignant," "chill-fever"—or just plain "the fever." Recurring fevers, chills, sweats and, often, death characterized the disease. Probably every man on the expedition suffered from its troublesome and tormenting symptoms. The disease was endemic to the Ohio, Mississippi and Missouri river valleys, and affected millions and killed thousands of Americans in 1803. Lewis had noted, as he was reaching the lower stretches of the Ohio River, its presence in his journal entry of September 14, 1803: "the fever and ague and bilious fevers commence their banefull oppression and continue through the whole course of the river with increasing violence as you approach it's mouth."

It continues to affect hundreds of millions of people and is still probably the leading cause of death worldwide. We know it today by one of the same names it was known by in 1803: malaria.[13]

Historically, few parasitic diseases have had such widespread and profound effect on civilization as malaria. In the 4th century, the Greeks noted an association between exposure to swamp water and the occurrence in victims of periodic fevers and enlarged spleens. The connection between swamps and the presence of mosquitoes, the disease-carrying agent, was not made until 1880. Although they hadn't understood the rationale behind their actions, the Greeks and Romans at least possessed the insight to drain their swamps in an effort to control the illness.

In the 20th century, well after identification of the one-celled protozoan, genus *Plasmodium*, which is carried by the *Anopheles* mosquito and injected into the victim's bloodstream via the mosquito's bite, immense efforts continued to attempt to control the plasmodium. This was done through a two-pronged attack. Medication attacked the plasmodia, and insecticides the mosquito. The program lasted for twenty-one years and cost billions of dollars. In spite of this huge outlay of money and effort, the program was declared a failure by the World Health Organization in 1976, due to developing resistance among plasmodia to the drug chloroquine, and among mosquitoes to the insecticide, DDT.

Although mosquitoes and other blood-feeding arthropods (mites, ticks, and insects other than mosquitoes) prefer to get their meals from other vertebrate animals including mammals, reptiles, birds or amphibians, humans have been an alternate source of food for these pests throughout the millennia. Only the female mosquito bites, and feeds every three or four days. They are chiefly attracted to their food through their sense of smell. The female mosquito lands on its victim, inserts its long hypodermic-like feeding tube through the skin, injects some of its saliva, and sucks up its dinner of blood. The human body generally reacts to the irritating substances within the mosquito saliva with localized swelling and itching, which can last for several days. (Male mosquitoes, as with all species, are the kinder and gentler sex, feeding only on nectar and other plant juices.)

Although it was not realized in 1803, when an infected female anopheles mosquito bites its human victim and starts to partake of its meal of blood, it can inject into the victim's blood stream a small unicellular protozoan that lives in mosquito saliva. This small parasite travels through the bloodstream and invades the victim's liver cells (hepatocytes), where it starts to reproduce within the living cells. Inside a week, the multiplying protozoans cause liver cells to die and rupture, releasing thousands of new malarial parasites into the victim's blood stream. These plasmodia now invade red blood cells, where they live and reproduce.

There are four types of malarial parasites that cause disease in humans: *Plasmodium vivax*, *Plasmodium ovale*, *Plasmodium malariae*, and, potentially the most serious form, *Plasmodium falciparum*. It is likely that all forms of the *Plasmodium* existed in early America, although *P. ovale* and *P. vivax* are more prominent in temperate zones such as most of North America.

Falciparum is by far the deadliest form of malaria. Unlike disease caused by *P. ovale* and *P. vivax*, which produce dormant liver stages and cause relapses, *P. falciparum* is not responsible for months of recurrent chills, fever, and other symptoms. A patient can be reinfected with *P. falciparum* on numerous occasions, because being infected does not produce immunity to further attacks.

Unlike many diseases of the early 19th century that have been conquered, or nearly so, since then, malaria continues to be an immense problem in much of the world, with 300 to 500 million cases per year, and as many as 2 to 3 million deaths annually.[14]

About a week to a month passes between the infecting bite and the

"Misqutrs" on the Ohio

resulting onset of malarial symptoms. With the less severe forms of the disease, the onset of illness is characterized by fatigue and a slowly rising fever for several days. This is followed by a shaking chills and rapid temperature elevation, with headache and nausea, which ends with the victim sweating profusely. This pattern is repeated every one to three days for anywhere from a week to a month, or perhaps longer. Recurrent bouts of fever, chills, etc., may occur irregularly for as long as six to eleven months if the patient is infected with *P. ovale or P. vivax* (or both).[15] Adults in highly endemic areas, who have been exposed to infective mosquitoes for years, may become tolerant through the effects of their immune systems and fail to exhibit outward signs of infection. If death results from the malarial infection, it usually comes from the *falciparum* species, and results from complications such as severe anemia, kidney failure, pulmonary edema (fluid within the lungs), or central nervous system (brain or spinal cord) involvement.

Since nearly the entire trip of the Corps of Discovery was spent on or around water where mosquitoes live and breed, it was an obvious environmental and occupational hazard for the men of the Corps to be exposed to numerous mosquitoes. From early April during the spring of 1804, when William Clark found it newsworthy enough to mention that, "I saw a Musquetor to day," to the first hard freeze in the fall, the men were frequently tormented by hoards of these bloodsuckers. Frequent entries occur in the journals during the warm months, describing the torment the insects provided such as "Musquetors verry troublesom," and Lewis's entry of July 30, 1805 along the Jefferson River in present-day Montana, "...having now secured my supper I looked our [around?] for a suitable place to amuse myself in combating the musquetoes for the ballance of the evening..." adding that he "layed down and should have had a comfortable nights lodge but for the musquetoes which infested me all night." The factors of tormenting discomfort and disease risk these six-legged vixens posed to the Corps can not be overestimated.

Mosquitoes make excellent food sources for fish and birds. I cannot attest to their flavor as I have never knowingly eaten one. But there are few environmental nuisances that have caused me more discomfort in the outdoors than mosquitoes. The worst I have ever seen was during a float trip in Lewis and Clark country on the Missouri River near Craig,

Montana. When evening arrived on the river, the mosquito dinner bell rang and there were clouds of humming pests around my face, ears and nostrils, landing and biting any exposed square inch of skin. My fishing ended and the swatting began. Itching and burning bites started to swell on my arms and neck. Such was the misery I have shared with Lewis and Clark.

In today's wilderness medicine, and available to the many expeditions that venture into endemic malarial areas, are several modern conveniences unavailable to Lewis and Clark. These tools attack the mosquito/malarial problem on various fronts. The key to modern malaria control is prevention. Eliminating standing or slowly moving water where the females lay their eggs can minimize mosquito breeding areas. If the eggs are laid, insecticides can help prevent their hatching. Preventing the disease can be aided by using modern insect repellants containing the chemicals DEET and/or permethrine. In 1993, according to the Environmental Protection Agency, there were 212 products in use as repellants, which ranged from pine tar oil to oil of citronella.[16]

One of the few really beneficial medications purchased by Captain Lewis during his shopping spree in Philadelphia was the fifteen pounds of powdered Peruvian bark. The bark is obtained from the stem and root of a native tree of South America, genus *Cinchona*. It is an amazing fact of creation that this tree can synthesize within its cells a chemical called quinine, an alkaloid (a pharmacologically active chemical produced by a plant) that works against the malarial organism. About a dozen species of the tree exist, but three in particular produce the highest percentage of the active alkaloid. The molecular structure of the present-day anti-malarial drugs—chloroquine, primaquine, and mefloquine—is similar to the naturally occurring alkaloid, quinine. Of course, the early users of this beneficial herbal medication, including Lewis and Clark, did not realize why it worked. However, their empirical observations noted that it did work against "autumnal fever" symptoms. It is believed today that quinine interferes with certain enzymes within the plasmodium required to sustain its life.

Medications possess the notorious quality of being double-edged swords. This is true for botanical medications as well as for modern synthesized pharmaceuticals. While they benefit the patient, they also pose risks of dangerous side effects. Such is the case with Peruvian

"Misqutrs" on the Ohio

bark. The dosing of the bark was a real guessing game. The alkaloids in the bark, quinine and quinidine, while attacking the plasmodia, also have the possibility of dangerous side effects by interacting with the nervous conduction system within the patient's heart, producing irregular heart rhythms, and lowering blood sugar. Quinine given orally can also cause a condition known as cinchonism, characterized by ringing in the ears, headache, nausea, and visual changes. As with hundreds of medically active plant products, great consideration has to be given to correct dosing. There are hundreds of so-called "natural" plant products that can kill and injure. If a little is good, a lot is not always better. One must consider how many patients died through the years, the victims of cinchona poisoning.

Time after time, when members of the Corps of Discovery started to exhibit symptoms of malaria over the next three summers, the captains probably administered a portion of the powdered bark, or made it into a tea. The taste of the concoction was bitter but could be flavored with some medicinal wine or with some of the cloves or cinnamon in the medicine chest. If the fever, shaking and pain were sufficiently bad, some laudanum could always ease the discomfort.

As Lewis and his small fleet made progress down the Ohio, the river gradually deepened, making for fewer episodes of towing the keelboat through the shallows. Lewis stopped for a week in Cincinnati beginning September 28. While there, his mind turned to another illness that shaped life on the frontier: smallpox. He wrote to Jefferson and, among other matters, added, "I would thank you for forwarding me some of the Vaxcine matter, as I have reason to believe from several experiments made with what I have, that it has lost it's virtue."[17]

With the addition of this substance, the Corps had hoped to become a travelling immunization clinic to protect themselves and Indians encountered from smallpox. But the kinepox that Lewis had taken along apparently failed to produce any reaction in those he immunized along the Ohio. Although Lewis realized at the time that the kinepox had become inactivated, and that the procedure using active kinepox helped protect, he had no idea why or how it worked, or of the tiny virus within the substance.

Leaving Cincinnati, the Corps floated another hundred miles downstream and finally pulled into Clarksville, Indiana Territory, on October 15. Undoubtedly it was a happy occasion for Meriwether Lewis as he jumped onto shore and had a reunion with his old friend and commander William Clark. Their time was probably filled with stories of old days in the army, discussions of their plans for the expedition, and introductions of the men that Clark had enlisted. Lewis certainly must have relayed stories about living and working in Washington, at the highest levels of power, and sitting at the fireside with President Jefferson, sipping wine. Sadly for us, Lewis apparently was not keeping his journal at the time. At least, no record of the reunion between Lewis and Clark survives.

After two weeks in Clarksville, the team set off down the Ohio and began covering the several hundred miles to its convergence with the Tennessee River. The current now ran deep and the boats easily floated downstream toward the Mississippi.

A few miles past the Tennessee lay Fort Massac, where they arrived on November 11, 1803, and added two more members. It was here that Lewis noted in his journal, "Arived at Massac engaged George Drewyer in the public service as an Indian Interpretter, contracted to pay him 25 dollards pr. Month for his services." George Drouillard was half Shawnee Indian and half French. He was a master of the Indian sign language and the most productive hunter the Corps would have. He was well worth the twenty-five dollars (compared to a private's five dollars) a month they paid him. Their trust began at once, it seems, because they immediately sent him to South West Point in Tennessee to guide another group of army volunteers to St. Louis.

On the 13th of November 1803, Lewis closed his journal entry, "raind very hard in the eving and I was siezed with a violent ague which continued about four hours and as usual was succeeded by a feever which however fortunately abated in some measure by sunrise the next morning." The following morning, rather than taking a dose of the barks that could have helped him, he displayed the influence of Dr. Rush and his love of purging. "I took a doze of Rush's pills which operated extremly well and I found myself much to my satisfaction intirely clear of fever by the evening." The fever probably would have left by evening anyway, but at least Captain Lewis wasn't constipated.

Lewis noted another effect of Rush's pills, writing that he "felt

"Misqutrs" on the Ohio

myself much better but extreemly weak." This was undoubtedly due to the effects of dehydration, or the muscular peristaltic movements produced by the potent jalap-calomel combination. In other words, Lewis was exhausted due to the massive bowel movements he had produced with the help of Rush's pills. Too bad for Lewis and the Corps that he didn't use more barks in treating his ague and fewer Thunderclappers. But intestinal purging was a treatment of choice for nearly everything in 1803.

At the junction of the Mississippi and Ohio rivers, where they camped for six nights, the captains first performed the time-consuming task of taking latitude and longitude readings with their brass sextant and expensive chronometer. Accurately measuring longitude was a problem that had vexed navigation for centuries, until an English clockmaker had been able to make a reliable timepiece portable enough to take on board His Majesty's ships during the 1700s. Now Lewis had his portable chronometer, and it would work if he could only remember to wind it. Establishing their position was of utmost importance to making accurate maps. Lewis spent a good deal of time and effort in Pennsylvania with American astronomer and mathematician Andrew Ellicott, and renowned mathematician Robert Patterson. The captain had practiced manipulating the sextant and the artificial horizon to take readings of the heavenly bodies, and making the needed calculations. His tutors had been patient, correcting his mistakes and suggesting how to improve his technique. But now he was on his own and any mistakes would go uncorrected.

On the third day here, the Corps encountered some friendly Shawnee and Delaware Indians near the mouth of the Ohio. Lewis was approached by one of the tribe, and wrote, "a respectable looking Indian offered me three beverskins for my dog and of course there was no bargan." Lewis loved Seaman, "prised much for his docility and qualifications generally for my journey." While the captains visited the Indians, the men practiced one of their favorite pastimes and caught a catfish weighing an estimated 128 pounds. Lewis took numerous measurements of this whopper fish, beginning his records of hundreds of species of North American flora and fauna that he would document for scientists back home.

On November 18, Lewis and Clark and eight of the men took off in either a canoe or one of the pirogues to visit the ground of abandoned Fort Jefferson, built by George Rogers Clark in 1780. They talked with a few frontier traders who had established themselves along the bank of the Mississippi to trade with Indians. On returning to the Corps' campground, they found that a number of the men had dipped into the whiskey and were drunk. Perhaps the captains wondered if this was a military operation or a group of hunting buddies out for a drunken weekend trip. Some of the men thought the latter. The captains obviously had some work to do to make this outfit into a legitimate military unit.

The inevitable finally came to pass, when on November 20 the relative ease of heading downstream ended, and the seemingly endless months of going against the current began as the boats turned up the Mississippi River. Their difficult progress made it apparent that more men—not a smaller party—would be needed to power the boats upriver. The long delay in waiting for the keelboat the previous August, as well as other delays that spring and summer, now put the group on a collision course with Mother Nature and approaching winter. They would be unable to sail farther than St. Louis for the season. There were another hundred-plus miles to go up the Mississippi before they could wrap it up for the winter and prepare themselves for the grueling voyage up the Missouri the following spring. Their progress upstream was at a snail's pace. The physical exertion of poling and rowing the smaller pirogues and the keelboat that had a draught of three feet was staggering.

They were usually able to progress upstream about ten to eleven miles a day. Lewis noted on November 22, "Set out at 1/2 after 6 A M. the current very rapid and difficult," adding that "we made soome soup for my friend Capt. Clark who has been much indisposed since the 16th…" For the previous six days Clark had been ill. We don't know his symptoms, so cannot guess the reason for his illness. Was it a recurrence of malaria? Was it some gastroenteritis from drinking the river water? Maybe it was both, perhaps neither. While Dr. Lewis attended to Captain Clark, Sergeant Nathaniel Pryor went out hunting. The rest of the enlisted men went to work.

The starboard bank was loaded with poplar and white oak trees, and Lewis estimated the width of the river, "including Islands at from 1 1/2 to 3 miles and the main chanel of it usually 1/2 mile wide." The Corps

"Misqutrs" on the Ohio

made thirteen miles that day and stopped for the night. They "lay upon a slate rock which here formed the beech." Imagine rowing and poling the boats for thirteen miles and then lying on a bed of slate for the night.

The next morning, Nathaniel Pryor set a precedent that would be followed by several other men during the next three years. Lewis wrote, "N. Pryor, the man who was hunting yesterday has not yet arrived, had several guns fired again and the horn wlown [blown]; waited untill half after 7 OC. And then set out without him."

By evening the Corps had arrived at Old Cape Girardeau where they stopped and Lewis called on the commandant of the fort. He was nowhere to be found but Lewis finally located him at a nearby horse race. There, "the seane reminded me very much of their small raises in Kentucky among the uncivilized backwoodsmen" adding in perhaps the spirit of his Virginia upbringing, that the people at the race track were "almost entirely emegrant from the fronteers of Kentuckey & Tennessee, and are the most dessolute and abandoned even among these people; they are men of desperate fortunes, but little to loose either character or property..." Lewis added that the commandant's Shawnee wife was "a very desent woman and if we may judge from her present appearance has been very handsome when young..." Showing his eye for the female form, Lewis added that the couple's daughter "is remarkably handsome & dresses in a plain yet fashonable stile or such as in now Common in the Atlantic States among the respectable people of the middle class," adding that she is "an affible girl, & much the most descent looking feemale I have seen since I left the settlement in Kentuckey a little below Louisville."

On return to the camp, Lewis noted without any elaboration that he "found Capt. Clark very unwell." No symptoms or treatments were recorded, so once again, we are left to pure speculation.

On the morning of the 24th, the group set out on the river at 7 A.M., and shortly thereafter heard a shout from the riverbank. It was Nathaniel Pryor, the wayfaring hunter who was "much fatiequed with his wandering and somewhat indisposed." For two days he had likely been without food. He had spent his nights away from the Corps campsite, and in later November, the nighttime temperatures were likely quite chilly. He was probably much relieved to get something warm to eat and drink and be back in the company of his comrades.

Four more days of upriver struggle and the group arrived at the army post of Fort Kaskaskia, where Clark's brother George had led a half-starved group of Continental soldiers marching on Detroit twenty-eight years earlier during the American Revolution. Undoubtedly Captain Clark shared with the Corps some of the early Illinois wilderness adventures that his elder brother had told him; tales of near starvation and unbelievable cold. The Corps would soon learn their own lessons about these hardships.

Now the captains split up for the first of many times. Clark edged his way with the men up the Mississippi, noting frequent caves in the rocks along the river and encountering various small populations of American settlers, many of French descent. Preparations for the winter camp across the river from St. Louis now went into full swing. Lewis went ahead on land to Cahokia, from where the postmaster, John Hay, and a French fur trader, Nicholas Jarrot, accompanied him the few miles upriver to St. Louis. In the old French town, Lewis, Hay, and Jarrot met with the Spanish governor who would exercise authority over the region for another few months before it became part of the United States. Clark and the men continued to struggle upstream in cold and rainy weather, noting that "the current is verry Swift." Clark and the Corps reached Cahokia on December 7, where they stayed until the 10th. The weather was anything but pleasant. The air was cold, with rain and strong winds pelting their little camp on an island in the immense river.

St. Louis in 1803 was the capital of Spanish Upper Louisiana, center of the Missouri fur trade, and about forty years old. The majority of its approximately one thousand citizens spoke French. The influence of French culture had been established in 1763 when France, which ruled the Louisiana Territory at that time, granted a French company exclusive rights to run the fur trade on the Missouri. Accordingly, the French moved in and established themselves as the dominant ethnic group. French fur traders had frequented the lower Missouri upriver from St. Louis, trading with local Indians and establishing their businesses. French men married Indian women, producing offspring, some of whom grew up and were now members of the Corps of Discovery.

With St. Louis being a hub of activity, the Corps would spend the winter nearby securing additional men to help row the canoes and keelboats as well as any further supplies they needed. The captains could search out men with knowledge of the river and the Indians who inhabited its banks, preparing for what lay ahead in the coming spring.

Clark located their winter camp on a tract of land across the Mississippi from St. Louis, near the mouth of Wood River. He arrived with the men and boats in a storm of violent wind, with alternating hail and snow, noting that the river waves "was so high." Upon their arrival, Clark observed an approaching Indian canoe that had come to check them out. The stormy river tossed the small Indian boat around like a cork and Clark feared that the canoe would soon capsize. But the tiny craft pulled up to the island and to Clark's surprise, he found that the Indians "were all Drunk." They were drunk but their canoe was dry. The hunters Clark had sent out earlier in the day returned with "Turkeys & opossoms" for dinner and a positive report on the amount of game in the region.

Along the frigid bank across from the Mississippi/Missouri confluence, the Corps of Discovery began to nest for the winter of 1803-1804. The men cut down trees, crafted logs and assembled them into structures suited to provide some minimal protection from the cold and howling December winds off the frozen rivers. The work of building log cabins was exhausting and Clark noted "the men much fatigued Carrying logs..." The carpenters and blacksmiths were rewarded with an extra gill of whiskey per day and were declared exempt from guard duty. On awakening to "hard frosty mornings," the hunters went into the woods and continued to provide ruffed grouse, "verry fat" turkeys, opossums, rabbits and deer which the camp messes roasted over the campfires while hungry and cold men eagerly awaited the warm meal and a break from their work. Fresh meat was supplemented with corn from Mr. Morrison's nearby farm and turnips courtesy of Mr. Griffeth and his garden. Shooting contests were held daily, with each contestant shooting one round, "at the distance of fifty yards off hand." The prize was an extra gill of whiskey.

On December 22, the gifted French-Shawnee hunter and interpreter George Drouillard arrived at camp with eight Army men he had been sent to collect from Tennessee. Three of the eight, Privates Hugh Hall, Thomas Howard, and John Potts would become permanent members of the Corps; a fourth, Corporal Richard Warfington, was the captains' choice to command the return keelboat party to St. Louis the following spring. The others didn't make the cut. One must wonder why. Were they in ill health? Or were they perhaps men, who like the horse racers in "Cape Jeradeau" were "dessolute and abandoned," men "of desperate fortunes," with "little to loose either character or property." Were they the cast-offs from another military command, or slackers and drunks? Whatever the reasons, they have vanished into history.

While the men labored and hunted, Lewis went shopping for supplies of flour, pork, lard, tools, and other goods from St. Louis merchants. He studied maps and interviewed men who had traveled the 1,600 miles farther up the Missouri to the edge of known settlement, the villages of the Mandan and Hidatsa Indians. He picked their brains for every detail that might be of some help in the coming year.

Christmas Day 1803 dawned cold and snowy at the Corps' camp on Wood River. Captain Clark was roused by a celebratory discharge of the men's rifles. Most of the Corps amused themselves during the holiday and "frolicked and hunted all day." Apparently deciding to celebrate in an alternative fashion, two men had a fight. Three Indians came to camp and Clark presented them with a bottle of whiskey as a Christmas present. Wild turkey, cheese, and butter formed at least part of the Christmas feast.

Boredom combined with a local trader's whiskey supply allowed John Colter, William Leakens, Hugh Hall and John Collins to get drunk on New Year's Eve. Captain Clark put a stop to these spur-of-the-moment parties and ordered the trader to stay clear of the men and the camp.

Environmental problems abounded. Winter temperatures sunk to as low as ten below zero. If the cold wasn't bad enough, collapsing dirt banks along the nearby Mississippi were a constant threat to the anchored vessels. Discovering that one of the boats had become scuttled, Clark awakened the men at midnight to walk into the freezing waters of the river and "right the boat."

On an early January day of 1804, Clark's wet feet "frozed to my

Shoes," which led to his feeling "verry unwell all day." He had repeated episodes of illness throughout January and February, writing, "I am verry unwell all day," without elaborating on any of his symptoms. Considering the season and the harshness of the living conditions, he could have had anything from a recurrence of malaria to bronchitis, pneumonia, or the flu. On February 3, after several days of illness, he wrote, "take some medisone without effect." On February 4 he added, "I am verry Sick." Exhibiting some typical thinking of his day, on February 5, Captain Clark sent Private Shields into the woods to get him some walnut bark to be used "for pills." Medicine and botany continued their synchronous paths. The next day he took his walnut pills and noted, "My Pills—work &c."

Black walnut had been used in Greek and Roman medicine in the treatment of fungal infections of the skin.[18] Other possible uses seem to ascribe to the walnut an all-around beneficial status for producing vomiting (emetics), purging, and as a "tonic to the system." It was also thought to be beneficial to a "weak and debilitated state of the bowels." (Does this sound familiar?) In addition, the green walnut rind was reported being useful in curing irritation of the membranes after treatment of syphilis with mercury.[19]

In February, Captain Clark arranged to hire non-military French voyageurs to aid in paddling and towing the boats up the Missouri River. Their expertise in negotiating the great river the first year would be crucial to the expedition, even though their civilian lack of discipline was opposite to the Corps' military aims.

One of the biggest threats to the success of any wilderness expedition is the potential disintegration of morale and/or discipline among the members of the group. When members begin to act as individuals and not as a team, the success of the endeavor is threatened. Thus the biggest trouble and threat to the cohesion of the Corps this winter came from the bad behavior of several men. Private Reubin Field was apparently encouraged by John Shields (the collector of walnuts) to refuse Sgt. John Ordway's order to stand guard duty. This brought a stern written rebuke by Lewis on March 3. The same rebuke included a ten-day sentence of confinement to camp for Colter, Boley, Peter Weiser and John Robertson, who "made hunting or other business a pretext to cover their design of visiting a neighbouring whiskey shop."

I wonder if Lewis's memory of his own drunken escapade as a young lieutenant softened his response to these young offenders.

With days lengthening, the eternal cycle of March's warming temperatures and melting snow and ice slowly warmed the continent, and the approaching spring started to peek over the shoulder of old man winter. Besides warmer weather, springtime would also make the Louisiana Territory the property of the United States. Lewis and Clark would soon begin their appointment as the explorers of the western lands. Everyone was getting anxious.

On the late winter day of March 7, at the St. Louis government house of the Spanish, probably with Captain Lewis looking on, the Spanish transferred authority over Louisiana to the French who in turn transferred it the following day to the new owners, the Americans. America now had 827,000 square miles of new backyard wilderness. It was full of unknown beauty, danger, riches, and adventure.

The Corps of Discovery was gearing up to push into its unknown and abundant bounty in fewer than three months. They were like young bulls inside a rodeo chute, kicking and rearing to be let loose. The anticipation of warmer weather and their departure helped to relieve the abundant boredom of a continued cold, windy, and snowy late-winter camp. The daily routine of getting food and trying to keep warm couldn't end too soon.

"Misqutrs" on the Ohio

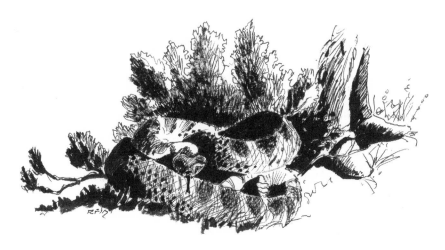

☙ 6 ☙

SNAKES IN THE GRASS
& BUGS IN THE RIVER

Rattlers and Diarrhea on the Missouri

*The secret of reaping the greatest fruitfulness and the
greatest enjoyment from life is to live dangerously!*
—Nietzsche

By the first of April 1804, spring had arrived along the Mississippi, and the spice bushes and peach, apple, and cherry trees were in full bloom. The block of ice in front of the camp once again became a river where geese and ducks swam, while cranes that had wintered on that portion of the Mississippi left for their summer homes in the north. Rain had replaced snow, and the men's patience was running thin.

That night the camp was treated to a phenomenon of nature that took place in the northern sky, the northern lights. This fascinating and beautiful display, also known as the aurora borealis, happens when major solar flares produce solar winds that carry electrons and protons to the earth's magnetic field. The magnetic fields become compressed and allow high-energy electrons and protons trapped in Earth's Van Allen belts (two donut-shaped regions of magnetism), to enter the polar atmosphere where the Van Allen belts are thin. These high-energy solar particles excite gases in the atmosphere and as these gases lose energy, that energy is in the form of visible light, which dances in the northern sky.[1] Since they had no knowledge of the underlying physics that produces this natural spectacle, we must wonder what the relatively enlightened Corps of Discovery thought about the origin of these lights.

Supplies were now being organized and stowed in the keelboat hold. Every square foot of space was valued, and the process of arranging and rearranging the materials for the lengthy trip ahead ate up several days. Each man who did not have his own flintlock had been issued an Army rifle from the United States arsenal at Harpers Ferry, Virginia. The barrels and wooden stocks were all hand made, as were the intricate lock mechanisms powering the cock (hammer). Multiple hand-forged springs within the lock provided the tension needed to power the cock that held the flint. When the trigger was pulled, the stored energy in the springs pushed the cock forward, moving the flint that struck the metal frizzen, producing a spark. The spark ignited the powder in the flash pan, which in turn ignited the charge in the barrel. The weapons required a lot of care; cleaning, oiling, and occasional fixing of broken parts. (The latter repair a job for a professional gunsmith.) The rifle was a decent weapon to hunt and protect oneself with, but certainly not comparable to the effectiveness of a modern big game rifle. In terms of relative importance to the expedition, if they were not the backbone of the expedition, the rifles were worth at least several vertebrae. The men would depend on them for their lives, their food, and their protection.

At 4 P.M. on the rainy Monday of May 14, 1804, the long awaited departure became a reality. All the pent up excitement and anticipation of the last several months was evident around the bustling boats. The little armada of explorers consisted of twenty-two men manning twenty oars on the keelboat, a sergeant and seven French boatmen in the large pirogue, and a corporal and six privates in the other pirogue. At departure, Clark's note in the journals tells the story: "men in high Spirits."

The first two days on the Missouri, the team covered 4.5 and 9.5 miles respectively. One of the pirogues was undermanned and continually lagged behind. The springtime river had "excessively rapid" current, and collapsing banks that threatened the boats with hundreds of pounds of falling dirt and mud. Submerged trees produced hidden hazards called "sawyers." They could topple a boat and were an ever-present danger.

On May 16, the men arrived at St. Charles, a village of "450 inhabitents Chiefly French." Clark added that, "those people apear pore, polite & harmonious." That evening, the captains were invited to the residence of Francois Duquette for dinner and appropriately were worried about the men's behavior in their absence. Warnings were issued that the Corps were expected to behave, as if from parents leaving some kids alone for the first time. How the men behaved is manifest in an entry of the following day: "3 men Confined for misconduct, I had a Court martial & punishment." While the captains ate dinner, William Werner and Hugh Hall left their post, and John Collins went AWOL and apparently sneaked into a ball in town and made himself obnoxious to the proper citizens of St. Charles. The charge read, "for behaveing in an unbecomeing manner at the Ball last night" and "for Speaking in a language last night after his return tending to bring into disrespect the orders of the Commanding officer."

A court-martial was held with Sgt. Ordway, Pvts. Potts, Richard Windsor, Reubin Field, and Joseph Whitehouse the jury. Werner and Hall pled guilty and were sentenced to twenty-five lashes "on their naked back," but the sentence was revoked by Lewis and Clark due to the court's recommendation of leniency. Private Collins pled guilty to the AWOL charge, but not guilty to the other two charges. "After mature deliberation & agreeable to the evidence aduced," the court found Collins guilty of all charges and sentenced him to fifty lashes, "on his naked back," to take place "this evening at Sun Set in the Presence of the Party." Fifty lashes with a leather whip would certainly do some significant damage to the skin and subcutaneous tissue of the offender's back as well as encourage better behavior. There is no record of the medical care given to the man punished, but whatever they may have put on the wounds, I doubt that the captains provided him with any laudanum or opium to relieve his pain. Tensing any muscle in his shoulders and back must have been excruciatingly painful for Collins. Rowing or poling seems hard to imagine under such conditions. After the whipping, it must have been a long couple of weeks for Private Collins. I hope the party was worth it.

Progress up the Missouri meant further contact with Indian tribes who lived along the river. On May 22, after camp was made, two Indians arrived with four deer that they presented to the men. The captains returned the good will and gave the Indians two quarts of whiskey. The same scenario was repeated the next day. The Indians would have been better off to keep the deer.

As the men rowed, towed, and poled the boats upriver, the intensity of the work must have been numbing. The strain of shoulder muscles, the wear and tear on hands tightly clamped around oars and poles for hours on end, make one ache to think about it. The pain produced probably made the evening gill of whiskey a welcome relief. The caloric intake needed to continue such work must have been in the neighborhood of five thousand calories per day.

Vital responsibilities were allotted to the three junior commanders. One sergeant stood guard at the helm of the keelboat, one in the center and one at the bow. The helmsman steered the boat and made sure all baggage was securely stowed. The center sergeant commanded the guard, managed the sails and made sure the men on the oars did their duty. He also had to ensure a timely departure, provide refreshment and breaks during the day, manage the "sperituous liquors," and take care of securing the campsites at night. The bow sergeant would look ahead for any sign of danger, either in the river or from potential enemies on the bank, and inform the center sergeant. The sergeants rotated their duties (and nightly guard duty) daily and were exempt from making fires, cooking, or pitching tents. John Ordway was the chief sergeant.

On May 25, Clark noted "rain last night." Let's take a look at the implications of his simple statement. The men were involved in mind-numbing work all day. They stopped for the evening, made their fires, and cooked and ate a warm meal. Rations were "lyed corn and grece, Poark and flour," or "indian meal and poark." No salt pork was eaten if fresh game meat was killed. Any man who preferred Indian meal to flour could have it. During the ascent of the Missouri, the men camped on shore sheltered by tents made of oiled linen.[2] The captains, at least on occasion, stayed onboard the keelboat. All probably slept in their clothing, covered by blankets. The rain started to fall, with most of it being shed by the oiled linen tents. But the guards on duty undoubtedly got wet, wet to the bone. If the rain was sufficient, run-off could have easily penetrated under the tent edges. The fire that they slept around was either put out or decreased by the shower. The men may have awakened or slept poorly during the rain due to the added noise. Water being the most efficient coolant known, the rain could rapidly cool the men's bodies and produce mild hypothermia, even in relatively warm weather. They awakened in the morning still tired, probably cold, very sore, but facing another day on the river.

By the end of May, Clark began to note the reappearance of the hated "Musquetors." On the 29th of May, Private Joseph Whitehouse followed the example set by Shields and got himself lost in the woods while exploring a cave.

Always needing fresh meat, four hunters were sent out into the countryside to get game. They were ordered to return by noon. In the evening the Corps camped on a muddy island and Clark noted the width of the Missouri as 875 yards. Much the same story was repeated day in and day out. The hunters provided some culinary variety, bringing in three black bears later that day. Following their practice of not wasting anything of use, they ate what they could of the fresh bear and jerked (cut into thin strips and dried) the rest for future use. York's athletic skill and ingenuity became apparent in early June when he "Swam to the Island to pick greens, and Swam back with his greens." Exactly what plant this was is unknown, but the addition of some fresh plant to their diet was surely welcome.

The same day Clark added, "I am verry unwell with a Slight feever from a bad cold caught three days ago." He would add on June 4, and again on the 6th, that he was "very unwell with a Sore throat & head ake." It provides some insight into Clark, that he thought himself, "verry unwell," even though he noted that he only had a bad cold. I don't mean to imply that Captain Clark lacked any intestinal fortitude, but it does strike me as curious that he evaluated his condition in that manner. Perhaps he had a strep throat or a sinus infection, either one of which can certainly make one feel "verry unwell." Whatever the condition, it seems to have been a bit more than an uncomplicated viral upper respiratory infection to elicit such a comment from Clark.

Arising from their extra-firm natural mattresses that Mother Nature provided each night, the men slogged upstream for a couple of hours before stopping to eat some of the cold food cooked the previous day. Probably many comments about bodily aches and pains that hadn't been there the night before could be heard as the men sat together at breakfast. Lively conversations in French and English, with frequent jokes flying back and forth, were probably part of the morning routine. The glue of rapport and trust that holds men together during difficult times was being poured and starting to set.

Travelling the springtime Missouri with its rising waters, strong current, and hidden snags was ever dangerous. On June 9, Clark wrote: "the Sturn of the boat Struck a log which was not proceiveable the Curt. Struck her bow and turn the boat against Some drift & Snags which [were] below with great force; This was a diagreeable and Dangerous Situation, particularly as immense large trees were Drifting down and we lay imediately in their Course." A precarious and potentially disastrous situation required quick action. "Some of our men being prepared for all Situations leaped into the water Swam ashore with a roap, and fixed themselves in Such Situations, that the boat was off in a fiew minits, I can Say with Confidence that our party is not inferior to any that was ever on the waters of the Missoppie."

Clark closed that day's entry with, "one of our French hands had a [complaint]— We Commsd Doctering." The captain/physicians were having "sick-call."

At camp the following evening, while the men erected their tents and set up camp for the night, Clark and Lewis walked about three miles into the surrounding prairie. Numerous white-tailed deer, spooked at their presence, shot their tails into the air as they sprinted effortlessly away. The countryside was lush and rolling. The captains found some wild plum bushes and probably regretted that it was only June, and the fruit was not yet ripe.

During the days, while Clark maintained command on board the keelboat, Lewis hiked the banks of the Missouri observing the plants, animals, and rocks for possible discoveries for the world of science and the members of the American Philosophical Society back in Philadelphia. Everything was proceeding in a splendid fashion, and Clark noted in early June, "our party in high Spirits." The high morale of their men has been music to the ears of every expedition leader in history.

On June 11, Clark noted that "my Cold is yet verry bad." After nearly two weeks with this ailment, it is highly likely that he was suffering from a complication of the ordinarily mild stuffy nose and scratchy throat of the common cold. He very likely had a bacterial sinus infection, which causes a good deal of pain in the facial sinuses, cough, possible fever, headache, and general fatigue. Today we could treat this condition with antibiotics, steroids, decongestants, and perhaps some pain medication. We must speculate about Clark's treatment of his condition—probably more purges with Rush's pills. He would still be suffering from the illness five days later.

The next day the sergeant at the bow shouted a warning of approaching boats from upstream, and both armadas pulled to shore for introductions to be made. The boats heading downstream for St. Louis were loaded with beautiful furs obtained upriver. Among their party was a gentleman named Pierre Dorion, who had lived with the Yankton band of the Sioux nation for more than twenty years. The captains talked with him about the Sioux, trying to gain information about this powerful and potentially dangerous tribe that they would soon encounter. His information was reliable, with Clark noting, "This man being a verry Confidential friend of those people…" The captains saw a great opportunity to ease their way into Sioux society, and asked Dorion to accompany them upriver. Dorion agreed to go and act as an intermediary in inviting the chiefs to go to Washington for a visit with their "new father." If a visit to the capital could be arranged, the powerful Sioux could be properly impressed with the might and "good will" of the United States government. In addition to the diplomatic negotiations, the captains bought three hundred pounds of buffalo grease and tallow, known as "voyageurs' grease." This multi-purposed fat product could be used either to make a foodstuff called pemmican or to provide some protection from the ever present mosquitoes.

Years of Indian intertribal warfare became apparent when the group discovered a former village of the Missouri Indians where as Clark noted, "at this place 300 of them were killed by the Saaukees." Historian Gary E. Moulton explains that the Missouris, once a large and important tribe, were all but wiped out during the later 18th century by Mississippi tribes, particularly the Sauk and Fox tribes.[3] Among the captains' prime objectives was to foster peace among the tribes, but they would not see much success.

At a campsite above a submerged sandbar that had nearly overturned the boat, while the fire crackled and spat sparks into the dark sky, Drouillard provided a bit of colorful storytelling. He spun a tale of an immense and "remarkable Snake inhabiting a Small lake 5 ms. below which gobbles like a Turkey & may be herd Several miles." George claimed to have heard the gobbling himself and, trying to flush out the turkey, had fired his gun, only to have the gobbling get louder. Apparently the Indians had also mentioned this snake, and another Frenchman attested to the veracity of the story. I wonder if George kept a straight face spinning that yarn.

At times the current of the Missouri was too swift to make any progress, even with all oars manned and a wind in the sail. On these occasions the ropes were brought out and the men acted as oxen, towing the craft upstream from the riverbank or in the shallows. But the river's current and its collapsing banks were only two of the problems the men encountered. By the middle of June, Clark would note, "the misquitoes have been troublesome" and the ticks were "numerous and large." Out came a supply of buffalo grease for the men to smear on their exposed skin in an effort to repel the insects.

The boats were now making their way along banks that were "well timbered," abounding with deer, elk, and bear. Several of the men's intestines started to cramp terribly as they ran for the bushes or just jumped into the river shallows where they could relieve their bowels. As they rowed or towed the boat, they would have to either leave their posts for the moment or go in their pants.

At the same time they had painful, pus-filled boils on their skin. The insides of their thighs, which continually rubbed together as they walked along the shore, became as sore as the soles of their feet. "The party is much afflicted with Boils and Several have the Decissentary, which I contribute to the water," Clark wrote on June 17.

A good water supply was a colossal and unsolvable problem for the Corps of Discovery. Today we have portable water filtering devices that can be taken into the field and provide excellent and thorough filtering for particles as small as a virus. But when the men on the Missouri in 1804 got thirsty, they drank directly from the muddy waters of the river.

Every mouthful of Missouri River water probably contained a combination of water, mud, algae, fungi, bacteria, possibly viruses, and a group of one-celled organisms we call protozoa, the last probably agents of gastrointestinal illness for the men of the Corps.

Protozoans don't categorically cause diarrhea. With virtually all of the water supply in the nation being untreated in 1803, probably all the men of the Corps had protozoans inhabiting their intestines much or all of the time, with very little illness occurring as a result. The men ingested these little "critters" in their drinking water. Many of these small organisms would pass through their intestines without manifesting illness, but the protozoan *Giardia lamblia* can cause diarrhea.

Giardia is endemic in fresh water supplies of the western mountains of the United States, but outbreaks have occurred in every region of the country.[4] The ingested giardia is in two forms: the mobile trophozoite, and the non-mobile, encapsulated form that is shed in the stool. If a member of the Corps drank water containing the trophozoite form of giardia, it would pass from his stomach into the first part of his small intestine where it would attach itself to the wall. An incubation period of from one to three weeks followed. Some of the trophozoites encapsulate themselves and are passed out of the body in the victim's feces. The probable sources of the giardia in nature are dogs, beavers, sheep, cats, cattle, and rodents. Only ten to twenty-five cysts are necessary to produce an infection, with more than twenty-five cysts causing infection in 100 percent of victims.[5] The cysts are also very resistant to extremes of the environment. They can live in cold water for two to three months.[6]

When the diarrheal symptoms start, they can either begin slowly or explosively. Explosive watery diarrhea accompanied by cramping, foul smelling gas, vomiting, fever, and malaise is common. This acute phase usually lasts three to four days and then subsides into a milder form, or what we call in medicine a "subacute" phase that can be manifest with fatigue, weight loss, and loss of appetite. The exact mechanism by which the giardia produces its symptoms is not known, but several hypotheses have been floated. Most victims' immune systems will respond appropriately and fight off the infection within three to ten weeks.[7]

Another bad actor that could have been in the Missouri and is capable of producing the diarrhea is the protozoan *Entamoeba histolytica*. Again, as with giardia, both a trophozoite and an encapsulated form of the amoeba exist. If this agent affected the Corps of Discovery it was probably transmitted by drinking water from the Missouri that had been contaminated by humans using the river as a toilet. It could have been obtained from food that had been prepared by dirty hands not washed after the person had a bowel movement. An infected human can shed 45 million cysts per day in their bowel movements. Flies and cockroaches that come in contact with infected feces could transfer the cysts to exposed food before it was ingested by humans. Most people who ingest this protozoan do not exhibit symptoms. If symptoms are present, they come from invasion of the intestinal wall by the amoeba. This can result in anything from bloody diarrhea that usually clears within a few days, to a chronic intermittent diarrhea, weight loss, stomach pain and lots of gas. Some unlucky victims may go on to have the amoebas spread through their blood and form liver, lung or brain abscesses. Complications occur in only 1 to 4 percent of cases and include rupture of the intestine and intestinal abscess.[8]

Modern medications can eradicate both giardia and entamoeba. But Lewis and Clark had a medication that may have helped solve these problems and it was in the form of their "Dr. Rush's Bilious Pills." These could definitely have decreased a large load of amoebas in the colon by their aggressive purging action, and may have helped cure the giardia as well. The mercury in the calomel portion of the Thunderclappers could have had a directly toxic effect on the organisms as well as having a strongly irritating effect on the lining of the intestine that gave it its potent cathartic action. The ipecacuan that was in the captains' medicine chest contained emetine, an anti-amoebic alkaloid. Of course the captains knew nothing about organic chemistry or the presence of emetine. Since they also had no concept of amoebas, any ipecac they may have used was the result of their seemingly never-ending luck.

There are other organisms that could have caused the diarrhea, including the protozoan *Cryptosporidium*, which is known to cause diarrhea associated with wilderness travel. Infecting wild animals such as raccoons, beavers, squirrels, and coyotes,[9] it is usually spread through animal feces that contaminate drinking water. Cryptosporidia live in the lining of the small intestine of humans and other mammals. If symptoms are present, they may include diarrhea mild to severe, with cramping, nausea, vomiting, and loss of appetite. The symptoms may last from several days to several weeks. Other bacterial organisms that can be spread via contaminated water and that cause diarrhea include the bacterial organisms, *E. coli*, *Shigella*, *Salmonella*, and *Vibrio*, as well as various viral organisms. These are usually spread through fecal contamination of food or water supplies. The men of the Corps drank water from the various rivers they encountered that amounted to a diluted cesspool—nature's cesspool.

Captain Clark's June 21 description of "Swift water over roleing Sands which rored like an immence falls" sounds like a prescription for disaster but, protected by the river-reading skill of men like pilot Pierre Cruzatte, the boats avoided the destruction awaiting them under the murky waters of the Missouri.

Due to the great turbulence of the churning, boiling, and sandy water, which had risen three inches overnight, some means of stabilization was needed to protect the keelboat. A long towrope was secured from the mast to men on the shore, and an anchor suspended in the water below the boat. This provided some stability for the heavy and awkward craft. During a particularly violent maneuver, one of the windows in the cabin of the keelboat was broken in a violent whirlpool. Numerous river obstacles were time and again successfully negotiated as the boats continued to crawl up the Missouri.

Fortunately for the men, the river provided something other than danger and endless toil. With afternoon temperatures in the high 80s, they frequently cooled themselves in the water. It was an irony of nature that the same body of water could produce such opposite effects on a constant and daily basis.

Captain Clark left his usual position onboard and took to the shoreline to spend the day walking on June 23. Strong winds prevented the boats from moving, so they never reached Clark. Deciding to stay out alone, he located a likely source of game for supper on a willow-covered island. As he made his way through the high brush, he became mired in an immense field of muddy goo. Crawling and now covered with silt, the captain made camp, started a fire, scraped and washed off the mud that covered him, and washed his clothes. He fired his flintlock hoping that the rifle shot might signal anyone of the party who may be in the area and prepared his bed by peeling some bark off a tree. He "geathered wood to make fires to Keep off the musquitor & Knats." George Drouillard, who had as usual been out hunting, heard the signal shot and came in to meet the captain, bringing along with him a fat deer and bear that he had bagged that afternoon. The two weary outdoorsman "feasted of meet & water, the latter we made great use of being much fatigued & thirsty." Clark slept in his hunting clothes on his bed of peeled bark with the mosquitoes and ticks as his bedfellows.

As Clark struggled through the mud of the Missouri island and Drouillard stalked his game on the Great Plains that afternoon, the great snow packs in the distant Rockies continued to melt and dwindle as they had for weeks in the summer sun. The effect of the steadily diminishing water supply in the mountains so far away had its ripple effect hundreds of miles downstream at Clark and Drouillard's camp—Clark noted the following morning that the river had dropped eight inches during the night.

At the end of June, the captains were noticing great quantities of "fine Coal" in the bank along the Missouri. Constant contact with wildlife on shore provided Joseph Field with a wolf pup that he brought into camp to try to tame as a pet. John Ordway found a spring that provided him with some water he described as the "best and coolest I have seen in the country." The fishermen in the group caught several large catfish. Lewis noted seeing "a great number of Parrot queets" one evening. The species was the Carolina parakeet (*Conuropsis carolinensis*), which is now extinct.[10]

On June 27, the exhausted party stopped to rest for four days. They had arrived at the confluence of the Kansas River with the Missouri. Clark drank of the Kansas and pronounced that the "waters of the Kansas is verry disigreeably tasted to me."

June 29 brought more trouble with the men. John Collins and Hugh Hall were called before a court-martial. Collins was accused by Sgt. Floyd of "getting drunk on his post this morning out of whiskey put under his Charge as a Sentinal and for Suffering Hugh Hall to draw whiskey out of the Said Barrel intended for the party." The captains must have been shaking their heads in disgust. Here they were in the middle of nowhere and their guards who are supposed to be watching over the group as it slept are dipping into the hooch. Collins pled not guilty. After what Clark noted was "mature deliveration on the evidence abduced &c...," the court came to the "oppinion that the prisoner is Guilty of the Charge exibited against him, and do therefore Sentence him to recive one hundred Lashes on his bear Back." Hugh Hall, probably very sheepishly, pled guilty and got fifty lashes. The punishment was to be carried out at 3 P.M. in front of the assembled Corps.

Every person who has ever crawled out of a tent or sleeping bag on a cold morning looking for something warm to eat can identify with Captain Clark's comment of June 30, 1804. "We opened the Bag of Bread" and "our Bacon...found Sound and good," adding that "a relish of this old bacon this morning was verry agreeable." We can almost smell it cooking and hear the grease popping. Raspberries found nearby added some much-needed vitamin C to the men's diet. The berries were "perple, ripe and abundant."

The party was in generally good health by the 1st of July, with the exception that many men had boils. Clark was either constipated or just wanted to clear his system out and noted, "I took Some medison last night which has worked me very much." The "medison" which acted overnight would certainly have been some cathartic. With the collection they had of laxatives, I can only wonder at how much they "worked" the captain.

During the night, as the exhausted men slept around the fires, the guards on duty roused them with shouts of alarm. The weary men staggered to their feet and reached for their weapons. Anticipation of attacking Indians probably raced through the imaginations of the disoriented men. But the perceived menace never materialized, and soon they all decided that the noise was that of "either a man or Beast, which run off." Irritated but relieved, the spent men lay back down and once again drifted into blessed insensibility for a few more hours.

The Fourth of July brought the group of forty-six men, four horses and a dog together for a celebration of Independence Day. The occasion was marked in part with a shot fired from the cannon mounted on the bow of the keelboat. They were in an area that Clark described as "Situated far removed from the Sivilised world to be enjoyed by nothing but the Buffalo Elk Deer & Bear in which it abounds & Savage Indi-ans." The surroundings were of "sweetest and most norushing" green grass. Intermittent groves of trees with springs and brooks of "fine water" and scrubs covered with ripe and delicious fruits dotted the landscape. Was it the Garden of Eden or the pristine American wilderness? Except for the mosquitoes, ticks, and diarrhea, they probably could have been one and the same. An extra gill of whiskey livened up the Fourth of July picnic, and the bow cannon was fired again at night, as Ordway put it, "for Independence of the U.S."

During the breakfast break along the bank that morning, Joseph Field had wandered along the shore enjoying a few moments of exploring. Suddenly he felt something hit his ankle. He gazed downward and was surprised to find a snake within spitting distance of his foot. Within seconds, the foot began to hurt and, as was noted in the journals, "the Side of his foot which Swelled much..." The snake is not identified, but was likely the prairie rattlesnake, *Crotalus viridis viridis*.

Field's ankle and foot responded in a typical fashion to envenomation by a rattler. The captains' medical response was application of a poultice of barks to the wound. The powdered Peruvian bark was probably mixed with some gunpowder, a popular method among frontiersman of the day.

Rattlesnakes are reptiles, belonging to the same taxonomic class as lizards, turtles, crocodiles, and alligators. Separated from the others into a more specific category, they are part of the pit viper family (Crotalidae), so named due to a small heat-sensing pit below each eye. In spite of being deaf, and having poor vision, the rattlesnake can locate warm-blooded prey with the use of this infrared sensor, even in the dark. This group of heat sensitive cells can sense differences in temperature as little as 0.003 degrees Celsius, but only within a range of about fourteen inches.[11] As Joseph Field walked on the shoreline, the snake felt the approaching vibration of his moccasined feet and may have smelled him with its flicking forked tongue, which brought Field's molecules to the smell detectors in the snake's head. The snake that bit Private Field was probably hiding in the shade, avoiding the hot sun and awaiting the cooler temperatures of the night to do its hunting.

When a rattlesnake strikes, it does so very rapidly, and usually only once, burying its long hypodermic-like fangs into the victim and injecting its venom. This all happens in an instant, in a matter of milliseconds. The snake's rattles, interlocking keratin rings, make a distinctive "buzz" but the snake does not always precede its strike with a warning rattle. After the snake bites and envenomates its prey, depending on the size, the prey may be immobilized and die within seconds or may take several minutes or hours to succumb. Non-envenomation bites do occur, and death for larger animals is by no means a certain outcome. The snake will then relocate the dead prey with its heat sensing pits and, size permitting, swallow its meal whole. The rattlesnake that the Corps of Discovery encountered most often was the prairie rattlesnake. Its venom has a potency that is approximately in the middle of the spectrum of rattlesnake venom.[12]

The venom of a rattlesnake is 90 percent water, with five to fifteen different enzymes (proteins that cause chemical reactions to occur). One of the first reactions of the injected venom occurs when short protein chains—of twenty to twenty-eight amino acids in length—attack the endothelial cells of vascular walls (the cells that line the blood vessels). This action results in the destruction of the membranes surrounding other blood vessel cells in the neighborhood. Blood cells (red and white), as well as the fluid portion of the blood (serum), leak into the surrounding tissue. Fluids that were contained within the ruptured cells around the blood vessels now accumulate within the tissues. These fluids in the affected tissues result in swelling (edema) of the involved area.[13]

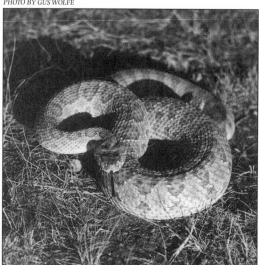

Western rattlesnake, commonly known as diamondback.

Important enzymes found in the venom inside Private Field's swelling leg were: proteolytic enzymes that damage muscle and other tissues, causing their death; hyaluronidase, which attacks connective tissue, aiding in the spread of the venom; and phospholipase A2, which attacks red cell membranes and muscle cells. Other cells in the victim's tissue contain the substance called histamine. These cells also rupture in response to the venom, causing yet more swelling and loss of blood volume.[14]

If the snake injects sufficient venom, enough tissue damage occurs and enough fluid is lost from the vascular system to give the victim hypovolemic shock—insufficient blood in the vascular system to maintain blood pressure. The victim's blood pressure falls, the brain is robbed of sufficient blood supply and the oxygen it carries, and the victim loses consciousness. Blood pressure is too low to supply other organs such as the kidneys, and consequently urine production stops. If the deadly spiral continues, death may result.

Problems involving the blood platelets, which function in clotting, can also occur, resulting in diffuse hemorrhage within the body. If the unlucky victim suffered a bite that penetrated a vein, resulting in direct injection of venom into the blood system, dangerous decreases in blood pressure (hypotension) and shock can occur rapidly.

Within minutes of being bitten by the rattler, Joseph Field's ankle and foot started to swell, which is the normal reaction to a rattlesnake bite with a "minimal envenomation." Pain accompanied the swelling. Field's symptoms apparently never progressed past this stage. A more severe envenomation would have resulted in symptoms such as nausea, vomiting, bruising around the bite site, and tingling around his mouth and in his extremities. A severe envenomation would also have included blood clotting disorders, muscle twitching (fasiculations), and multisystem failure, with possible shock and death. Severe envenomations may require surgery to relieve the extreme pressure that may result in various muscle compartments due to the swelling of the tissue, a so-called "compartment syndrome." This can cause the loss of blood supply to the muscles, resulting in great pain and ultimately death of the involved tissue. If Joseph Field had suffered a severe envenomation, he probably would have died along the Missouri.

Modern treatment of rattlesnake bites involves calming the victim, immobilizing the bitten extremity, and getting rapid medical attention; no tourniquets and cutting of the fang marks and sucking out the poison like you saw on all those Saturday morning cowboy movies. Once the patient is at a hospital, antivenin is administered and samples taken for laboratory tests to check on organ function and clotting mechanisms, all of which help to determine the bite's severity and how aggressively to treat it. The key to successful treatment is prompt intravenous administration of antivenin that neutralizes the venom.[15]

Given the calmness of Lewis and Clark, they probably reassured Joseph Field as they applied the poultice of Peruvian bark, which probably had no beneficial pharmacologic effect at all. Quinine and the other alkaloids in the bark act against the malarial *Plasmodium*, but not against rattlesnake venom. But the "barks" in 1804 were a tonic and a "cure-all." If it worked for the fevers of ague, why wouldn't it work for the sickness caused by a rattlesnake bite? The captains did what they could. They used what they had. They treated their patient with concern and did what they thought proper.

Field's leg continued to hurt and be swollen for several days. Private Patrick Gass noted on July 9, that "The man that was snake bitten is become well." In honor of Private Joseph Field and his battle with the rattler, Captain Clark named the site "Joseph Fields Snake Prarie." I can't help but believe that there was a lot of laughing among the Corps at that announcement—laughter and thanksgiving that Field was alive and well.

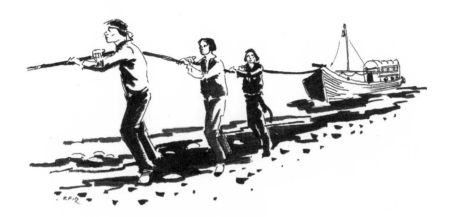

⚜ 7 ⚜

THE SUN AND DYING YOUNG

A Lucky Streak Ends

The hero is strangely akin to those who die young.
—*Poet Rainer Maria Rilke*

As the hot and humid days of July dragged on, the Missouri River undoubtedly seemed endless. Every turn brought another view of the endless muddy water and the forebodings of backbreaking labor required to conquer it. The day-time heat and the ever-present mosquitoes sapped the energy and threatened the health of the Corps. The boatmen sweated profusely, their bodies trying desperately to cool down while at the same time depleting themselves of needed fluids and minerals. William Clark noted the severity of the effect, and wrote, "Those men that do not work at all will wet a Shirt in a Few minits & those who work, the Swet will run off in Streams." Clark thought that the profuse sweating might be the result of some mysterious property of the Missouri's water. His logic was a probable extension of the same 18th century thought process that attributed malaria to the inhalation of swamp gases. Occasionally a welcome rain provided a cooling shower during the day, but the same shower became a vexation in the evening when the men were trying to make a camp.

A potential disaster brewed for one member of the Corps of Discovery on the afternoon of July 7. Private Robert Frazer, a probable native of Virginia, was under the command of Sgt. Charles Floyd. Apparently, Frazer had found the early days with the group difficult and had misbehaved in some manner, because the captains noted in April that he "has don bad." But Frazer was now in some potentially deep trouble on the boat in the middle of the Missouri. Clark's simple entry about Frazer, "one man verry Sick, Struck with the Sun, Capt. Lewis bled him & gave Niter which has revived him much," may have recorded anything but a minor incident. Frazer was suffering from either heat exhaustion or possibly the life-threatening problem of heat stroke.

As already noted, the boatmen were working in great heat and direct sunlight while rowing, towing, or pushing the boats upstream. As Frazer exerted his muscles, one of the byproducts was heat that was dissipated by the body in part by the cooling action of sweat. As sweat evaporates from the body it carries heat away. As the body loses water in the form of perspiration, chemical sensors within us monitor this and stimulate our brain to tell us to "Drink!" If the work is not severe and prolonged, we can drink enough to replenish the lost sweat and stay out of trouble. But if the work is severe and performed in hot weather, the body's temperature rises and fluids lost through sweat cannot be replaced fast enough by drinking. While Frazer's body tried to cool itself by sweating for a prolonged period of time, he became dehydrated. He became nauseated and weak, and likely vomited. He may have fainted.

Certain factors contribute to heat-related illness, including fatigue, lack of sleep, loss of electrolytes (sodium, potassium, chloride) contained in perspiration, dehydration, high air temperature and humidity, and wearing impermeable clothing such as buckskin or wool.[1] One result is reduced appetite that further worsens the picture, with the victim not wanting to take in extra food or fluid to replace the lost fluid and electrolytes. Frazer was undoubtedly experiencing fatigue and lack of sleep that hot day in July of 1804, and if he was one of the unlucky guys to have diarrhea he was probably dehydrated at the onset of the day's activities. Summer in the Midwest, and particularly on the river where humidity probably approached the 90 percent range, made heat dissipation from the body very difficult indeed. As the sun rose and the air got hotter and hotter, sweat poured, Frazer got thirsty and had insufficient water intake that led to dehydration. The poor guy got very sick and the problem progressed. The sequence of events took their toll.

In periods of heat and body exertion, the brain commands glands in the skin to produce sweat. A world-class runner was monitored producing 3.71 liters per hour of sweat in a 1984 experiment.[2] To replace the lost fluids, an equal amount would have to be taken into the stomach. But the maximum rate of gastric emptying is only about 1.2 liters per hour, much less than the maximal sweating rate.[3] The math is easy; in severe conditions, we cannot take in enough fluid by mouth to keep ourselves from becoming dehydrated.

Modern treatment of heat related illness involves reducing the body temperature and rehydrating the patient. The victim must stop exercising. Cooling measures, such as removing clothing and placing ice bags in the armpits and groin, help to cool the overheated blood. Spraying water and fanning the body reduce its temperature by carrying away heat through the processes of evaporation, conduction, and convection. Intravenous rehydration is often helpful.

The treatment administered to Frazer by Dr. Lewis was not one of Lewis's shining medical moments, but he followed the thinking of the day. Lewis noted that Frazer was weak and faint. He probably took Frazer's pulse and, due to the man's dehydration, the pulse was probably somewhat weak and rapid. The rapid pulse was produced by his dehydration and the resulting decreased amount of blood in Frazer's vessels; in order to maintain an adequate blood pressure, Frazer's heart had to increase its output of blood by increasing the rate at which it beat. The best treatment would have been to replace the lost fluids within Frazer's body. But the accepted method of treatment in that era, and following Dr. Rush's philosophy, was to bleed the patient. This is exactly what Frazer did not need. The act of bleeding only complicated his illness and put him further behind by further decreasing his blood pressure and body fluids. Fifty years later Oliver Wendell Holmes pretty much summed up what physicians of the era of Lewis and Clark thought about bleeding when he said, "The lancet was the magician's wand of the dark ages of medicine." In addition to the bleeding, "niter," or saltpeter (potassium nitrate), was given to Frazer. This chemical is listed in old materia medica books as a diuretic, or medication that increases urination. Urination would of course further reduce the amount of fluids within the body

Most otherwise-healthy patients will recover from non–life-threatening illnesses in spite of what the physician does. The healthy human body has an amazing resilience, as witnessed by Clark's comment that the dehydrating treatment of Frazer, "has revived him much." Probably the simple act of lying down on the boat and drinking some fluids was responsible for Frazer's "revival." Frazer recovered in spite of, not because of, the treatment he received.

Lest we citizens of the early 21st century start feeling arrogant about our position in history and our relative societal sophistication, there still exist in our modern world examples of stupidity and ignorance that would make Lewis and Clark and Benjamin Rush look like cutting edge scientists! For example, in a case that defies common sense, in 1976, a young boy in Australia was treated for a health problem by an herbalist, by "immersion in a heap of fermenting horse manure for forty minutes." The boy subsequently died of heatstroke.[4] Football coaches, at least in my day, used to force players to keep their helmets on along the sidelines, not allowing needed cooling of the head and body to occur. We unfortunately still hear periodically about some poor athlete who was run to death on a hot day by an ignorant coach trying to toughen him up. At least Lewis probably allowed poor Frazer the luxury of resting and drinking on board the keelboat.

It is interesting to note that the captains recorded that five men were sick the following day with violent headaches. In light of the extreme heat and probable dehydration of more than just Frazer, these men were probably suffering some symptoms of dehydration and heat-related illness.

As the Corps approached the end of July they also approached the mouth of the Platte River, just a few miles south of present-day Omaha, Nebraska. This was Plains Indian territory, and the group anticipated making contact with some of the locals, hoping for a friendly reception and ears that would be open to their message of American sovereignty and their desire to trade. Clark's experience in dealing with Indians was the greater of the two captains, and it is said that he genuinely enjoyed the company of Indians.[5] The many gifts and trade items the Corps had stored and tried to keep dry for months would now be used as diplomatic tools. Items of cloth, fishhooks, tobacco, sewing needles, knives, brooches, and colored beads, as well as medals with Jefferson's likeness on one side, and two hands shaking in friendship on the other would soon be presented to various tribes. All these precious commodities were lying in wait, neatly packed away in the hull of the keelboat, waiting for their first opportunity to be of use.

Perhaps Lewis and Clark started to review the list of anthropological questions that Dr. Rush and others had given them. These were inquiries designed to gather information on the Indians' health and society, such as whether crime or suicide existed among them, and what the Indians used to produce intoxication. How did they bury their dead and what were their objects of worship? How long did they live and what were their vices? At what age do Indian women begin and cease to menstruate? Do the Indians sacrifice animals in their worship? And, surely from Dr. Rush, "Are artificial discharges of blood ever used among them?"[6] Besides being explorers, cartographers, hunters, boatmen, commanders and physicians, the captains would also soon become ethnographers.

It was well known by the American government prior to the expedition's departure that some Sioux Indians made life difficult for traders ascending the Missouri. The Sioux exerted control over the river by blocking the passage of any trader headed upstream, demanding payment to pass or at times simply just robbing them of their goods. Other tribes such as the Arikaras and Omahas had on occasion joined in the fun of exacting tribute from white men on their way up the Missouri.

There existed within the greater tribe of Sioux several distinct bands. The Brule, Oglala and Miniconjou bands were collectively known as the Teton Sioux. Other Sioux bands included the Sisseton and Yankton. These groups shared a common language and culture but oftentimes lived separately.

Political intrigue and economic considerations were as much a part of Plains Indian life as they were with white politicians in Washington,

D.C. The numerous tribes of the Missouri River valley had developed complex societal and trading relationships along the river. The Teton Sioux enjoyed their position of control along the middle Missouri. Obtaining the white man's trade goods from the North West Company posts on the Des Moines and St. Peters rivers, the Tetons would in turn trade these items to the Arikaras, who were famous for raising corn. As long as the Tetons controlled the incoming goods, they controlled the region's economy. The Tetons did not want traders coming upriver, looking to trade directly with other tribes they viewed as their customers. This in part was what led to the frequent clashes between river merchants and the Teton Sioux.[7] In contrast were the Yankton Sioux, who had on occasion been friendlier in their interactions with the white man.

On July 28, while out hunting, Drouillard found a lone Missouri Indian, whom he convinced to come to visit the captains. The Missouri tribe had been nearly wiped out by smallpox, and surviving members now lived with the Oto tribe. The lone native told Drouillard through the sign language that the Otos were out hunting buffalo on the plains.

The next day the captains sent the Indian and a French and Oto speaking engagé (hired boatman), back to the Indian village in an effort to coax them to come to a meeting with the captains. The Corps' plan was to continue upriver for a couple of days and then wait for the diplomats and their Indian guests to arrive.

That day the men caught three large and fat catfish, and saw a swath of fallen timber across a considerable part of the riverside. Some of the trees were as large as four feet in diameter and had fallen from the apparent effects of a tornado that had cut its roaring path of destruction through the area in recent weeks. The catfish were sliced up for food, and a quart of oil was rendered from excess fat on one of the fish.

Private Alexander Willard continued his string of mistakes. Several of the journal writers in the Corps, including John Ordway and Joseph Whitehouse, thought the latest incident interesting enough to record it. Willard, who had been a blacksmith with an artillery company in 1800, had been court-martialed two weeks earlier for sleeping while on guard duty. He could have been executed, but instead was given a hundred lashes, well laid on his bare back. The morning of July 29, he had been sent back to the camp of the previous night, to pick up his forgotten tomahawk, and while crossing a creek, had dropped his rifle into its depths. He reached into the waters but had no luck in recovering this irreplaceable necessity. He must have been frustrated, to say the least. He returned to the group and got Reubin Field to go with him back to the creek. Willard pointed out the spot where he had dropped the rifle, and Field made a salvage dive. Reubin found the weapon and brought it topside. It would take Willard a few hours to disassemble all the parts, dry, and oil them. But at least one bright light shown for Alex Willard that afternoon, and he and Reubin Field probably became much better friends.

August 1 was Captain Clark's thirty-fourth birthday. While resting and waiting for the upcoming summit, an impromptu party was organized. Clark wrote, "I order'd a Saddle of fat Vennison, an Elk fleece & a Bevertail to be cooked and a Desert of Cheries, Plumbs, Raspberries currents and grapes of a Supr. Quallity." The fierce hoards of mosquitoes detracted from the enjoyment of his birthday feast, but a restful birthday was nonetheless a welcome event.

After an anxious wait, a group of thirteen Oto and Missouri Indians, along with a French fur trader living with them, arrived in camp. That of "diplomat" could now be added to the captains' growing list of titles. At times their diplomacy would be naive and foolish, at times profoundly wise and insightful. At nightfall on August 2, at the site they named "the Council Bluff," the captains sent the visiting dignitaries some fresh meat, salt pork, flour, and meal. The Indians sent back some "Water millions," Clark's term for fruits and vegetables of that general shape. The encounter's tension could not be disguised with the food, however, and every man was "on his Guard & ready for any thing."

The next day, the formal affair took place. The site was an elevated area surrounded by a "butifull Plain both abov and below." The Corps displayed their military precision with a dress parade. The American flag was posted and gift packages were put together for the chiefs. The Indians arrived and prepared for what historian James Ronda wrote was "something like a Lewis and Clark Medicine Show." Lewis delivered a long-winded speech that outlined the power of the United States that now governed the area, and encouraged the Indians, whom Clark referred to as "thos Children of ours," to be obedient, and to "Cultivate friendship & good understanding." A probably less than professional translator did his best to translate the speech from English to Oto. The chiefs were presented with some gifts and agreed, according to Clark, to "prosue the good advice and Caustion" given them by their "new father who gave good advice" and who could "be Depended on." All the chiefs then asked for some gunpowder and a "Drop of Milk [whiskey]." Clark was generous, giving them "50 balls one Canister of powder & a Dram." Captain Lewis wound up the dog and pony show by astonishing the Indians with a few firings of his compressed-air–powered gun. American diplomacy was on its way.

Private Moses Reed had had enough. Enough hot days on the river and enough nights on guard duty; enough cold meals and too many sleepless nights in the rain and wind. The Corps continued to move farther away from civilization every monotonous day on that damned river, with nothing to look forward to but more campfires and more Indians. Whatever Moses thought he would find by joining the Corps, he didn't find it and he had had enough. He packed his powder and lead balls, shouldered his rifle, and left. His ruse was needing to go downriver to retrieve the knife he had lost there, and the captains gave him permission to go. Three days later he still hadn't returned. The knife was either very well hidden or Moses Reed had flown the coop. The captains believed the latter to be true.

The captains sent out four of their best men on August 7. Reubin Field, William Bratton and Pvt. Francois Labiche, as well as hunter/tracker George Drouillard were charged to take the "Deserter reid with order if he did not give up Peaceibly to put him to Death." I wonder if Captain Clark refused to capitalize "reid" on purpose? Clark was a bad speller but he didn't fail to capitalize other last names. Maybe it was his way of heaping contempt on the deserter in writing. That same day, Sergeant Floyd wrote that Reed "made that [knife] an excuse to Desarte from us with out aney Jest Case." I sense a note of disgust and surprise from Floyd.

On August 18, the posse returned to camp with their quarry. Reed confessed to his desertion and was sentenced to run the gantlet four times, running through the men, who had formed two lines, while they stuck him with switches. He probably was struck about five hundred times, and must have been a sore and awful mess. He was also kicked out of the Corps of Discovery and ordered to return to St. Louis the following spring along with the members already designated for the return party under Corporal Warfington.

The first serious glitch in the cohesiveness of the Corps had just been punished. But a desertion would be a significant psychological blow to the others who had lived, slept, and worked with Private Reed. They had trusted him to guard their lives at night while they slept, and now he had let them down in a big way.

Those who study the psychology of group travel list certain predicting factors that will influence the success or failure of any outdoor expedition. Member personality attributes such as attitude, sense of humor, and previous success or failure in an expedition situation, predict behaviors that contribute either to the success of a group, or to its failure. Success is also highly dependent upon the group's leadership. According to Tuckman's theory of group development, expedition members go through four stages from initiation to successful completion of an expedition. First, *members establish the structure of the task for which they convene.* For Lewis and Clark, the structure was a military unit, with well-assigned tasks, duties, and leadership. The goal was clear. In a nutshell, the Corps was to travel up the Missouri River, over the Rockies to the Pacific and return, while exploring, mapping and collecting, as well as doing numerous other chores. Secondly, Tuckman states that members will *emotionally react to the demands of the task.* With several courts-martial already under their belts, there seemed to be a lot of this going on. While most of the men seemed to be in high spirits much of the time, the stresses of the environment and living conditions were certainly causing emotional reactions. Thirdly, members will, *negotiate intra and inter group roles to develop group cohesion.* At this time in the Lewis and Clark Expedition, these roles were still evolving. But the nature of a military command limited negotiation about defined roles of the enlisted men. The enlisted men were there to be laborers. Fourth, and lastly: *members will resolve role conflicts and move on to the successful completion of the task.*[8]

Many members of the Corps had already accomplished this task. Nearly all of the hard heads of the group had been weeded out. Leadership and discipline would continue to be established and fine tuned. Future hardships and recreation, as well as a very real sense that they

The Sun and Dying Young

were in this together, that they would sink or swim as a group, provided the glue that kept the Corps together.

On August 11, the Corps reached the burial site of Blackbird, chief of the Omahas, and a victim, along with about four hundred of his tribe, of smallpox four years earlier. Sergeant Floyd wrote, "the nathion Goes 2 or 3 times a year to Cryes over him." It was now apparent that the Indians desperately needed the kinepox that Lewis had hoped to provide, but sadly it was unavailable. Apparently the replacement batch Lewis had requested nearly a year ago never arrived. As the group stood overlooking the memorial to those struck down by the foreigners' disease, the beauty of the area seemed in stark contrast with the reality of the situation. From the 300-foot-high cliff they were standing on, they had a spectacular view of the river to a distance of sixty or seventy miles.

On the 18th, the Corps received a delegation of Otos and Missouris, who stayed for a council the next day. Clark noted that one of their chiefs joined the captains for breakfast naked the next morning. The chief wanted one of the ninety-six lenses, or "sun glasses" bought in Philadelphia. Practicing a little Great Plains bargaining, he pleaded for more gifts, including whiskey, to give his young warriors, to keep them from going to war with the Omahas. While the captains were busy with their diplomacy, and also Reed's court martial, a disaster started to brew deep within the bowels of one of the nine young men from Kentucky.

Sergeant Charles Floyd was, in the words, of Captain Lewis, "a young man of much merit." He was only twenty-one years old by August of 1804, but was one of the three sergeants in the Corps. Like the others in the group, he was tough and used to abusing his body with the rigors required during the trip.

The sudden pain in his abdomen doubled up Charles Floyd. This was certainly no ordinary stomach ache. The pain was so incapacitating that every man who was keeping a journal made note of his illness. Clark wrote, "Sergt. Floyd was taken violently bad with the Beliose Chorlick and is dangerously ill." Ordway observed that "Sgt. Floyd taken verry Sudenly Ill this morning with a collick." Gass wrote, "This day sergeant Floyd became very sick and remained so all night. He was seized with a complaint somewhat like a violent colick." Private White-house noted, "Sergt. Floyd Taken verry ill this morning with a collick."

In an 1804 version of a wilderness emergency room, the captain/physicians went to work. "We attempt to relieive him, I am much concerned for his Situation—we could get nothing to Stay on his Stomach a moment." All the men attended to him, especially York. Clark wrote, "he gets wordse and we are muc allrmed at his Situation, all attention to him."

Floyd was in pain all night. His commanding officers stayed up with him, trying to render treatment that was beyond them to deliver. In the morning of the 20th, the group loaded the boats, and transported Floyd into one of the craft. "Sergeant Floyd much weaker and no better." On this morning, which was to be his last, he was "a[s] bad as he can be to live the [motion?] of his bowels having changed &c.&c. is the Cause of his violent attack &c. &c." The specific treatments Clark employed were not recorded. Did they bleed him? Probably. Did they purge him with some of Rush's pills? Maybe. But it is doubtful that anything could have been given to Floyd orally, as he couldn't keep anything down. Whatever they tried, it did not work and probably only made Floyd worse.

The boats continued upriver until around noon when the captains—desperate to do something, anything—decided to land and make a warm bath for Floyd, "hopeing it would brace him a little."

As a medical student, I was taught that if a patient has a sense of impending death, the physician should take the patient's fear seriously. I have often wondered if prior to exiting this life, we catch a glimpse of what is beyond or, as some have put it, we see our entire life in a moment. I wonder if Charles Floyd had that experience on the prairie two centuries ago. One thing for sure, he certainly had the sense that he was not going to recover from this illness.

Clark wrote this pathetic and sad last wish of a dying young man: "before his death he Said to me, 'I am going away, I want you to write me a letter'." Before they could get him into his hot bath, Charles Floyd slipped away and stopped breathing. As Clark noted, "Floyd Died with a great deel of Composure." Gass wrote, regretfully, "Floyd died, notwithstanding every possible effort was made by the commanding officers, and other persons, to save his life." Whitehouse described the event: "The disease which occasion'd his death, was a Bilious cholic, which baffled all medical aid, that Captain Lewis could administer."

The most popular opinion through the years of continuing speculation is that Sergeant Floyd died from the complications of appendicitis. Although this is a leading candidate, it's not an iron-clad diagnosis.

The appendix is a two- to three-inch-long, finger-like extension of the first portion of the large intestine, just below where the small intestine empties into the colon, or large intestine. If something—say a small hard bit of stool, or possibly parasites (including amoebas)—or a tumor blocks the cavity of the appendix, bacterial invasion of the tissue will result in inflammation, leading to swelling of the appendix. Pain is the result, but during the early course of the disease the victim might sense the pain as being around the belly-button and not in the usual location of the appendix, in the lower right part of the abdomen.

The swelling and inflammation that occur prohibit fresh blood from supplying the appendix, and that tissue begins to die. Nausea and vomiting are common, diarrhea is less so. A mild fever is possible. If the process continues, the appendix may break open (rupture), and spill the infected contents into the victim's abdominal cavity, causing a life-threatening infection called peritonitis. If untreated, peritonitis would likely result in shock, with its resulting loss of blood pressure, decreased kidney function (resulting from the decreased blood supply), coma, and death. The disease is most common among males, from the ages of fifteen to twenty-five.[9]

Modern diagnosis of this problem includes laboratory tests, including a complete blood count, various chemistries and a urinalysis. After the vampires (lab technicians) get done with the patient, an exam by a surgeon would be in order, and a possible CT (computerized tomagraphy) scan of the patient's abdomen, which gives the surgeon an incredible view of the area without having to look inside via cutting. Modern treatment for uncomplicated appendicitis includes a usually straightforward surgery, to remove the infected tissue. The patient is encouraged to walk soon after the anesthesia wears off, and usually recovers quickly. If peritonitis has occurred, aggressive antibiotic treatment is instituted along with other supportive treatments. Some bacteria that contribute to peritonitis have become highly resistant to antibiotics and can cause serious and life-threatening infections. But the vast majority of patients with this complication still recover through the use of multiple intravenous antibiotics.

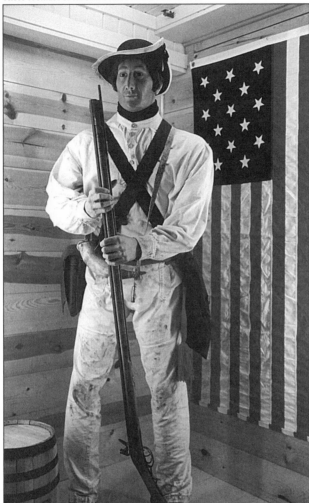

When Sgt. Charles Floyd's body was reburied in 1895, a plaster cast was made from his skull. Modern forensic science was used to reconstruct this life-sized image of him, on exhibit in Sioux City, Iowa.

What you do *not* want to use in treatment of appendicitis are cathartics and enemas. They could contribute to rupturing an intact but weakened appendix, thus leading to peritonitis. Remember the most popular treatment for symptoms of abdominal pain in 1804? Bleeding and purging were probably in the top three. The unknown treatments rendered by the captains could have included inducing Floyd to vomit or purge, both leading to rupture of the appendix. Bleeding would have decreased his blood pressure as well as the available red blood cells to carry oxygen and the white cells to fight infection. About the *only* thing the captains had which would have helped Charles would have been the laudanum, an alcohol/opium combination first introduced by the iconoclastic physician of the middle ages, Paracelsus. At least this would have helped Floyd's pain and probable anxiety.

Parasites can lead to the obstruction of the appendix, which sets off this disastrous cascade. It is certainly possible, but less probable, that Charles Floyd's problem could have been precipitated by an infection of *Entamoeba hystolitica* that he obtained from drinking Missouri River water. The protozoan parasites could have affected his appendix, blocking it to the point that the dominos started to fall.

It is also possible that Floyd had an underlying stomach ulcer that eroded through the wall of his stomach, resulting in a case of peritonitis. Again this is less probable, but certainly not beyond the scope of possibility.

Another remote possibility is an extremely nasty infection called tularemia, which Floyd could have obtained from the drinking water or from handling or cleaning infected meat, particularly rabbits. The organism, a bacterium named *Francisella tularensis*, inhabits about one hundred different mammal and blood-sucking arthropod species (mosquitoes, fleas, ticks, deer flies). Cottontail rabbits, squirrels, and beavers are all reservoirs of this infection.[10] Deer and bears have also been sources of the disease. Human-to-human transmission does not occur.

It is believed the organism enters the victim's body through unbroken skin from the flesh of an infected animal (but may, in fact enter via small, unapparent wounds), or via the bite of a tick or deer fly. This results in an ulcerating skin lesion that lasts for weeks, the so-called "ulceroglandular" form of the disease. An "oculoglandular" form, resulting from contaminated fingers touching the eye, causes a severe form of conjunctivitis, infecting the membrane that covers the insides of the eyelids and much of the eye—a form the captains would see later. Another manifestation of tularemia is a severe lung infection that may be either a primary infection from inhaling the bacteria—or a complication of other forms of the disease.[11] A gastrointestinal form can also result from the same two causes. Contaminated water or food can result in "oropharyngeal" tularemia, which causes severe sore throat.

Numerous nasty symptoms of tularemia may include fever, chills, headache, cough, skin ulcerations, diarrhea, abdominal pain and, rarely, peritonitis and appendicitis. Most victims will recover within weeks, and surviving an attack will generally confer immunity to further infections,[12] but prior to the antibiotic era, the death rate was as high as 33 percent.[13] Wearing gloves while cleaning wild game could have protected the men from one form of this disease, but knowledge of this organism and its method of transmission did not exist in 1804.

Whatever it was that ended our young hero's life, the respect that his fellow explorers had for him was apparent. Floyd was buried with the honors of war, with Captain Lewis reading the funeral ceremony, and giving a eulogy. The sergeant was buried on a high bluff overlooking the Missouri River. A simple red cedar head marker was placed on the grave: "Sergt. C. Floyd died here 20th of August 1804." Clark praised the fallen youth in his journal, writing, "This Man at all times gave us proofs of his firmness and Deturmined resolution to doe Service to his Countrey and honor to himself."

It was a blow to the morale of the men to lose Charles Floyd so abruptly—but the frequency and ease of death on the frontier had touched them all before the day they watched their teammate slip into eternity. Many of them had lost parents, siblings, and fellow soldiers, and Floyd was just the latest unlucky fellow to fall victim to the Grim Reaper who hid around every bend of the river. The remaining men were at least glad that it hadn't been them.

Four days after Floyd was laid to rest, the chronometer stopped just after Lewis had wound it. He feared he would not be able to fix it, and that his celestial readings (and mapping) would be impossible. But it was a false alarm, and the next day he was casually noting times in his journal. If the timepiece did fail, that was not life-threatening, but so much information the Corps was to take home depended on this one instrument.

The captains and a hiking party of eleven others took off toward a "High Hill Situated in an emence Plain" (today's Spirit Mound) on the morning of August 25. This hill had a great reputation with area Indian tribes, who believed that it was "Supposed to be a place of Deavels or that they are in human form with remarkable large heads and about 18 inches high; that they are very watchfull and ar armed with Sharp arrows with which they can kill at a great distance: they are said to kill all persons who are so hardy as to attemp to approach the hill; they have a state that tradition informs them that ma[n]y indians have suffered by these little people and among others that three Maha men fell a sacrefice to their murceyless fury not meany years since— so much do the Mahas Sioux Ottoes and other neigbhbouring nations believe this fable that no consideration is sufficient to induce them to approach this hill."

When they arrived at the hill, they noted large numbers of birds hovering over the top, where they were eating hoards of swarming flying ants that, as Clark approached, "bit me very sharp," injecting their tiny amounts of burning formic acid into the captain's skin.

Clark offered his explanation of the Indians' fear of the little devils. "One evidence which the Inds Give for believeing this place to be the residence of Some unusial Spirits is that they frequently discover a large assemblage of Birds about this mound—is in my opinion a Suffient proof to produce in the Savage mind a Confident belief of all the properties which they ascribe it."

Captain Lewis's and others' thirst and fatigue cut the visit short, and they walked three miles to a creek, drank and then crossed the waist-deep water and gorged themselves on "great quantities of the best largest grapes I ever tasted." They arrived back at the boats at sunset, with York exhausted, tired and thirsty. Dr. Clark's diagnosis was that York's fatigue was because he was "fat and un accustomed to walk as fast as I went." In other words, Clark had walked poor York's butt into the ground.

On August 26, the men held an election to recommend a replacement for the fallen Sergeant Floyd. The men's choice was accepted by the captains, who expressed every confidence in the nominee's continued faithful service. Private Patrick Gass became Sergeant Gass. Poor Floyd was now officially gone.

With the close of August, the group made contact with the Omahas and then the Yankton band of the Sioux nation. The captains were preparing for their first meeting with the Sioux, a much awaited and anticipated event. Speeches encouraging peace among Indian nations were written and rewritten, and the medicine show was put into gear. Presents were readied. Sergeant Pryor and interpreter Dorion were sent out as advance men to the Sioux, who offered to honor them by carrying them on buffalo skins into their village. Pryor was presented with a meal of roast dog, of which he "partook hartily and thought it good & well flavored."

On August 27, the expedition made contact with the Yankton band of Sioux at Calumet Bluff, near the present-day city of Yankton, South Dakota. With the Corps taking a several-day break here, the usual diplomatic formalities preceded the council, after Yankton musicians led their people to the meeting. Dorion translated as the captains described their exploration, mentioned setting up a U.S.–Yankton trading system, and encouraged the Yankton not to war with their Indian neighbors. Dorion in turn gave the captains the Yankton requests for trade items, including guns and ammunition. The captains, while not providing the Indians with what they really wanted, did present some medals, knives, beads, corn, tobacco, and other items. Chiefs White Crane and Weuche said they would cooperate with the new white father and the planned trading empire along the Missouri.[14]

One chief, Half Man, warned that his Teton Sioux cousins farther upriver would probably not be as cooperative, and he warned the captains, "I fear those nations above will not open their ears, and you cannot I fear open them." Half Man certainly knew something that the captains did not, and his insights would prove to be good ones.

George Shannon had begun his personal tradition of losing either himself or something that belonged to him on August 27, while out hunting for the group's horses. Men were sent ahead to try and catch up with him, as Shannon was without food. Days melted into a week and there was still no sight of young Shannon. The captains had more to worry about than trying to find the wayfarer, but they grew ever more concerned and sent John Colter first, then George Drouillard, to chase down Shannon. The young private was apparently moving upriver trying to catch up with his mates who were actually downriver.

Sixteen days after Shannon left, the Corps found him sitting weakly along the bank, out of ammunition and starving, probably thinking that he was prematurely homeward bound on the next trade boat to come along. He had been living on wild grapes for twelve days. Buffalo had wandered within thirty yards of him, but he had no ammo. As Private Whitehouse described it, "his balls ran Short."[15] Shannon had been able to kill a solitary rabbit by "shooting a piece of hard Stick in place of a ball," but those few hundred calories were long gone by now. Clark marveled: "Keeping one horse for the last resorse,—thus a man had like to have Starved to death in a land of Plenty for the want of bulletes or Something to kill his meat."

On September 28, the Corps met the most notorious Indians on the Missouri, the Teton band of the Sioux. The meeting took place near present-day Pierre, South Dakota. Because of warnings from the Yank-tons and white traders about the Tetons' violence against river traffic, the Corps, in Clark's words, "prepared all things for action in case of necessity." Anticipating trouble, and having no one who spoke Sioux fluently, kept the meeting tense.

The Sioux nation was the seat of power on the American plains of 1804, and Jefferson's instructions to Lewis were clear: "On that nation we wish most particularly to make a friendly impression, because of their immense power, and because we learn they are very desirous of being on the most friendly terms with us." They could not be avoided. All of the diplomatic and military might of the United States was now in the hands of the captains. That the Corps was going upriver to make contact with the enemies of the Sioux—the Mandans and Hidatsa tribes—did not escape the powerful Teton leaders Black Buffalo, the Partisan, and Buffalo Medicine.

On first meeting, a tense situation developed involving the Sioux chief's dissatisfaction with the gifts presented by the captains. The Tetons wanted the Corps to ante up more tribute for going upstream. Attempts at intimidation from both Indian and white led to cocked and aimed rifles and river banks lined with armed Sioux on the brink of attack. By Ordway's account, Clark warned the Sioux that "we were not Squaws, but warriers." Black Buffalo threw the threat back at Clark, warning that "he had warriers too and if we were to go on they would follow us and kill and take the whole of us by degrees."[16] Clark disdainfully told the Teton chief that he had "medican on board that would kill 20 Such nations in one day," according to Whitehouse.[17] The crisis was defused, and Black Buffalo and some warriers spent the night aboard the keelboat.

Two more days of posturing and thinly veiled intimidation were coupled with apparently friendly visits to the tribe's village. Feasts were cooked and the Americans were treated as honored guests who participated in ceremonial smoking of the pipe and tribal singing and dancing. Corps members honored the singers and dancers with tobacco. Tribal chiefs offered the captains Indian women to take with them for the night. The captains refused. The offer was repeated the following night, with the admonition for the captains to "take her and not dispise them." The women were being offered as agents of diplomacy, as a sign of good will. The Sioux leaders were bewildered at the captains' continued refusal.

On the night before the Corps' departure, another tense and nearly bloody moment erupted. A pirogue had struck and broken the keelboat's anchor cable, causing the keelboat to swing dangerously in the river current. When Clark shouted to his men to attend to the boat, they responded quickly. The Sioux, expecting attack, responded with the drawn bows and firearms of two hundred warriors. More angry words were exchanged, and then this situation was defused with a simple request for tobacco from the Sioux chief, and Lewis's finally finding it prudent to part with a little tobacco.

The Arikara village with its dome shaped lodges made of sticks and mud, where the gardens grew pumpkins, corn, beans, squash, and tobacco,[18] was a week up the river. Empty Arikara villages, evidence of the impact of smallpox epidemics in the 1780s, stood as silent and ghostly monuments as the Corps rowed their way past the eerie scenes. A population of twenty to thirty thousand Arikaras had been reduced by 75 percent during the epidemic of 1780-1781. Another epidemic in 1803-1804 further diminished the tribe's strength, from around eighteen villages down to an anemic three.[19]

It was in the Arikara village that the Corps of Discovery of North America would take on another new member. Leaving this Indian society that boasted a friendly and organized agricultural and trading system, the men would soon find themselves living with a new recruit. They would ultimately curse his existence and live to regret their association.

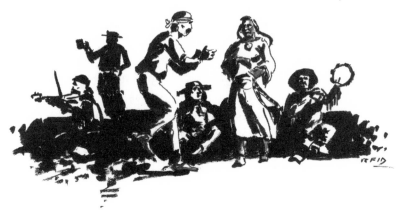

〰 8 〰

THEY SHOULD HAVE
DANCED ALL NIGHT

"Louis Veneri" Joins the Corps

Two minutes with Venus, two years with mercury.
—American physician J. Earle Moore

He wasn't Italian, although you might think so by reading his name, or by listening to the French—who said he was Italian or maybe Spanish. But the Italians wouldn't claim him either; they said he was a Frenchman. No one knows for sure where he came from, but it is said that he came from an old European family dating back to the 15th century. Some said he was a shepherd boy before he joined the army. The force of his personality was strong and he never met a person on whom he didn't have a major effect.

No one really liked Louis very much. In fact, one could say that whoever had contact with him hated him. Two of the reasons for Louis' success in life were his diversity, as well as the company he kept. No one could accuse Louis of snobbery, as he willingly rubbed elbows with the high and mighty as well as the lowest members of society.

You might say he was a "hanger-on," one of those guys who go through life with little good or winsome about themselves to make them attractive to others. In fact, most would say that Louis had no personality at all and, in many ways, he was downright dull. Louis's key to success was to seek out acquaintances with whom he could associate, who had some influence in society, or whose pleasant personalities could bring him an opportunity to bask in their spotlight. Louis was that kind of guy.

But Louis had a dark side. In fact, he was a real back-stabber. Through the years, he had gone on numerous explorations and been a member of numerous army outfits. He came into contact with many, pretending to be their friend, only to end up killing them. But he didn't do it quickly; he did it slowly, day by day, month by month, year by year. Their energy sapped, at times their bodies disfigured with their faces eaten away, his friends were rendered hideous and disgusting monsters.

In the fall of 1804, Louis joined up with the Corps of Discovery during their stop at the Arikara villages. At first the men treated him with nonchalance, but they soon learned to hate him. Some tolerated him as a necessary member of the group. The captains even tried to get rid of him, but another of Louis' attributes was his perseverance. He was there to stay. Louis was also known by another name, *lues venerea*, Latin for "disease, sickness or pestilence." Another alias, given to Louis in 1546 by the Italian physician Girolamo Fracastoro, was "Morbus Gallicus," or the French disease. Another was the "Great Pox." Today we just call him syphilis.

Few diseases have enjoyed the mystery and attention that syphilis has through the ages. Although controversy still swirls around the origins of the disease, it is known that the grand coming-out party for "Louis," the time that he made his first great impression on society, was at the end of the 15th century in Europe. The disease then spread from Europe to India, China, and Japan, and on to the rest of the world.[1]

Early medical thought was that the French army brought it to Italy during their attack on Naples in 1495. Others thought that it was in Naples first, where it was contracted by the French. The French army was in fact mercenary, with members from Germany, Switzerland, England, Hungary, Poland, and Spain. So many French soldiers came down with the disease that they had to call off the war. The army disbanded, and the various nationalities went home, taking "Louis" back with them to their respective homelands.[2]

It is also possible that the crew of Christopher Columbus picked up Louis during their first trip to America. Upon Columbus' departure from Haiti in 1493, he took along ten native men from the West Indies. The natives were dispersed in the Spanish cities of Seville and Barcelona. When Columbus's crew disbanded, some believe that the infected sailors became soldiers and marched with the Spaniards, who were part of the French army that attacked Naples, Italy. The infected West Indian natives remained. Many medical historians believe this scenario, but controversy surrounds the entire topic to this day.

Another theory of the origin of syphilis has "Louis" coming to Spain and Portugal through importation of African slaves, a large number of whom were sent to the West Indies. This theory's supportive evidence comes from the fact that there exists in Africa a common disease known as yaws, which is caused by a bacterium, genus *Treponema*, similar to the one that causes syphilis. The organism that causes yaws has a slightly different genetic makeup, which is responsible for its different disease manifestation. Yaws is not spread through venereal (genital) contact, but through skin-to-skin transmission, generally in very unclean and unhygienic conditions, especially among children who often play together. It produces skin sores similar to those made by Louis, but does not progress.

Whatever the source of the disease was, there is no disagreement about the tremendous influence it has had throughout the centuries since its appearance in the 1500s on the stage of human suffering. And, on some October afternoon in 1804, inside Arikara lodges when some unknown members of the Corps responded to the Arikara women's love of "carressing," Louis became a permanent part of the Corps of Discovery.

Syphilis is known in medicine as "the great imitator" for its numerous symptoms that mimic other diseases. It is usually spread by sexual contact and is characterized by five distinct phases of the illness: incubating, primary, secondary, latent, and late syphilis.[3]

The disease is caused by a helical bacterium called a spirochete.

Usually within hours after sexual intercourse with an infected person, the bacteria penetrate the mucous membrane lining of the penile urethra or vaginal mucosa, spreading into the lymphatic or blood system, then spreading throughout the body. Any organ in the body can be invaded, including the central nervous system. Incubation, that time from when the bacteria enter the body until the onset of symptoms, takes around three weeks, but ranges from three days to three months.

At the site of bacterial infection, and during the primary disease stage, there usually appears a painless skin lesion that lasts from two to eight weeks. The secondary stage is characterized by diffuse skin rashes, low-grade fever, fatigue, sore throat, loss of appetite and weight, achy joints, and highly infectious lesions on the lips, mouth, and vaginal lining or penis. Up to 40 percent of victims will have involvement of the brain or spinal cord, with headache and stiff neck common for those unfortunates. Bones can also become infected, along with any other organ of the body including kidneys, liver, or eyes.[4]

Syphilis may then go into its latent phase, when there are no clinical symptoms, but the disease continues to progress. This can last up to four years. Relapses of the secondary stage may recur during the latent phase, mostly during the first year.[5]

Late syphilis is a slowly progressive phase and can affect the nervous system, with manifestations of personality changes such as marked mood swing or paranoia, megalomania, delusions, and hallucinations, and decreased memory, and poor judgment and insight. It can cause vision loss, slurred speech, or deafness. Syphilis can also attack the walls of the body's main artery, the aorta, causing it to weaken and forming a bulge, an aneurysm. A significant syphilitic aneurysm can lead to the aortic heart valve becoming incompetent, which in turn results in either very poor exercise tolerance or even death. Late syphilitic manifestations can take from three to twenty-five years to develop, and occur in 10 to 20 percent of those who are untreated[6] or—in the case of the Corps of Discovery—who were inadequately treated.

Through the centuries, the medical profession had attributed syphilis and other venereal diseases to all kinds of things; gout, bladder stones, exposure to dampness, the overuse of spices, snuff, or the cutting of a tooth. One physician wrote a six-volume treatise on venereal diseases in the 1760s, and blamed the diseases on horse riding, drinking strong beer, and "immoderate venery, though pure." Some believed that intercourse during menstruation could lead to a severe case of gonorrhea, as could having intercourse too often over a short period of time. Even eight decades after Lewis and Clark, Dr. Henry Lyman noted in his book, *The Practical Home Physician*, that young newlywed husbands would call on him for advice concerning possible sexually transmitted disease. The good doctor would reassure the husbands that it was just due to "the youthful husband's impetuosity," encouraging them to slow down a bit.

Equally unbelievable advice as to the proper treatment of these social diseases included an early 1800s concoction called "Davy's Lac-Elephantis," a "medicated elephant's milk," which promised to cure the venereal diseases if taken orally within twenty-four hours of an "illicit connexion." Other preventives were lotions, urethral injections of mercury solutions, water, or spirit of niter, and washing the genitals either before or after intercourse with lemon juice, vinegar, white wine mixed with turpentine, camphor, or urine. Gum tragacanth (a Lewis and Clark medicine), mixed with calomel (mercurous chloride), could be applied to the penis prior to the deed. The 16th century Italian physician Fracastoro suggested a post-coital lemon juice wash; the noted Dutch physician Hermann Boerhaave liked lemon juice and salt. Applying these acids was thought to constrict the urethral opening enough to disallow the "contagion" from entering the penis.[7] It would seem that such application should have been pre-coital, thus removing all desire for sex and preventing the contagion from entering the urethra.

If the preventative measures failed and the amorite contracted symptoms of venereal disease, treatments available throughout the centuries could probably fill volumes. Marshmallow roots, salve of lard and tar, tincture of guaiac, sarsaparilla and sassafras, Epsom salt purges, linens soaked in acetate of lead (another Lewis and Clark med), opium and henbane pills, prunes and figs, leeches—and, if all else fails, a good bloodletting—have been considered beneficial treatments through the ages. My personal favorite was undoubtedly highly effective in preventing syphilis and would surely provide such negative reinforcement that no recipient would ever want to have sex again: pouring scalding water over the genitals! That treatment probably had very few proponents and even fewer recipients.

The most popular treatment for syphilis through nearly three centuries (1500-1800) was mercury. Paracelsus, a Swiss physician and alchemist of the 15th century, was an early proponent. At times a patient was treated with a combination of mercury and chalk, calomel, or "corrosive sublimate" (bichloride of mercury). Mercury achieved the status as the "Samson of the Materia Medica," in part by being the foremost treatment for syphilis. "Keyser's Mercury Pills," a popular 18th century syphilis treatment, even boasted a poem written in its honor, praising the power and virtue of the miracle medicine. A few of the lines suffice to allow the reader to appreciate the medication's efficacy as well as the poet's ability:

> Illustrious Keyser has at length restor'd
> The beauteous Sylvia to my longing Arms!...
> You've conquer'd—the fell Monster reigns no more.
> Now each glad Hour Love's Raptures we repeat;
> Our warmest Praise attends on Keyser's name![8]

But the administration of mercury to cure a nasty problem was a very sharp double-edged sword. The mercury was toxic to the causative organism of syphilis, but the mode of administration was uncertain, some thinking that intestinal purging action was the way to go, others believing that topical application was the ticket. The side effects of the mercury could cut nearly as deep as the syphilitic bacteria. Salivation was thought to be the end point of mercury treatment, signaling that the body was expelling the poison that caused the disease. Salivation is now a well-known sign of mercury poisoning. There was a thin line between salivation and sloughing of oral tissue, producing a cure that was nearly as bad as the disease. The early 18th century saw heroic doses of calomel being administered to syphilitic patients, resulting in the mouth turning brown, breath smelling of mercury, and teeth falling out. Mercury was administered via pills, or ointments applied to armpits at night, or rubbed on the syphilitic rash. Lewis and Clark carried both versions. The ointment regimen was followed for several weeks, until the salivation appeared.

Although intestinal absorption is only 10 to 15 percent of the amount ingested, poisoning with mercury is most easily achieved through orally administering a mercury salt (calomel or bichloride of mercury).[9] Application to the skin results in slower and less intense absorption, and thus slower manifestation of side effects. Oral mercury produces severe local inflammation to the mouth, throat and intestines, causing pain, nausea, vomiting, and world-class bowel movements. Chronic exposure to mercury salts can produce red body rash and sweating, lessen appetite, increase heart rate, and cause constipation or diarrhea.[10] Mercury concentrates in the kidneys, poisoning the cells that filter urine and control the reabsorption of electrolytes from the urine that is forming and flowing through the kidney's filtration system. This produces mercury's effect of increasing urination (diuresis), an effect for which it was used medicinally for years. Toxic doses can wipe out the kidneys, leading to a cessation of blood filtering, no urine production, and death.

Chronic exposure to elemental mercury, the non-salt form, as used by Lewis and Clark in their mercury ointments, takes a bit longer to rear its ugly head. Salivation, irritation of the mouth and gums, diarrhea, and neurologic manifestations such as tremors or difficulty walking and speaking, are common. Neurologic damage can also be evident by personality changes of excitation, irritability, apprehension, withdrawal, or depression. All are signs of chronic poisoning of metallic mercury, which could have resulted from prolonged or repeated use of the mercury ointment that the captains used to treat their men who contracted the syphilitic bug.

Although it is not documented, gonorrhea could have been another contracted venereal disease for Lewis and Clark's merry band of men. Caused by another bacterium, *Neisseria gonorrhea*, its clinical appearance is more obvious, with males having severe pain with urination for up to eight weeks, along with a penile discharge of green or yellow fluid. After the pain and discharge are gone, the bacteria may still live inside the urethra and be a source of infection to other sexual contacts. Females may have frequent or painful urination, vaginal discharge and/or abnormal menstrual bleeding. In the female, the infection can involve the cervix, extending into the fallopian tubes in 15 percent of cases. It can contribute to an illness called Pelvic Inflammatory Disease, which will be but briefly mentioned for now. This pelvic infection could result in marked lower-abdominal pain, nausea, vomiting, and possible pelvic abscess formation. If the woman recovers, her fertility can be permanently impaired in 15 to 25 percent of cases. The bacteria may also involve the female's liver, causing abdominal pain in the upper right abdomen.[11] Long after meeting the Arikaras, the captains would face dealing with a possible victim of this disease.

The captains had taken along treatment for the "clap," or gonorrhea, in the form of four special syringes used to rinse out the penile urethra with a solution of some medication popular during that time, possibly the balsam of copaiba, camphor, or lead acetate. There is no documentation in the journals that they used them. The threat of such a pleasant treatment would be enough to keep many a man's mouth shut, even if he had the symptoms.

Today, a shot of penicillin or other antibiotic and a course of oral medication would solve nearly any of the problems associated with either syphilis or gonorrhea. Advanced syphilitic disease is virtually never seen any more in this country.

So, as the men in the Corps, at least those who decided to take advantage of the "amorous damsels" that they met along the middle Missouri, came down with the "Louis Veneri," the captains broke out their supply of mercury. Unaware of the extensive consequences of the mercury treatment and the numerous complications supplied by "Louis," at least some of the men continued to, shall we say, be remiss in virtue. One must wonder if they had known of all the information we have just discussed, it would have made a difference. Although I am inclined to say perhaps for some it may have, my years of practice tell me otherwise. I think that most of them would have continued to visit those Indian lodges regardless of any warning. The temptation and availability of some eager and willing females coupled with some good old-fashioned denial, was just too much for some of the men. So goes human nature and the influence of testosterone.

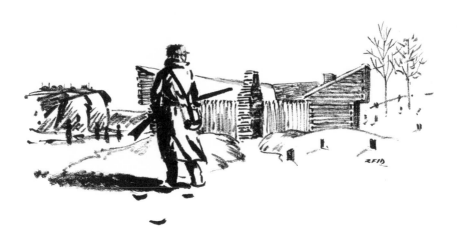

◢◣ 9 ◢◣

COLD TOES AND A BABY BOY

Winter with the Mandans

I enjoy convalescence. It is the part that makes the illness worthwhile.
—*George Bernard Shaw*

The end of October 1804 was seeing the sunrise over the prairie around 7:30 to 8:00 A.M., with crisp mornings and occasional snow flurries. On the morning of October 25, the ground and tents were covered with snow as the men lay inside their flimsy linen fortresses, shrouded in their inadequate clothing with a blanket or two to cover them. The insides of the tents were coated with frozen breath, and the heat of the past summer was just a distant memory. Afternoon temperatures were tolerable, but as the sun moved farther down the southern sky, the air started to cool off by mid-afternoon. It was now getting dark and chilly by 5:00 P.M.

Perhaps the combination of cold nighttime temperatures with the

Corps' strenuous daytime exertion started to produce aches and pains that hadn't seemed so common during the hotter weather. Exertion and lying on the cold ground at night with the earth conducting away body heat was at least partially responsible for the aches and pains that were beyond the normal daily routine the men suffered. Captain Clark became the victim of one of these episodes when he awoke abruptly on the "verry cold" night of October 25 at 1 A.M., with severe pain and stiffness in his neck, unable to turn his head at all. In his own words, the pain was "So violent I could not move." Captain Lewis, awakened by the probable commotion, crawled out of his bed and fetched one of the warm stones from around the campfire, wrapped it in some flannel and returned to their lair, placing the hot stone to the neck of his friend. This frontier physical therapy provided Clark with some "temperry ease" of the pain, but the spasms in his neck muscles lasted for days. Rheumatic pains started to strike other members of the Corps. Clark wrote, "R Fields with Rhumitisum in his Neck, P. Crusat with the Same Complaint in his Legs."

At least they knew that traveling would soon end. The Mandan and Hidatsa villages they aimed for were well known among whites. French fur trappers and English traders had been visiting and living among the Mandan tribe since 1738, when a Frenchman with a name nearly as long as the Missouri, Pierre Gaultier de Varennes de La Verendrye, ventured into the village in search of some legendary "white Indians" who possessed an array of precious metals.[1]

Although their skin was lighter than that of some neighboring tribes, the Mandans were not white. Nor were they rich. There were also many fewer of them than in the old days, ever since a devastating epidemic of smallpox swept through the villages in 1781. Weakened in numbers, they were forced to move north, away from their enemies the Sioux and Arikara, to form an alliance with the Hidatsa tribe. The alliance wasn't a marriage—it was more like two step-siblings who really didn't get along very well, trying to live together in order to survive. Through the years, their settlements became the center of Northern Plains trading, and numerous tribes, including the Cheyenne, Assiniboine, Crow and Arapaho, made yearly journeys to trade their horses, mules, leather clothing, and guns for Mandan and Hidatsa corn, beans, squash, and tobacco.[2]

Cold Toes and a Baby Boy

As soon as the Corps encountered a party of Mandans that included a chief, he was invited onto the keelboat. The captains introduced an Arikara chief they had convinced to come along from his village; Lewis and Clark were to mediate peace negotiations between the then-warring tribes. They hoped to help forge an alliance between the Mandans/Hidatsas and the Arikara, effectively removing the Arikara from Sioux influence, and weakening the Sioux control of the middle Missouri. The two chiefs now met with formal greetings and ceremonial smokes.

Thinking about his own brand of diplomatic business, John Ordway noted that the Mandans "had Some handsome women with them." The Corps encamped among friendly Mandans who came to call. While the fires blazed in the cool evening air, the son of a deceased great chief of the Mandans walked into camp. The captains noted that two of his fingers were missing and he had been pierced in many places over his body. Through an interpreter they asked the young Mandan about his wounds. Clark "was informed that it was a testimony to their grief for Deceased friends, they frequently Cut off Sevral fingers & pierced themselves in Different parts, a Mark of Savage effection."

Several friendly introductory visits, including lots of tobacco smoking, passed between the men of the Corps and their Mandan hosts. During late October and the early days of November the men became familiar with their hosts, who included Frenchmen living with the Indians and married to Mandan women. One such fellow was Rene Jusseaume, a trader who had been with the tribe for fifteen years. His knowledge of the Mandan language made him a natural for the captains to hire as an interpreter.

The Mandan chiefs were fascinated by the Lewis and Clark travelling circus. The keelboat was a big attraction, with Clark noting that they viewed it "as great medison." In the words of Nicholas Biddle, the first editor of the journals, "whatever is mysterious or unintelligible is called great medicine." York, with his black skin, was viewed with at least as much awe as the boat.

Five and a half months of travel were finally over. The rowing and towing were over—at least for the winter—and the men rejoiced! As Clark put it, "our men verry Chearfull this evening."

Natural disaster struck on the afternoon of October 29, when a nearby prairie fire became a raging inferno. A man and woman of the tribe, who had been out on the prairie, were overtaken by the rapidly moving flames and, in spite of attempts to escape, burned to death. A half-white boy escaped by hiding under the hide of a freshly killed buffalo. His survival was more evidence to the Mandans and Hidatsas of the protection the presence of the whites afforded, believing that "all white flesh is medisan," citing that the grass around the boy was not even burned. The fire swept by the Corp's temporary camp at 8 P.M., as the men stood in unison watching the roaring wall of crackling flames, a view that "looked truly tremendious."

In several diplomatic meetings with the Mandans, Hidatsas, and visiting Arikara chief, the captains encouraged peace and cooperation among these nations. A Mandan chief accepted the idea, stating that he would send envoys to the Arikara to parley and smoke in honor of the proposed peace deal. He said the Mandans had never wanted war with the "Ricares," but had been forced into it, stating that the Arikaras had killed their chiefs, "killed them like the birds."

By November 2, the captains had reconnoitered the area and decided on a spot for the winter encampment about two miles below the southernmost of five Indian villages north of the Missouri River. The Indian villages were situated on the Knife River, where it ran parallel to but a few hundred yards west of the Missouri. The lower two villages were Mandan, and the upper three each held a different band of Hidatsas. The fort was closest to the two Mandan villages, and six to nine miles downriver from the Hidatsas.[3]

The men's struggles now changed from wrestling the Missouri to cutting down the immense cottonwood trees, which would be used to fashion a triangular log fortress to protect them from the brutal northern plains winter already blowing its frigid winds upon them. Cottonwoods are extremely heavy due to their high water content. During one day alone, two men cut themselves with their axes. The wounds were probably wrapped up in cloth bandages. As the logs were shaped and piled up, and the winter home took shape, Captain Lewis wrote on November 2, "This place we have named Fort Mandan in honour of our Neighbours."

The Corps' new interpreter, Rene Jusseaume, along with his wife and children, moved in with the white men. By November 13, the day of the "grand opening" of Fort Mandan, the ground and air were full of blowing, biting snow. The men continued to put finishing touches inside their fort, working until 1:00 A.M. on the 15th. The next day, they were chinking spaces between the logs.

On the 19th, the Corps' hunters returned with a feast of thirty-two deer, twelve elk and a buffalo, while the rest of the men moved into their huts. Warm fires and cooking meat held a new and added attraction, and some temporary relief and comfort from the dropping temperatures.

The captains became policemen on November 22, stopping the murder of an Indian woman by her enraged husband. Two days earlier he had beaten her and stabbed her three times. The man told the captains, through an interpreter, that his wife had run away, and he accused one of the sergeants of having had sex with her. He "would give her to him" if the sergeant wanted her. Interestingly, Captain Clark responded that "not one man of the party had touched his wife except the one he had given the use of her for a nite, in his own bed." Clark forbade any Corps member from further relations with this woman, and placated the husband with a few gifts. After this intervention, Clark became the first white marriage counselor among the Mandans, and "advised him to take his Squar home and live hapily together in future."

By the 25th of November, many men had bad colds, and some had "Rrumitism." But at least the huts were now finished as the long, cold winter began. The fort served as the official ambassadorial residence of this diplomatic delegation from the United States. Daily visits with the Mandans resulted in trading as well as research by the captains into the tribe's language and customs. Parties were held. The men sang and danced, celebrating the end of months of hard labor. The Indians were benevolent hosts, providing and trading their corn for beads, handkerchiefs, arm bands, paint, cloth, fishhooks, and other items.

On November 29, Sergeant Pryor was working on the keelboat, and reached up with his arm to secure the mast and take it down. Upon wrestling with the mast, the bone in his upper arm (humerus), pulled away from its normal attachment to a bony extension of the shoulder blade (glenoid) and dislocated. Pryor's arm hung abnormally (and very painfully) at his side, and he was unable to lift it.

Most such dislocations are caused by a trauma that forces the humerus forward, tearing its supporting ligaments and joint capsule. Pryor had probably suffered the original injury in a fall, months or years previously, resulting in chronically stretched or torn ligaments and an unstable shoulder joint. Unfortunately, once ligaments tear, they never naturally resume their original tightness, and sloppy and loose shoulders that may more easily dislocate in the future.

Today, a shoulder dislocation would be treated by giving the patient some narcotic for pain and perhaps some medication to reduce the tension and spasm of the supporting shoulder muscles. Once the patient is relaxed, manual force is applied to the arm, and with some manipulation the humerus will usually return or "pop" back into its proper position. If the problem recurs, an orthopedic surgeon can perform a surgical procedure to repair the defective shoulder capsule.

Perhaps the captains gave Pryor some opium or laudanum for his pain and perhaps not. They did not record any meds being given, but they did record the four attempts that it took them to reduce the dislocation. It reads a little like a chamber of horrors. Overcoming the strength of the shoulder muscles of a man who had just ascended 1,600 miles of the Missouri must have taken a lot of pulling and strain. This problem would continue to bother Pryor on the rest of the trek, and worsen in years to come.

The captains demonstrated the latest in technology by firing the airgun and using a magnifying glass to start a fire. These Caucasians certainly had mysterious powers. Even the Corps' great hunting ability was thought to be "big medicine" by the Indians. The positive interactions between the two cultures led to a trust built between men of two radically different societies. Cooperation on hunts, and the subsequent sharing of meat obtained, added to the rapport developed over the winter.

And then there was the "black white man"—York. Indian children were amazed at the sight of him, and enjoyed his teasing. When he danced with the others, he was surprisingly light on his feet for his large size. Warriors and chiefs alike had pronounced him "big medicine." One Hidatsa chief, Le Borgne, had spat on his finger and rubbed York's skin, thinking he was a painted white man. When York showed Le Borgne his scalp (where one didn't paint), the great chief's astonishment knew no bounds.

The temperatures of December frequently dipped below zero, with the coldest reading yet occurring on December 17, when the thermometer reading was -45 degrees F. Numerous men suffered frostbite of their ears, feet, and hands. The air temperatures were so brutal that the guards outside the huts had to be rotated on an hourly schedule. There were no Goretex boots, no goose down or Fiberfill among the men. Undoubtedly York was not wearing underpants that would have provided some compressive effect with its added warmth to his genitals, when he suffered some frostbite of his penis. Hypothermia (systemic injury from cold) and frostbite (local injury from cold) were probably the rule rather that the exception. Oh, for some of those hot days of the previous summer!

Frostbite was certainly not something new in the area of medical history; none other than the "father of modern medicine," Hippocrates had described some of its symptoms. The American revolutionary army suffered greatly during the winter of 1777-1778, while they huddled in their tents and log shelters at Valley Forge. Similar to the medical practice of the captains, the "proper" treatment of that time was rubbing the cold extremity with snow or ice, or immersing the cold body part in some cold water. Heat was thought to produce gangrene.

The human body is much better at losing heat then it is at retaining it, which in a cold climate means either getting indoors where it's warm, or protecting oneself with adequate clothing. The men had the former to some degree, and the latter to a lesser degree. Air, being a poor thermal conductor, does not have a great ability on its own to produce hypothermia or frostbite except in extremes of temperature. In other words, cold air alone is not as dangerous as cold, *wet*, and/or windy conditions that can rapidly damage human tissue. Windchill can make an air temperature of 20 degrees F. feel like -40 degrees F. when accompanied by a wind of 45 miles per hour. Wet clothing can conduct body heat away at an alarming rate, as water is a twenty-five-times better coolant than air. Prior cold injury increases the risk of worse injury during subsequent exposures to cold. All the factors were there in Dakota of 1804—cold, wet, and windy weather, with inadequately clothed and sweating men who had probably been frostbit before.

Simply put, frostbite is the result of freezing most of the water inside and outside the cells of the skin, when the skin's temperature reaches 24.8 degrees F. This is below the level of the freezing of pure water, due to the underlying radiation of heat from the lower layers of the body, and the chemical makeup of cellular fluid. When skin temperature reaches this point, local blood vessels spasm and fluid from the blood leaks out of the vessels into the tissues. The circulation of blood to the skin slows and ultimately ceases, clots form in the tiny vessels, and the skin's oxygen supply is ended. Cells die and severe frostbite has occurred. Mild frostbite occurs with milder exposure and without loss of tissue.[4]

The first sign of skin injury from frostbite is redness and numbness. The skin then swells a bit and, with further injury, blisters form. If the injury continues, deeper blisters appear, colored purple with blood-containing fluid. The last and most serious degree of injury is if the entire skin freezes, and layers of tissue underlying are frozen, including bone and muscle. This will produce "mummification,"[5] or what occurred to a young Indian boy during extreme cold weather on January 10, 1805. Clark recorded:

"[L]ast night was excessively Cold the murkery this morning Stood at 40 below 0 which is 72° below the freesing point…The Indians of the lower Villages turned out to hunt for a man & a boy who had not returnd from the hunt of yesterday, and borrowd a Slay to bring them in expecting to find them frosed to death about 10 oclock the boy about 13 years of age Came to the fort with his feet frosed and had layen out last night without fire with only a Buffalow Robe to Cover him, the Dress which he wore was a pr of Cabra [pronghorn] Legins, which is verry thin and mockersons— we had his feet put in Cold water and they are Comeing too…"

Today's treatment of choice for this unlucky but extremely tough kid would be to rapidly rewarm his feet and avoid refreezing. With the extent of his injury it may not have made much difference, but immersing his feet in cold water was not the best treatment. He had, without question, an extremely painful several weeks after he came to the Fort Mandan Hospital, with throbbing pain starting two to three days after the feet rewarmed. The pain probably lasted for weeks. In addition, it is common for burning and electrical current–like sensations to last for up to six weeks after rewarming. This boy must have suffered greatly, and one hopes the captains gave him some of their laudanum or opium to help relieve his pain.

Over the next few weeks, the boy's injury started to declare itself

Cold Toes and a Baby Boy

more fully. Dead tissue "demarcates," that is, shows an obvious boundary between itself and living tissue. This occurs usually from between twenty-two and forty-five days after the initial injury. The dead tissue of the boy's feet started to turn black. Sixteen days after the injury, on January 27, Captain Lewis, "took of[f] the Toes of one foot of the Boy who got frost bit Some time ago." He undoubtedly accomplished this feat of surgery with a good deal of hesitancy and anxiety. His tools were probably a sharp knife or the elementary surgical tools he had purchased in Philadelphia. Imagine having to take off dead skin and subcutaneous tissue and then cut through the bones and ligaments of the involved toes without having done this before. It may have been done prematurely, as the toes could have likely undergone a process of automatic amputation in several more weeks without the intervention. But in Lewis's mind, the frost-injured tissue was infected, which it may not have been. Just because the toes were black did not mean they were infected. Four days later, however, more of the boy's toes were "sawed off."

Whatever the captains did, whether right or wrong, their patient survived and left their little hospital on the prairie on February 23, 1805. Clark's note summed it up; "The father of the Boy whose feet were frose near this place, and nearly Cured by us took him home in a Slay." The proof is in the pudding. The boy got well.

Another Indian woman had brought her child for treatment by the white men with "big medicine" on December 21. The child had an abscess, or localized tissue infection characterized by a swollen, red, pus-filled sore. The anxious mother pathetically offered the captains "as much corn as She Could carry for Some medison." The treatment of choice for an abscess is to cut it open and drain the pus, then fill the cavity with packing cloth and allow it to heal over a period of a couple of weeks. It is unclear what Lewis did, with Clark's brief note stating only that, "Capt. Lewis administered &c."

Beginning in November, Louis Veneri had started to come calling again, the result of frequent sexual encounters between the Corps and the Indian women. Clark noted in January that one man was "verry bad with the pox," meaning syphilis. At the end of March the men were healthy "except the—vn. [veneral]—which is common with the Indians and have been communicated to many of our party at this place—those favores bieng easy acquired."

One fascinating Indian ritual involved the ceremonial lending of a wife for the express purpose of sexual intercourse. The Mandans believed that the power and hunting abilities of the recipient could be transferred to the husband through sex with the same woman. This act was also thought to guarantee the arrival of large buffalo herds that would provide the food necessary to sustain the tribe. The men of the Corps were invited, and participated. As Stephen Ambrose notes in *Undaunted Courage*: "One unnamed private made four contributions."[6]

With the cold weather and deep snow of winter, and the close contact it forced among the men, respiratory infections were probably passed around with ease, contained in the infectious drops of viral-filled mucus expelled through coughing and sneezing. It was probably one of these infections that led to a bad case of pains in the chest for one of the men on January 26, 1805. Dr. Clark diagnosed the problem as "Plurisee."

Pleurisy is the medical term for an inflammation of either the outside lining of the lungs or the inside lining of the chest cavity. There are two layers of pleurae, thin membranes within the chest. The membranes normally allow for frictionless movement of the lungs as they expand and contract against the chest wall during the breathing process. But when the pleural membrane lining the inside of the chest cavity becomes inflamed, as it could with an infection involving the lungs, it becomes painful with every breath or coughing spell. (The pleural layer surrounding the lungs, called the visceral pleura, has no sensory nerves and therefore is not a source of pain. Its counterpart, the pleura that lines the thoracic cavity, the parietal pleura, does have sensory nerves, and can be a source of pain.) Infections could come in a variety of ways, with the most common being either bacterial or viral. The onset of the problem is usually sudden and painful. The underlying disease needs to be treated, perhaps with antibiotics, perhaps with supportive care and some pain relief. Generally the problem is painful but not necessarily dangerous.

Captain Clark treated this man with a good blood letting and "remedeis Common to that disorder." These could have been topical applications to the chest of some grease or camphor, or poultices of the omnipotent Peruvian bark. George Drouillard came down with similar pleuritic symptoms five days later and was treated with bloodletting and some sage tea. Both men improved rapidly.

With nine inches of snow outside, most of the time the men were probably inside their huts. On the days when the men left the shelters and ventured into the snow-covered terrain to hunt or to walk the two miles up to the Hidatsa villages, they encountered an invisible enemy that left their eyes painful and red. The Indians had some insight into the cause of this problem and also had a novel approach to its treatment. Clark wrote on February 15, "one Chief of the Mandans returned from Capt Lewises [horse-seeking] Party nearly blind—this Complaint is as I am infomd. Common at this Season of the year and caused by the reflection of the Sun on the ice & Snow, it is cured by 'jentilley Swetting the part affected by throweng Snow on a hot Stone'."

The irritation to the eye was caused by ultraviolet light reflected off the white surface of the snow and striking the surface of the eye. Ultraviolet light cannot be seen with the human eye, as the wavelengths are too short to be perceived by the retina's light-detecting cells. (Its wavelength is around 300 nanometers [nm], with visible light having wavelengths of 400nm for the blues to 700nm for red. 1 nm=10-9 meters.) The clear part of the eye that overlies the pupil is called the cornea, and it has sensory nerves as everyone who has ever had a foreign body in the eye can testify. The cornea absorbs ultraviolet radiation with wavelengths below 300nm that, when concentrated, can burn the cornea surface within an hour. (Longer wavelengths penetrate the cornea into the lens, over periods of years contributing to cataracts.) After the cornea is burned, pain gets severe in about six hours, and the victim's eyes become red, tearful, scratchy, and very sensitive to light. Corneal burns can be miserable.

The cornea has an incredible ability to heal itself rather quickly, usually within twenty-four hours of this type of injury. Pain can be controlled today with local anesthetic eyedrops and oral pain medication, and possible patching the involved eye. I sometimes see welders who have this injury from a momentary glance at an extremely bright flame, or people who have not worn ultraviolet-absorbing sunglasses on a day out in the snow or on the water.

The Indians' approach to treatment was interesting and helpful. The steam from the snow thrown on hot rocks probably moisturized the eyes, providing some momentary relief. The rapid natural healing of their eyes could have been erroneously attributed to the steam's limited efficacy.

It is also interesting that this problem seemed to be novel to Captain Clark. It seems that where he had always lived, there never was enough snow for long enough, with bright sunlight, to produce similar problems.

It is impressive to realize what amazing relief my little bottle of anesthetic eyedrops could have provided to those people two hundred years ago. It would have been very, very big medicine.

During the winter with the Mandans, the captains recruited an additional interpreter who spoke French and Hidatsa. He was a French fur-trapper/trader who had conducted business with the North West Company and had lived with the Mandan/Hidatsa clan for several years by the time the Corps arrived in town in 1804. He presented himself to the captains on November 4, and through the help of one of the French/English speaking privates, offered to hire on as an interpreter. His name was Toussaint Charbonneau.

Charbonneau's real attraction to Lewis and Clark was not only his language abilities, but also those of two of his three wives, who happened to be Shoshones. The captains could pay Charbonneau and get his wives' services thrown in for free. The Shoshone factor was a card that was enormously advantageous. By now, the captains knew that they would be travelling through Shoshone country during the upcoming year and would need to obtain horses from them to cross the Rocky Mountains. The presence of natives who could smooth their way into Shoshone culture and provide language skills would be a major boost to their chances of success.

About four years earlier, the younger Shoshone wife, then around twelve, had been busy doing her chores with several of her tribe near the Missouri River's headwaters and the present-day town of Three Forks, Montana. Her people, the Lemhi Shoshone, lived to the west but came here annually to hunt buffalo. The Shoshones had it rough. They had been forced into the mountains to live and hide, leaving the relative bounty of western Montana valleys behind due to the ever-present danger of the Blackfeet. Armed with guns obtained from traders in the north, the Blackfeet roamed the plains and valleys of western Montana with impunity. The Blackfeet aimed for a monopoly on the area and were not about to share it with the Shoshones. The Hidatsas also traveled to the headwaters area from their homes hundreds of miles to the east. They came to hunt and raid, looking for buffalo to eat and Shoshone horses to augment their herds. For the Shoshones, the valleys of western Montana were beautiful but dangerous.

Fate would have it that this small group of Shoshones, minding their own business, fell victim to a band of Hidatsas that day around 1800. Several were murdered, and more were taken prisoner. The Hidatsa took the captured Shoshones along with them, back the hundreds of miles down the Missouri, where they could be kept to do the work. Such was the fate of the young girl named Sacagawea, who later was given in marriage to Charbonneau. Sacagawea was pregnant with their first child in late October 1804. By the time February rolled around, the baby was ready to make his appearance into the new United States territory.

I can still recall the first child I ever delivered. I was a student on duty in a hospital in Los Angeles, with another medical student on her OB/GYN rotation. We were both green, she a little bit more than I. A woman had gone into labor and had been taken into the delivery suite and readied for the birth of her child. Everything was great, except…her obstetrician wasn't there. He had been paged, but had not arrived. I was elected to do the delivery. As I scrubbed my hands and forearms with the foaming betadine sponge, and knowing that I had

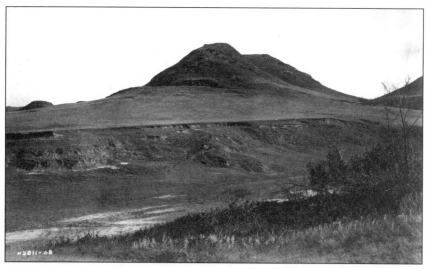

Edward Curtis's early 20-century photograph of the one-time site of the Hidatsa villages in North Dakota. LIBRARY OF CONGRESS, LC-USZ62-96184

absolutely no desire to go into obstetrics, my irritation slowly built and I found myself thinking, *"Where the hell is this lady's doctor?"* Realizing at that moment that I was this lady's doctor, I felt an extra shot of adrenaline pump into my blood. The scrubbing done, I slipped into a paper gown and pushed my hands into the latex gloves held by the scrub nurse. I sat down in front of the now properly positioned woman, and did a brief exam, noting that the baby's head was crowning, or appearing in the birth canal. I again wondered, this time with a more irritation, "WHERE THE HELL IS THIS LADY'S DOCTOR?" I took the hypodermic syringe filled with local anesthetic and ran the long thin needle into the perineum (the tissue between the rectum and external vaginal opening), and injected the lidocaine as I slowly withdrew the needle. As the contractions continued and the baby's head started to forcibly separate the vaginal walls, I made an episiotomy incision with special scissors along the perineum. "Where is that OB?" started to fade in my mind, as the head came out first...then the arms...and, amazingly, the legs. I suctioned the child's mouth and nostrils as he lay on my lap, and clamped the umbilical cord in two spots and cut between them. The child was put into warm blankets and put on top of Mom's chest. Everybody was happy, and I thought exultantly, "I'm this lady's doctor!" As the thought passed through my mind, the new mother's official obstetrician walked into the delivery room. I should have billed him.

On the cold winter afternoon of February 11, 1805, probably sometime around 4 P.M., Dr. Lewis was called to attend the birth of his interpreter's child. A few weeks earlier he had been a surgeon, amputating necrotic frostbitten toes. Now he was expected to be an obstetrician.

It is frequently seen that a first time pregnancy results in a prolonged and difficult delivery. The uterus of the mother, having stretched far beyond its normal size for the first time, often has some difficulty in contracting sufficiently to quickly deliver her offspring. Hours of intermittent and severe pain can occur. The great comedian Bill Cosby has likened it to pulling your upper lip over your forehead.

At sixteen, Sacagawea found herself inside an earthen lodge in the middle village of the Hidatsas on the Knife River. The weather was pleasantly fair for a mid-winter day on the northern plains, with a breeze coming from the northwest. But any pleasantries were wasted on Sacagawea, as she found herself on her back on the floor, unable to

Cold Toes and a Baby Boy

do much of anything but experience the pain of childbirth. There was no lidocaine to numb, no episiotomy to make the delivery easier. As Dr. Lewis put it, "as is common in such cases her labour was tedious and the pain violent…"

In the present day, with a prolonged and difficult labor, the uterus can be stimulated to contract with the intravenous administration of oxytocin, a hormone produced in the body that stimulates the contraction of smooth muscles of the uterus. If the fetus is in distress, a Caesarian section can be performed to get the child out quickly. However, in 1805, there would be no such thing. In 1805, the next best thing would be…a rattlesnake rattle.

You may ask justifiably, "A rattlesnake rattle?" Mr. Jusseaume, Charbonneau's fellow interpreter, was at the delivery of his buddy's baby. (I wonder what modern women would think about having their husbands' friends around at such a time.) Mr. Jusseaume, in the words of Meriwether Lewis, "informed me that he had freequently adminstered a small portion of the rattle of the rattle-snake, which he assured me had never failed to produce the desired effect, that of hastening the birth of the child; having the rattle of a snake by me I gave it to him and he administered two rings of it to the woman broken in small pieces with the fingers and added to a small quantity of water. Whether this medicine was truly the cause or not I shall not undertake to determine, but I was informed that she had not taken it more than ten minutes before she brought forth."

Rattlesnake rattles are made out of a substance we call keratin. Keratin is also found in fingernails, horns, and hair. It is insoluble in gastric juices, and therefore I doubt that it had any effect whatsoever on the delivery. But it makes a great story.

The baby would be baptized Jean Baptiste Charbonneau, but Clark nicknamed him "Pompey." Although oblivious to it all, he was a popular and important part of the exploration team. Amazingly, he would make the entire remaining portion of the trip to the Pacific and back here to his home. Shannon was now replaced as the youngest member of the Corps of Discovery.

As the winter days slowly lengthened, and the temperatures slowly increased, the desire to renew the quest for the Pacific started to bud along with the willows growing on the banks of the springtime Dakota creeks. The winter had been a great time for the men of the Corps. The Indians had been friendly, their quarters were tolerably comfortable and they had enough fresh buffalo, deer and Mandan corn and squash to be pretty well content. It is also probable that some of them didn't look forward to leaving the relatively easy life they were living and renewing the endless days of towing and rowing the boats upstream. At least that beast of a tub, the keelboat, would be gone. Corporal Warfington and a group of men would take it, along with plant and animal samples, official maps, records and correspondence, back down the Missouri to St. Louis. Riding along would be deserter Moses Reed and mutineer John Newman, who had been drummed out of the Corps.

The captains had met at least some of their directives. They had made lists of Indian vocabulary, encouraged peace among the Indian nations, and gained a greater understanding of Indian cultures. Their good rapport with the Indians had furthered the causes of American diplomacy in the newly acquired Louisiana Territory. They had also learned from the Hidatsa about some of the geography that lay to the west of them and what to expect and look for along the path. They had been told of a great waterfall they would find on the Missouri. They knew of the Shoshone and their horses that they needed. The acquisition of the horses would be smoothed with Sacagawea's help and then they would have a smooth ride over the Rocky Mountains. Once over the mountains they could catch a river on the other side and float down to the Pacific.

Clark and Lewis had also increased their skill and confidence level as physicians. Medical confidence is built only with individual stones of experience. As army officers of the time, the captains already had been required to know how to treat wounds, set broken bones, and reduce dislocated joints. Their list of medical procedures had grown to include amputating dead toes, treating various fevers and pains, soothing burned corneas, and more. Their skill with the lancet was becoming second nature, as evidenced by the small pools of dried blood on the grounds of Fort Mandan, the result of their "therapeutic" bloodletting. They were in the middle of their unsupervised medical internship.

In the months to come the men of the Corps of Discovery would remember Fort Mandan and long to return. With any luck at all, they thought they would be back by next winter.

Cold Toes and a Baby Boy

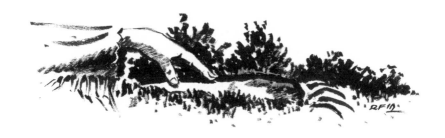

ॐ 10 ॐ

WILD TIMES IN OLD MONTANA

Act One: May-June, 1805

*Of course I realized there was a measure of danger. Obviously I faced
the possibility of not returning when first I considered going. Once
faced and settled there really wasn't any good reason to refer to it.*
—Amelia Earhart

The winter was over. Old Jack Frost had put away his topcoat and
retreated into his cold storage in the Southern Hemisphere. The
Great Plains rejoiced, with blades of green grass poking their heads out
of the dark wet earth, meeting the warming rays of sunlight that had
been far too absent for the last five months. The singing birds, the melting snowbanks and the rising waters of the Missouri, all joined together
with the excitement of the men to produce one great ethereal shout of
anticipation. But early April warmth on the northern plains can easily
give way to cold blustering winds that carry more than a few

snowflakes. April warm spells often last just long enough to deceive the overly optimistic.

The Corps now divided into two separate armadas. The keelboat, under the command of Corporal Warfington, would descend the Missouri to St. Louis, while the flotilla of six canoes and two larger pirogues would ascend the Missouri under the captains' command. The latter group included York, Drouillard, Charbonneau, Sacagawea, Pompey, the three sergeants, twenty-two privates, and Seaman the Newfoundland wonderdog.

Leaving the middle Missouri River area, the Corps of Discovery would become true to their official title. Except for a few fur traders who had ventured a ways up the Missouri, the departing group now ventured into unknown and uncharted territory—perhaps the home of active volcanoes and the still elusive megalonyx, the extinct creature that some scientists thought might survive out there.

Meriwether Lewis was as excited the first week of April as he was efficient. His love of the wilderness and of rambling that carried back to the days when he roamed the Virginia woods as a kid, was now an empty bag he could fill up with new wilderness adventures and discovery. His boyish anticipation can be felt in his entry of April 7, 1805.

This little fleet altho' not quite so rispectable as those of Columbus or Capt. Cook were still viewed by us with as much pleasure as those deservedly famed adventurers ever beheld theirs; and I dare say with quite as much anxiety for their safety and preservation. we were now about to penetrate a country at least two thousand miles in width, on which the foot of civillized man had never trodden; the good or evil it had in store for us was for experiment yet to determine, and these little vessells contained every article by which we were to expect to subsist or defend ourselves. however as this the state of mind in which we are, generally gives the colouring to events, when the immagination is suffered to wander into futurity, the picture which now presented itself to me was a most pleasing one. entertaing as I do, the most confident hope of succeading in a voyage which had formed a da[r]ling project of mine for the last ten years, I could but esteem this moment of my departure as among the most happy of my life. The party are in excellent health and sperits, zealously attatched to the enterprise, and anxious to pro-

ceed; not a whisper of murmur or discontent to be heard among them, but all act in unison, and with the most perfect harmony.

Shortly after the departure, with hundreds of Mandan and Hidatsa Indians lining the banks to see them depart, one of the canoes tipped into the current and flooded, ruining "half a bag of bisquit" and some thirty pounds of gunpowder. In an effort to save the gunpowder, the men unloaded it and spread it out to dry. While this minor catastrophe occurred, Captain Lewis, unknowing, marched along the muddy riverbank to the upper Mandan village where he visited and had a farewell smoke with the Mandan chief, Black Cat.

On the second night out, Sacagawea's experience with regional foods paid off for the team when she located numerous edible roots, with Lewis commenting that in flavor, "this root resembles that of the Jerusalem Artichoke," which it, in fact, was. The roots might have been passed by—missed for dinner or scientific collection—without the help from the young Shoshone mother.

The maple, elm, and cottonwood trees that lined the river began to bud, pronghorn kept their usual wary distance from the men, and with the warming weather the hated mosquitoes started to make their unwelcome presence known once again.

As the boats continued up the churning, swirling current, they caught up with a group of three French trappers who had ascended the river ahead of the Corps. The Frenchmen, going to the Yellowstone River, were taking advantage of the protection the Corps provided from Assiniboine warriors who might be hunting here. The highly productive trapping waters, on previous trips without the benefit of an armed escort, had proved dangerous waters indeed. The chance of losing their hair or their lives was as good as their chances for finding beaver—both, very real possibilities. They had already taken twelve beavers, which Lewis described as, "by far the best I have ever seen."

Lewis noted a white substance along the banks, and in a tribute to his native curiosity if not his common sense, he tasted a small amount of the substance, "which tastes like a mixture of common salt and glauber salts." He noted the "purgative effect" of surrounding springs "impregnated" with the stuff. Just what they needed—another cathartic.

During the past winter, information gathered from the Hidatsas had traveled through the interesting translation chain of Charbonneau, who translated the Hidatsa into French, to Private Labiche, who translated the French into English for the captains. It was during one of these games of "Operator" that the men began to hear terrifying stories about a species of bear that awaited them up the river. The Indians along the Knife River tried their best to warn the white men of the dangers these furry monsters posed. The captains listened intently but, shall we say, failed to fully appreciate the warnings.

It was now spring and, as the men ascended the Missouri on April 13, the bears had awakened from their long winter naps and were now frequenting its muddy shores, making up for all those months without food and leaving large foot and claw prints behind as testaments to their size. Lewis noted on the 13th, "we…saw many tracks of the white bear of enormous size, along the river shore and about the carcases of the Buffaloe, on which I presume they feed. we have not as yet seen one of these anamals, tho' their tracks are so abundant and recent."

Lewis added further comments on the dangers these animals had posed to the Indians.

> the Indians give a very formidable account of the strengh and ferocity of this anamal, which they never dare to attack but in parties of six eight or ten persons; and are even then frequently defeated with the loss of one or more of their party. the savages attack this anamal with their bows and arrows and the indifferent guns with which the traders furnish them, with these they shoot with such uncertainty and at so short a distance that they frequently mis their aim & fall a sacrefice to the bear. two Minetaries were killed during the last winter in an attack on a white bear. this anamall is said more frequently to attack a man on meeting with him, than to flee from him. When the Indians are about to go in quest of the white bear, previous to their departure, they paint themselves and perform all those superscicious rights commonly observed when they are about to make war uppon a neighbouring nation.

In a serious display of unfounded overconfidence, Lewis commented, "the men as well as ourselves are anxious to meet with some of

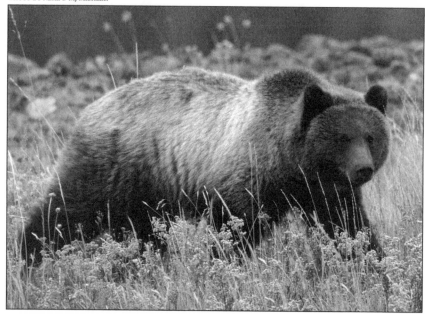

Grizzly bear.

these bear." He would soon experience otherwise and his anticipation would turn to anxiety.

The grizzly bear, also referred to by Lewis and Clark as the "white," "yellow" or, sometimes, "brown" bear, had an immense territory 250 years ago, covering nearly the entire western United States. They even lived in Southern California, with my home town of Santa Barbara and its neighboring village of Montecito having grizzly bears that slept in the chaparral thickets of the foothills. Over the last 200 years, the advance of civilization has pushed the grizzlies into about 20,000 square miles of the mountains of Idaho, Montana, Washington, and Wyoming.

Humans' problems with grizzlies have been well documented throughout the history of the western North America. Cases of human predation have occurred, as when grizzlies started eating dead victims of a smallpox epidemic among the Assiniboine tribe of Alberta, Canada, in 1865, and then started eating the living ones as well. Problems have usually arisen as the result of a sudden and close encounter with a surprised bear, or if the bears "decided" that a human was a threat to itself or its young. There can be no mistake: Grizzlies are powerful and potent killing machines if they want to be. Along with numerous other animals that once roamed the Great Plains, they have found it impossible to occupy the same areas as human populations. Civilization had its own ideas about what to do with the land, and none of those ideas involved grizzly bears.

On Friday, April 26, the Corps arrived at another great landmark. From the south, the mighty Yellowstone River dumped its vast supply of water into the eastward flowing Missouri, combining to make its way to New Orleans and the Gulf of Mexico. Joseph Field was dispatched up the river and told to explore it to the extent that would allow him to return that evening. The Yellowstone's possibilities would shape the captains' plans for next year.

On the morning of April 29, 1805, somewhere in today's far eastern Montana, the captains and their men got their wish for an introduction to a grizzly. Let's let Captain Lewis give us the report:

> *about 8 A.M. we fell in with two brown or yellow bear; both of which we wounded; one of them made his escape, the other after my firing on him pursued me seventy or eighty yards, but fortunately had been so badly wounded that he was unable to pursue so closely as to prevent my chargin my gun; we again repeated our fir and killed him.*

They butchered it and estimated its weight at three hundred pounds.

The encounter left Lewis a little shaken and impressed with his newfound species. "...it is a much more furious and formidable anamal, and will frequently pursue the hunter when wounded. it is asstonishing to see the wounds they will bear before they can be put to death."

In an amazing show of bravado, making comments which I find hard to imagine, Lewis added, "the Indians may well fear this anamal equiped as they generally are with their bows and arrows or indifferent fuzees [muskets], but in the hands of skillful riflemen they are by no means as formidable or dangerous as they have been represented."

Eastern Montana was a wide-open, dry land, with rolling hills interspersed with vast and dramatic gorges. There were few trees, except for the cottonwood groves that stood as oases at intervals along the Missouri, absorbing the thousands of gallons a day of water that they require. The surrounding prairie lands were typically dry and covered with low-growing and closely spaced blue-green sagebrush, with occasional stands of pine on surrounding hilltops. The prairie air was filled with the scent of the sage. Except for the presence of the predators, it was the Garden of Eden for browsing animals like deer, elk, and buffalo. Without the Missouri, however, it would have been a wasteland.

On the 30th of April, as Captain Clark, Sacagawea, and Charbonneau walked and explored along the banks, the pronghorns were thick and there was a "scattering" of elk, deer, buffalo, wolves, geese, ducks, and crows. Clark noted that "the Countrey on both Sides have a butifull appearance." The Corps found more and more beaver, which Lewis noted was "esteemed a delecacy among us." One beaver made a meal for two hungry men, and the tail was particularly tasty.

With the trees budding and prairie flowers in bloom, the 3rd of May surprised Clark with a morning temperature of 26 degrees F., a quarter of an inch of ice on the water kettle and an inch of snow on the ground. "A verry extroadernaley Climate" was the comment from Clark. Lewis sent Reubin Field to explore a "bold running stream," thirty yards wide, which they named "2000 mile Creek," in honor of its believed geographical position from the mouth of the Missouri. (Today it is Redwater River.)

The country was spectacular! Lewis reported on May 4: "...in the after part of the day we passed an extensive beautifull plain on the Stard. side which gradually ascended from the river. I saw immence quantities of buffaloe in every direction, also some Elk deer and goats [pronghorns]; having an abundnce of meat on hand I passed them without firing on them; they are extreemly gentle the bull buffaloe particularly will scarcely give way to you. I passed several in the open plain within fifty paces, they viewed me for a moment as something novel and then very unconcernedly continued to feed."

Some of the idyllic scene was broken when Joseph Field came down with a "high fever" and "disentary." Lewis responded with the Glauber's salts, another in his potent armory of oral cathartics. These various saline laxatives operated through the principle of osmosis. When the highly salted fluid entered the large intestine, the normal function of the large intestine in reabsorbing fluids from the liquid stool was dimin-

Buffalo bull.
MONTANA HISTORICAL
SOCIETY, 945-841

ished. The high salt content counters this process, with the stool remaining liquid, and thus has a laxative or cathartic effect. The dysentery was apparently accompanied by some remarkable abdominal cramping, and Lewis supplied pain relief for the private in the form of "30 drops of laudnum." The opium would also have decreased the diarrhea by slowing the transport of the fluids through the intestines. Again, our speculation can run wild. Was it food poisoning from a bacterial or parasitic source? Or perhaps it was some amoeba or other protozoan from the water?

Ever since beginning their ascent of the Missouri, it had been the men's practice to eat wild game whenever it was available. For the most part, this meat was from animals such as buffalo, elk, deer, and pronghorn, that graze to obtain their food, and then digest their grassy diet in a series of stomachs. The men ate bear meat on occasion, and ground squirrels, coyotes, wolves, and, as we have just noted, beavers. Many of these animals may have been infected by a variety of intestinal and/or muscular parasites. When the men ingested any piece of poorly cooked meat, skinned an animal, or drank contaminated water, they set themselves up for the possibility of serious, although not necessarily life threatening, infections.

Tapeworms from the genus *Taenia* could have been found in wild populations of animals that the Corps of Discovery utilized for food. It is documented that the tapeworm *Taenia ovis krabbei* has been found in modern-day Montana grizzly bears, mule deer, and moose.[1] During part of the life cycle of this parasite, the organism is found within the muscle tissue of infected animals that obtained the parasite by eating infected wild meat. Once inside the host's intestine, the worm is liberated from the muscle tissue, attaches to the intestinal lining, and begins to grow and reproduce. As the host has bowel movements, parasite eggs are passed into the environment and then ingested by other animals that then become infected. Eating poorly cooked meat from infected game animals could have produced an intestinal infection in the men with symptoms of abdominal pain, diarrhea, weight loss, irritability, and nausea. The adult tapeworm attaches to the intestinal wall of its victim helping itself to a continuing source of digested food. Many of these infections are asymptomatic but on rare occasions they can become such a problem as to even produce a blockage of the appendix, resulting in appendicitis as we have already seen.

Echinococcus, a 2.5- to 9-millimeter tapeworm, causes cystic lesions in the host's liver or lungs and comes from infected dog, wolf, fox, or coyote meat—or, in the case of humans, from ingesting the parasite's eggs passed in their feces into the environment.

Trichinosis is a disease of predators, a parasitic disease caused by the 1.5- to 3.5-millimeter-long parasitic nematode, *Trichinella spiralis*. Within one to seven days after eating infected meat, the victim begins to have fever, nausea, vomiting, sweats, and possible red blotchy rashes on his trunk and extremities. The trichinella larva then migrates through the intestinal wall of the victim and burrows into muscle cells causing generalized pains and swelling, with possible involvement of the heart muscle and lung tissue. The parasite is present in bear, wolf, coyote, dog and rabbit meat, particularly in the western states.

Trichinella is present in approximately 60 percent of the grizzly bears now living in the state of Montana, and approximately 11 percent of black bears in the state. It is present in up to 70 percent of Montana cougars.[2] The predator ingests the trichinella worm by eating the raw and infected meat of its victim. The larvae present in the meat are released during the process of digestion, and then make their way from the predator's intestine into the muscle, where they form cysts containing the live organism.

Rather than being a remote possibility, the threats to the Corps' health from these parasitic infections were a very real and daily experience. Five days before Joe Field's case of dysentery on May 3, a grizzly was killed, butchered, and probably eaten. There were no USDA stamps of inspection on the steaks eaten by the Corps of Discovery. Dozens of other potential parasitic infections could have been ingested in the wild meats. Cooking the infected meat until its temperature reaches 150 to 170 degrees Fahrenheit for approximately five minutes can generally kill these parasites. Did the cooks in the three messes consistently do this with their infected game? Hot campfires and famished men do not lend themselves well to slow and thorough cooking. If they boiled the meats, the temperature of around 212 degrees Fahrenheit, taking off a few degrees for elevation, could have killed the parasites. Slow cooking over embers could have accomplished a slow roast and dead parasites. We don't know how they prepared their meat, but even if they routinely cooked their meat "well done," a possible infection was just a bite away in a portion of undercooked meat. It is highly likely that many or perhaps all of the men had parasitic infections during the trip.

Clark, walking along the blooming bank and hillsides adjacent to the river on May 5, found a den of young "wolves," which Lewis described as between the size of a fox and a dog, with "deep sea green" eyes, a pale reddish-brown coat, and a tendency to retreat to their burrows when pursued. Their bark was "precisely that of the small dog." This was the first scientific description of a coyote.

That same day, Lewis catalogued another species of wolf. It was larger in stature than the coyote, but smaller than wolves of the East. Its coat was a "grey or blackish brown and every intermediate from that to a…white." This wild canine never retreated to a burrow. They hunted in packs, and Lewis added that "we scarcely see a gang of buffaloe without observing a parsel of those faithfull shepherds on their skirts in readiness to take care of the mamed & wounded." This animal, probably a type of gray wolf, didn't yip like its smaller cousins, but howled like the true wolf it was.

But the catch of this day was a furry brown monster that lay dead on the wet sand and stones of a Missouri River island as the men gathered and captains carefully measured from the nose to the tip of the hind paw that was stretched to its limit. "Eight feet, seven and a half inches," Lewis breathed. The cloth was now stretched around the chest of the beast and "5 F. 10 1/2 Inch" was penned on the journal page. The official weight was estimated by Clark to be five hundred pounds, which Lewis thought was at least a hundred pounds too low. Each talon was four and three-eighths inches in length. It was the biggest grizzly that the Corps had yet seen, and it was a "tremendious looking anamal," according to Captain Lewis.

Clark and Drouillard had stalked the animal after it was spotted on the Missouri's "sand beech," and the bear immediately became the combination of menu item and scientific specimen. They wounded the animal with several rounds from their single shot flintlocks. The bear, roaring from the instant the first lead ball entered his chest, fled into the Missouri and swam for a sandbar to escape from the flying lead. Several more rounds were pumped into his half-dead carcass while he swam across the river, roaring as he went. Upon reaching the sand bar, the bear crawled on the mud and continued to roar for at least twenty minutes, until his powerful life force slipped away and he went wherever good grizzly bears go when they leave this earth.

The men took to their canoes and paddled to the sandbar. They measured him, then butchered and divided the carcass among the messes. The captains instructed the cooks, ordering that the bear fat be boiled and saved for a future use. During the meat cutting, they counted ten wounds, five of which penetrated the lungs and left them a hemorrhaging pile of airsacks. There were five more in other parts of the carcass. A formidable animal indeed.

The following day, another grizzly was spotted swimming across the river, upstream from the boats. The men paddled hard in pursuit, but the bear escaped. Perhaps twenty-four hours of reflection about the events of the previous day began to shape Meriwether Lewis's consciousness. The thought of all those lead balls hitting the bear with seeming impunity, and close inspection of the creature's size, had put a little respect in him for this great beast. He wrote, "I find that the curiossity of our party is pretty well satisfyed with rispect to this anamal, the formidable appearance of the male bear killed on the 5th added to the difficulty with which they die when even shot through the vital parts, has staggered the resolution of several of them, others however seem keen for action with the bear…" Some folks learn slower than others.

With the men eating as much as eight to nine pounds of deer, elk, buffalo and grizzly apiece, daily, the diet was I am sure monotonous. It was the "Low Carbohydrate Diet of the Plains"—a 19th-century version of the popular American fad diet of the early 21st century; the Lewis and Clark weight loss plan through physical adversity and dietary denial. But Charbonneau shortly came to the rescue with his recipe of what he called "boudin blanc," or "white pudding." Charbonneau took about six feet of the large intestine of a buffalo and, as Lewis said, that "is the first mo[r]sel that the cook makes love to," and using his fingers he slowly pushed out the contents, what Lewis astutely noted "is not good to eat." The prime cuts of buffalo, including the tenderloins and the muscle along the back of the shoulder blade were sliced and diced along with a generous portion of fat from around the kidneys. Salt, pepper and flour were added. With one end tied, the large intestine, with its exterior fat, was then turned inside out, and the steak mixture was stuffed inside. Greatly stretching the intestine, the other end of the tube-like organ was tied off. Lewis then said that, "it is then baptised in the missouri with two dips and a flirt, and bobbed into the kettle; from whence after it be well boiled it is taken and fryed with bears oil untill it becomes brown, when it is ready to esswage the pangs of a keen appetite or such as travelers in the wilderness are seldom at a loss for." It is certainly a possibility that those intestines contained some type of parasite, but the high temperatures involved in its preparation undoubtedly killed them.

Grizzlies weren't the only thing that the captains and the others were worried about along the river. They occasionally found abandoned campsites that Sacagawea identified as probably Assiniboine. Lewis noted on May 10, that informants had said "as they are a vicious illy disposed nation we think it best to be on our guard."

"Boils and imposthumes [abscesses] have been very common with the party Bratton is now unable to work with one on his hand" was the medical report from Lewis the same day.

Boils, also called "furuncles," are superficial skin infections. They result from infection of the skin by *Staphylococcus* bacteria, which normally live on human skin. Problems can arise with staph infections, particularly in the case of the Corps, when small wounds occur with retained foreign bodies (splinters, dirt). Mosquito bites, deer-fly bites, and burns would all predispose the men's skin to invasion and infection by staph germs. Hair follicles could have also frequently become the site of staphylococcus infection with frequent rubbing and chafing of oars, cloths, etc. The captains treated the boils with "emmolient poltices." "Emollients" are drugs or substances that soften and protect the skin and other tissues. Poultices are externally applied substances (possibly combinations of grease, camphor, barks, wild onions, bear's oil or beeswax),[3] held in place by cloth, whose contents either penetrate or are thought to penetrate the skin and provide their therapeutic action. The men recovered from these skin infections probably more as a result of their immune systems than due to the "emollient poltices."

Some have written about the presence of scurvy among the Corps. Scurvy is a disease resulting from the prolonged dietary deficiency of Vitamin C. Most animals can synthesize their own supply of vitamin C from glucose. Humans (as well as other primates, and guinea pigs), are missing only one enzyme (L-gluconolactone oxidase) in the needed chain to do this.[4]

Vitamin C is required in our bodies for several reasons, most importantly for the proper synthesis of collagen, a major component of connective tissue, cartilage, and bone. Another function of vitamin C is its function in iron metabolism, which greatly influences the health of red blood cells. The total body pool of vitamin C varies from 1.5 to 3 grams, with up to a maximum of 4 percent depletion per day of that quantity. So, even in a diet totally devoid of vitamin C, it would take about one to three months to produce symptoms of scurvy.[5] The most common symptoms would be a tendency to bruise easily, poor healing of wounds, hemorrhage into the muscles of the arms and legs or the joint spaces, and bleeding, sore, and swollen gums. Alterations in iron metabolism can adversely affect the blood, resulting in anemia, which in turn would result in poor exercise tolerance, fatigue, and possibly other symptoms.

Foods that contain vitamin C are fruits, vegetables, milk, and some meat (kidney, liver, and fish). The Corps, without question, did not have sufficient fruits or vegetables to eat what we would consider a well balanced diet. But they ate fish, corn, wild fruits when available in season, wild "vegetables" (leaves, stems, and roots), and probably ate some of the organ meats made available in the vast amount of wild game they killed. A poorly balanced diet was a fact of life among the men, but it is a bit of a stretch to diagnose them with scurvy.

The men started to suffer from sore and irritated eyes, the result of frequent and hard winds and the increasing amount of reflected ultraviolet radiation as the days lengthened and the sun's angle continued to rise. Rather than using the Indians' steam cure of last winter, the captains answered this problem with a pretty good remedy. They made up an eyewash solution from an ounce of water, with two grains of "white vitriol" (zinc sulfate) and one grain of "sugar of lead" (lead acetate). Zinc sulfate has been used through the years as an antiseptic, astringent (a substance which causes contraction of tissue, arrest of secretions, or control of bleeding), solution for treatment of urethral gonorrhea, and even an emetic. Lead acetate, listed in Latin on the captains' original medication list as "Sacchar. Saturn. opt.," is another astringent. The mild solution provided some relief from irritation and pain. It would have been a slightly effective treatment for eye infections that may have resulted from environmentally caused inflammation of the conjunctiva, (the membranes overlying the eye as well as the insides of the lids). As sun and wind irritated their eyes, the men would likely have unconsciously rubbed them with dirty fingers, a set-up for a case of "pinkeye," or conjunctivitis. Treatment today could have included various antibiotic eye drops. But the captains did well for their time.

On May 11, there was more trouble with a grizzly bear. Since Bratton had an infected hand, Captain Lewis allowed him to get some shore time, and he spent part of the day walking along the banks. At 5 P.M., Lewis saw someone in the distance, running toward the river, waving and yelling, "as if in distress." The canoes were pulled over and

Bratton, so severely out of breath that he couldn't speak, finally blurted out his story. It was a great one.

As he made his way through a grove of trees a mile and a half downriver, he first saw, and then shot a grizzly, which after being wounded by the lead ball turned on Bratton as the source of its trouble, and chased him for a "considerable distance." Bratton was able to keep away from the bear due to the severe nature of the beast's wound. Bratton kept running all the way to the river, showing good sense in not going back to see what had happened to the bear.

Captain Lewis "immediately turned out with seven of the party in quest of this monster, we at length found his trale and persued him about a mile by the blood through very thick brush of rosbushes and the large leafed willow; we finally found him concealed in some very thick brush and shot him through the skull with two balls; we proceeded dress him as soon as possible, we found him in good order; it was a monstrous beast..."

Bratton wounded the bear through "the center of the lungs" and, in spite of this wound, the bear chased him a half mile and then turned and ran another mile in the opposite direction, dug a two-feet-by-five-feet-deep bed, and "was perfectly alive when we found him" at least two hours later.

Meriwether Lewis was finally impressed on a personal level with the strength and tenacity of the great bears. His comment, in which he finally includes himself, says it all. "...these bear being so hard to die reather intimedates us all; I must confess that I do not like the gentlemen and had reather fight two Indians than one bear; there is no other chance to conquer them by a single shot but by shooting them through the brains, and this becomes difficult in consequence of two large muscles which cover the sides of the forehead..." The skin of the grizzly took two men to carry, and the carcass yielded eight gallons of oil for future use.

The following day, Lewis added further to his newfound wisdom. He walked on the shore alone, except for his rifle and his spear-like espontoon. His confidence in his "skillful riflemen" and modern weaponry slightly shaken, Lewis decided to "act on the defencive only, should I meet these gentlemen [grizzlies] in the open country."

In an event that could only be called one of the highlights of the entire trip, grizzly mayhem broke out on the afternoon of May 14, 1805. This encounter made the others looked like trained bear acts in a circus. As the Corps rowed up the Missouri, in an area that is now under the water of today's Fort Peck Reservoir, in Valley County, Montana, a few miles above Snow Creek,[6] things got wild—very wild!

Captain Lewis tells the story:

> In the evening the men in two of the rear canoes discovered a large brown bear lying in the open grounds about 300 paces from the river, and six of them went out to attack him, all good hunters; they took the advantage of a small eminence which concealed them and got within 40 paces of him unperceived, two of them reserved their fires as had been previously conscerted, the four others fired nearly at the same time and put each his bullet through him, two of the balls passed through the bulk of both lobes of his lungs, in an instant this monster ran at them with open mouth, the two who had reserved their fires discharged their pieces at him as he came towards them, boath of them struck him, one only slightly and the other fortunately broke his shoulder, this however only retarded his motion for a moment only, the men unable to reload their guns took to flight, the bear pursued and had very nearly overtaken them before they reached the river; two of the party betook themselves to a canoe and the others seperated an concealed themselves among the willow, reloaded their pieces, each discharged his piece at him as they had an opportunity they struck him several times again but the guns served only to direct the bear to them, in this manner he pursued two of them seperately so close that they were obliged to throw aside their guns and pouches and throw themselves into the river altho' the bank was nearly twenty feet perpendicular, so enraged was this anamal that he plunged into the river only a few feet behind the second man he had compelled take refuge in the water, when one of those who still remained on shore shot him through the head and finally killed him...

When the postmortem was performed, "they found eight balls had passed through him in different directions."

I have read this passage at least a hundred times, and have never done so without an increase in my heart and respiration rate. What a show!

Clark added his own report, albeit one much briefer and somewhat understated: "Six good hunters of the party fired at a Brown or Yellow Bear Several times before they killed him, & indeed he had like to have defeated the whole party…"

An impromptu celebration was held around the campfire that night, a celebration of victory over the furry monster with its long claws, and for their intact bodies. In the Lewis's words, "we thought it a proper occasion to console ourselves and cheer the sperits of our men and accordingly took a drink of grog and gave each man a gill of sperits." Having enjoyed many retellings of exciting hunting incidents around dinner with friends in elk and deer camps, I can sense the men's excitement and wonder as they marvelled at the bear's size, speed, and ferocity. I would love to have been in the cottonwood grove that night around the snapping fires and heard the toasts the men offered and the laughter born from a narrow escape of a violent death. They appropriately named the area, "Brown Bear Defeat Creek."

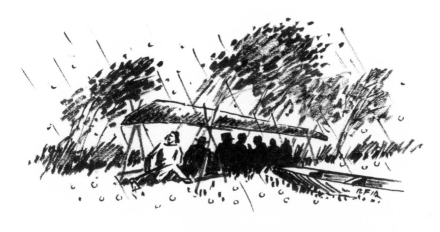

〰 11 〰

WILD TIMES IN OLD MONTANA

Act Two: May-July 1805

> *When you are all in trouble together, it becomes a party.*
> *—Advice given to the author during his first*
> *weeks of medical school by Nadir Khan, Ph.D.,*
> *Professor of Microbiology, Western University*
> *of Health Sciences, Pomona, California*

By mid-May, the daytime temperatures were warm but not yet hot and the river current was strong enough to require use of the towrope. Men lined up on the shore and in the shallows, and pulled the boats upstream like the beasts of burden they had become. They continually slipped and fell into the river, or bruised their feet on the rocky riverbed.

Captain William Clark narrowly escaped the bite of a prairie rattler on May 17. A similar one killed at that night's campsite was two and a half feet in length and had seventeen buttons on his rattle. Clark noted that his snake was small but fierce.

They pitched camp and built fires while Sacagawea erected the buffalo skin teepee that had provided shelter for herself, Pompey, her husband, the captains, and Drouillard since their departure from Fort Mandan. While the band of explorers drifted off to sleep, a catastrophe brewed.

"Fire!" the sergeant of the guard shouted. Jumping up quickly, the dazed group of five snatched the baby boy and ducked through the portal in the skins just in time to see a tree that was directly over their lodge becoming engulfed in flame and already dropping incendiary bombs onto the buffalo skin tent below. The winds were howling and embers from the tree were flying everywhere, seeding new areas of conflagration around the camp. They quickly pulled down the lodge, moving it a safer distance from the burning tree. Within minutes a large, heavy portion of the burning tree broke off and crashed down on what had just seconds before been their beds. All the men were now up, stamping their feet and going for water. The focus of the problem exploded into a great torch, snapping, popping, and roaring into the springtime sky. But the wind was too much and the embers too many, and the spreading fire moved out into the surrounding area and ignited a stand of dead timber, making it impossible for the early American smokejumpers to extinguish. No one was hurt, but the captains' tent was significantly damaged.

More encounters with Mother Nature's little irritations came the way of the Corps on May 20, with hordes of blowflies that "infest[ed] our meat while roasting or boiling" and made life something less than pleasant. In addition, small living pincushions in the form of prickly pear cacti were scattered over the ground, making those on shore vigilant in placing their moccasined feet. The one- to two-inch-long spines caused extremely painful foot wounds.

Above the confluence of the Musselshell River, which flowed in from the south, the Missouri had turned from its muddy brown at Fort Mandan to a slightly more transparent white. The river was wide, 222 yards by the captains' estimate, with a calm and gentle current. The surrounding hills, naked except for sage, prickly pear and grass, extended to the north as far as the eye could see.

The capricious weather amused itself by freezing the kettle of water sitting in the fire ring, as well as the edges of the river, on the night of May 24. The frost destroyed the green spring foliage on the cotton-woods, making the ancient trees bud once again in late spring. The wind for once played a pleasant tune for the Corps, and blew upstream, allowing the men to deploy the boats' sails and spend the day in passive progress. The air was crystal clear, so clear that "mountains and other elivated objects appear much nearer than they really are…we sent a man…to explore the country he returned late in the evening and informed that he had proceeded ten miles directly towards these mountains and that he did not think himself by any mean half way."

Somewhere in this Missouri Breaks area the next day, Drouillard, Clark, and Bratton each killed a bighorn sheep, the first seen on the trip. Lewis noted that the animals preferred to live among the cliffs and rocks "where the wolf nor bear can reach them and where indeed man himself would in many instancies find a similar deficiency…" Lewis provided a lengthy and precise description of the beast only recently known to science, and the animals provided some meat for the dinner table. Lewis also lamented the growing scarcity of buffalo, stating that "I begin to fear our harvest of white puddings are at an end."

The 26th was a momentous occasion for the Corps. For years they had heard tales of the distant and mysterious "Stony Mountains" that had been seen only by Indians, who had described them to French fur trappers. The French relayed the stories to their post at St. Louis and, from there, numerous white traders had dispersed the yarn to the edges of the U.S. frontier. The men of the Corps expected to find the Rocky Mountains, they just didn't know when. For a while they thought today was the day.

Clark, walking on shore, saw "mountts. on either side of the river at no great distance…I also think I saw a range of high mounts. at a great distance…" He was probably looking between the Judith Mountains and the Bears Paw Mountains to the 7,600-foot Highwood Range (around five thousand feet above his elevation on the Missouri). All are outliers of the Rockies. After Clark informed Lewis, the latter climbed "one of the highest piunts in the neighborhood…

"I thought myself well repaid for any labour; as from this point I beheld the Rocky Mountains for the first time." Lewis was looking on the sparkling snow that still blanketed the peaks about fifty air miles to the southwest. He was excited and satisfied, and also more prescient than he guessed:

> *while I viewed these mountains I felt a secret pleasure in finding myself so near the head of the heretofore conceived boundless Missouri; but when I reflected on the difficulties which this snowey barrier would most probably throw in my way to the Pacific, and the sufferings and hardships of myself an party in them, it in some measure counterballanced the joy...*

His attempted note of optimism followed: "but as I have always held it a crime to anticipate evils I will believe it a good comfortable road untill I am compelled to beleive differently."

Another brush with death came by way of hooves, supporting a half-ton of buffalo during the night of May 28-29. While the men slept, a lone buffalo entered the shallows on the opposite shore of the Missouri and swam the river, emerging on the bank below the camp. Finding his path blocked by an anchored pirogue in which the captains slept, he simply climbed over it and onto the shore. The buffalo proceeded to run up through the campfires, stomping potentially lethal hooves a few inches from the skulls of the sleeping men. Seaman, the magic Newfoundland dog, sprang up and diverted the charging behemoth. In another bizarre and amazing stroke of luck, the only things broken in camp were a blunderbuss in the pirogue and the stock of one of the rifles that lay on the ground.

During the day, the men were up to their armpits in the still cold springtime waters of the Missouri, towing the boats upriver. In some areas there was no bank on which to walk, the cliffs coming down at near 90-degree angles into the river. They walked over sharp rocks that bruised and sometimes cut their bare feet. The mud was as thick and slippery as oiled ice. "In short," wrote Lewis, "their labour is incredibly painfull and great, yet those faithfull fellows bear it without a murmur."

At the end of May, for a period of several days, the Corps passed through an area of bizarre and fascinating geological marvels. It is known today as the White Cliffs region of the Missouri. Lewis described the surrounding banks of whitish shale and sandstone as hav-

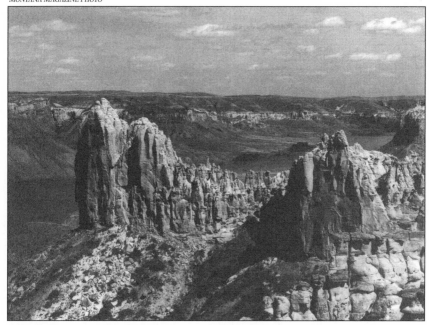

In the Missouri River Breaks.

ing "a most romantic appearance," adding that the rock formations formed a view of "visionary enchantment," with thousands of geometric, architectural and gargoyle-like formations. His journal entry consists of more than two pages of his flowing descriptions of the details of this incredibly picturesque area.

The Hidatsas had given the Corps a pretty good geographical scouting report to this point in their journey. It was not until June 3 that the men were surprised by an unknown "fork" in the river. The similarly sized streams led to a disagreement about which branch was the Missouri. If they took the wrong one, precious travel days of summer would be lost, and with an unknown distance yet to travel before the brutal winter once again beset them, the proper choice was essential. Reconnaissance teams were formed with Drouillard, Pryor, Shields, Windsor, Cruzatte, and Lepage to accompany Lewis up the right fork, and Clark, York, the Field brothers, Gass, and Shannon to go up the left.

On the 4th, Lewis took off over the high plains adjacent to the north fork amid a "great abundance of prickly pears which are extreemly troublesome; as the thorns very readily perce the foot through the Mockerson; they are so numerous that it requires one half of the traveler's attention to avoid them." There were even more buffalo on the plains than there were prickly pears.

The night of June 6, rain fell "almost without intermission," leaving Lewis's men with little sleep. The water penetrated only to a depth of about two inches and, as Lewis noted, resulted in walking on a surface of wet clay that is "precisely like walking over frozan grownd which is thawed to small debth and slips equally as bad."

On several occasions I have walked on these hillsides in the same weather conditions, and without warning have found myself going from a seemingly stable standing position to being flat on my back in an instant. As Lewis walked along a bluff, he too slipped, and without the aid of his espontoon, would have fallen down a "craggy pricipice of about ninety feet" and into the river. Lewis struggled to his feet with the aid of the espontoon and then heard a voice shouting in panic. "God! God! Captain! What shall I do?" He turned around to see Private Windsor, fallen, with his right arm and leg over the edge.

Expecting to see Windsor fall at any instant, and carefully disguising his alarm, Lewis "spoke very calmly to him and assured him that he was in no kind of danger, to take the knife out of his belt behind him with his wright hand and dig a hole with it in the face of the bank to receive his wright foot which he did and then raised himself to his knees; I then directed him to take off his mockersons and to come forward on his hands and knees holding the knife in one hand and the gun in the other this he happily effected and escaped." I believe that after the incident, Richard Windsor was one of Captain Lewis's biggest fans.

Meanwhile, Clark's group hiked thirteen miles up the left-hand river fork, camping at an old Indian lodge of "sticks and barks." Both parties encountered more grizzlies along the way, with Joseph Field nearly getting mauled. Field was saved at the last moment when shots directed at the bear by his mates set the grizzly to flight.

Lewis and his comrades returned to base camp on June 8, after ascending the north fork for sixty miles, but the maps that Lewis consulted provided a dilemma. They had been made by a surveyor for the Hudson's Bay Company, based on second-hand information he obtained from a chief of the Blackfeet Indian nation who lived in and hunted the area. The distances and locations of geographic landmarks had not been accurate, and the confusion created was apparent in the captains' struggle to decide which fork of the river to take.[1]

They decided that the northerly flow of the river they explored would not allow it to cross the Rocky Mountains, which lay farther to the west. Lewis thereby determined that the south fork was the true branch of the Missouri. Clark returned from his fifty-five-mile foray and agreed that the south fork was the one to take. The very experienced Pierre Cruzatte, a riverman for years, still thought the north fork to be the true Missouri. But the captains knew from the Hidatsas that there was a great waterfall on the Missouri. Clark, in spite of his going so far, had not discovered the falls. Now Lewis, being the more talented hiker, decided to hike the south fork until he found the landmark. He chose Drouillard, George Gibson, Joseph Field, and Silas Goodrich to accompany him. They would leave the following day. Cruzatte pulled out his fiddle, and the men danced and sang the evening away.

The following morning, prior to their departure, the captains decided to lighten the loads by caching the red pirogue, some excess provisions, and botanical and zoological specimens. Pierre Cruzatte, familiar with the construction of underground "caches," dug the pit and stored the goods. The supplies would be retrieved on the return trip—whenever that might be.

The morning of Lewis's proposed departure came and went with nobody leaving. Lewis had a case of "disentary," and he decided to wait for the following morning to depart.

Another major medical crisis was forming on the horizon, and this time it involved Sacagawea. The drama commenced with the terse observation by Lewis: "Sah-cah-gah, we a, our Indian woman is very sick this evening; Capt. C. blead her."

The next morning, the 11th of June, Lewis and his men departed despite the captain's feeling "somewhat weakened by my disorder." While the five men disappeared into the southwest, Dr. Clark's medical skills would be tried by fire.

That night of the 11th saw Sacagawea's condition worsen. From the following day's journal we can surmise that she suffered from lower abdominal pain, vomiting, and fever. Clark's treatment was in agreement with what the best physician in early 1800s America probably would have done, were he in the captain's position. Clark bled her, which he thought "appeared to be of great Service to her."

But she became still sicker. Clark started to worry and moved her from her sun-exposed position on the pirogue into a shaded portion in the rear. In addition to Sacagawea's ills, one of the men developed an abscess on his fingertip, and another got a toothache. When it rains it pours and, with Lewis gone, Captain Clark was the physician in charge.

On the morning of the 13th, at present-day Bird Coulee—a barren, sagebrush-filled gulch about eight miles downriver from Carter Ferry, Montana—Clark's group awoke to find a still worsening Sacagawea. Clark wrote twice in his journal entry that day, "the Indian woman verry Sick." Believing her condition to be brought on by, or at least con-tributed to by "costiveness," or constipation, Clark decided that provid-ing the young woman with a good bowel movement would relieve some of the pain. So Dr. Clark gave her a dose of cathartic salts. On the 14th, although noting that she had been "complaining all night & excessively bad this morning" and "that her case is Somewhat dangerous," she was put into the white pirogue and the men started upstream.

By the next day, with the bleeding and the dose of salts apparently not helping, Dr. Clark decided to try something new on his patient. He now put together a poultice containing some powdered Peruvian bark and applied it to the source of her pain, her lower abdomen and pelvic region. She apparently improved, because Clark noted that the poultice "revived her much." But the improvement was short-lived, and later that day he noted, "the Indian woman much wors this evening, She will not take any medison, her husband petetions to return &c." Charbon-neau was worried. Clark sent Joseph Field, who had arrived with a note from Lewis the previous afternoon, back up the river to get Lewis for an emergency call.

At about 2 P.M. on June 16, Lewis arrived back at the base camp and "found the Indian woman extreemly ill and much reduced by her indis-position." Lewis's compassion was kindled while observing the failing young woman and her baby, and his concern came through in his jour-nal entry: "this gave me some concern as well for the poor object her-self, then with a young child in her arms." In addition, he expressed concern for the success of the expedition if it were to continue without the Shoshone girl who promised to be a diplomatic and linguistic liaison between her tribe and the Corps, in its effort to obtain horses to cross the Rockies.

Lewis went into action and decided to try some sulfur-containing water he had discovered in a nearby spring. He also administered doses of the barks and some laudanum. The opium apparently helped with some nervous "twitching of the fingers and leader of the arm," and the mineral water helped to relieve her dehydrated system. Sacagawea complained of pain in her lower abdomen, and Dr. Lewis decided that her problem "originated principally from an obstruction of the mensis in consequence of taking could."

Despite a temporary setback associated with some dietary indiscretion encouraged by her husband, the young woman continued to improve. The barks and laudanum were continued with the addition of a general tonic of the day: fifteen drops of "oil of vitriol," or a diluted solution of sulfuric acid. I am not aware of any benefit that this diluted acid solution would have provided.

Of the treatments the captain-physicians used on Sacagawea, the only ones I see any benefit in are the pain relief of the opium and the rehydrating effects of the spring water; the beneficial effect from minerals in the water would be minimal and certainly not equivalent to modern intravenous fluids. The barks, though likely not harmful, probably did no good, and the bleeding and cathartics were indeed harmful. By bleeding, the red blood cells that function in oxygen transport, and the white blood cells that are part of the immune response in fighting off infection, would have both been compromised. Both the bleeding and the cathartics would have contributed to dehydration and possible loss of important minerals such as potassium and sodium.

Rather than having an obstruction of the menses from taking cold, as Lewis believed, the young Indian woman may have had a pelvic infection. There are numerous possibilities. P.I.D., or pelvic inflammatory disease, would be a top contender. Given the fact that Sacagawea was one of Charbonneau's three wives, and given the sexual practices among the Mandans and Hidatsas, it is highly unlikely, even ridiculous, to think that Charbonneau hadn't picked up sexually transmitted diseases (either gonorrhea or Chlamydia) and passed them along during his life on the Knife River in North Dakota. Sacagawea was probably one of the unlucky recipients of Charbonneau's "gift." This disease can strike the cervix, uterus, fallopian tubes, or ovaries. Symptoms include fever, lower abdominal pain, and discharge of pus-like fluid from the vagina, frequently with nausea and vomiting. If untreated, it could result in death, and frequently it results in scarred tubes that cause infertility. Modern treatment involves the use of antibiotics that can effectively and quickly solve the problem, along with advice to be very careful about sexual partners.

Another very real possibility is that Sacagawea's sickness was the initial symptoms of an infection from the parasite *Trichinella*. When we examine the journals, we note that grizzly bears were killed during the first week of June 1805. Since the bears were used as food, it is likely that Sacagawea ingested some grizzly meat during that time. Systemic symptoms of trichinosis may start from seven to fifteen days after eating the infected meat and include nausea, vomiting, abdominal pain, and fever.

There are other less likely possibilities, such as a severe urinary tract infection, as well as the numerous things that could have caused fever, vomiting, and severe lower abdominal pain: intestinal infections from parasites other than trichinella, or other disease-causing microorganisms.

Miles away from the base camp back on June 11, while Clark was busily cutting into Sacagawea's veins, Lewis had declined a gourmet feast of elk marrowbones, due to his high fever and a "violent pain in the intestens." He made himself a bed of willow branches and lay down to rest. He had not brought any of the store-bought medicine on this hike, but his mother's training gave Lewis an idea. He

> resolved to try an experiment with some simples; and the Choke cherry which grew abundantly in the bottom first struck my attention; I directed a parsel of the small twigs to be geathered striped of their leaves, cut into pieces of about 2 Inches in length and boiled in water untill a strong black decoction of an astringent bitter tast was produced; at sunset I took a [pint] of this decoction and abut an hour after repeated the dze by 10 in the evening I was entirely releived from pain and in fact every symptom of the disorder forsook me; my fever

abated, a gentle perspiration was produced and I had a comfortable and refreshing nights rest.

Lewis probably did not know it at the time, but he was playing with a plant that had potentially fatal side-effects if taken improperly. The chokecherry tree (*Prunus virginianus*) grows in abundance in the valleys of present-day Montana. Its fruit, about the size of a pea, is rather bitter to the taste, but makes a great jelly, wine, or syrup.

The genus Prunus is typified by the presence of a potentially deadly chemical compound known as a cyanogenic glycoside. Amygdalin is the name of this cyanide-containing sugar molecule. When plant cells containing amygdalin are crushed (particularly seeds of this genus), other enzymes in the plant come into contact with the amygdalin and break it down into a deadly compound, hydrogen cyanide. Amygdalin in its intact form is not particularly toxic to animals. Its toxicity depends on the co-ingestion of certain enzymes that would break down the amygdalin and produce the cyanide.[2] The bark portion that Lewis used contained smaller amounts of this compound than the seeds, and the boiling action of the brewing could have inactivated the enzymes that would have produced the cyanide.

The key to its non-toxic use was that Lewis probably did not use the unripened cherries and their seeds in his potion. What the herbal substance was that made Lewis feel better is not as readily identifiable, but this plant was a well-known herbal medication on the frontier for treatment of diarrhea and other ailments. The next morning Lewis drank another dose of his chokecherry tea and set out on a little stroll of twenty-seven miles. Along the way he helped kill two grizzlies, three mule deer, a buffalo, and a pronghorn that he and his men ate for the day's three meals. The rest they hung in trees along the river for the use of Clark's contingent that was slowly making it way up the south fork. Not yet being fully exhausted, Lewis went fishing with Goodrich and caught a slew of whitefish.

On the 13th, Lewis walked across a vast and nearly flat plain, viewing mountains far to the west, south and east. Late in the morning, he struck out in a southwest direction, and soon heard "a roaring too tremendious to be mistaken for any cause short of the great falls of the Missouri." At noon he arrived on the edge of a 200-foot rocky cliff and peered into the gorge. There he viewed a "sublimely grand specticle," adding that the Great Falls were "the grandest sight I ever beheld." He added copious descriptions of various aspects of the falls and the underlying rocks, ultimately expressing his dissatisfaction with his attempts to convey his amazement with the written word. What nature had perfected and presented to his eyes that afternoon was difficult for Lewis to put on paper.

The next morning, Captain Lewis sent Joseph Field downstream with a letter to Clark, describing how falls cut into the bluffs and made shoreline travel impossible here.

Then Lewis struck farther up the Missouri on his own and encountered more in a series of impressive falls. He wrote, "I now thought that if a skillfull painter had been asked to make a beautifull cascade that he would most probably have presented the precise immage of this one…" Comparing the second falls, "Crooked Falls," to the Great Falls, he described this one as "pleasingly beautifull," while the other was "sublimely grand."

Walking on through prairie that contained thousands of buffalo and passing three more falls, Lewis reached the mouth of present-day Sun River, which the Mandans/Hidatsas had described. From a nearby rise, he observed the Missouri with "vast flocks of geese" feeding in the "delightfull pasture" on either side. He decided to shoot a bull for his supper, and camp rather than return to his men that evening. "[A] few sticks of drift wood lying along the shore…would answer for my fire…" and a scattered of cottonwoods would do for shelter.

Lewis selected his supper and "shot him very well, through the lungs." As he stood with his unloaded rifle, watching the "poor anamal" die, Lewis failed to notice a grizzly that approached him from behind "within 20 steps before I discovered him…" Pulling up his rifle to shoot, Lewis immediately realized the gun was empty. Every outdoor survival skill he had ever mastered raced through his mind in an instant. There were no trees within three hundred yards, and the bear continued to advance. Lewis immediately turned and raced toward the river, about eighty yards away, with the bear "open mouthed and full speed" gaining on him fast. The captain scampered into the river to waist depth and turned, pointing his spear-like espontoon at the huge predator to defend himself to the death. Surprisingly, the fierce animal

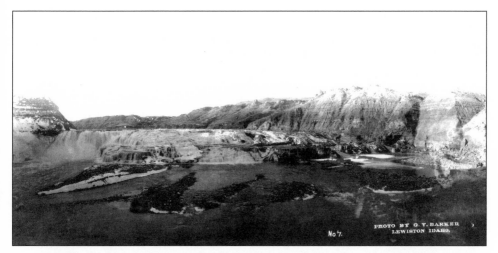

The first of the five Great Falls, now covered by Ryan Dam at Great Falls, Montana, as it looked in 1910. MONTANA HISTORICAL SOCIETY, 949-561

"wheeled about as if frightened, declined the combat on such unequal grounds, and retreated with quite as great precipitation as he had just before pursued me." The bear ran at full speed, occasionally stopping to "look behind him as if he expected pursuit."

Joseph Field reached the main party at 4 P.M., and the next morning Clark sent him back to collect Lewis for the consultation about Sacagawea.

Reunited, the Corps of Discovery had to dodge rattlesnakes as they established a base camp (their "Lower Portage Camp") on the east side of the Missouri River near the mouth of present-day Belt Creek. From here originated their epic eleven-day, sixteen-mile transport of the canoes across the plains, to an area upriver from the five waterfalls. Consideration was given to the idea of having the men carry the canoes across the plain, but the distance made that impossible. Six men were commissioned to cut down cottonwoods and saw them up to make wheels, tongues, couplings, and bodies for crude wagons to ferry the canoes across the hot, dusty, rattlesnake-ridden prairie. The white pirogue was unloaded and the captains decided to stash it, with other supplies, at Lower Portage Camp, to be picked up on the return trip. The five canoes were pulled 1.75 miles up "Portage Creek" (Belt

Creek) and then allowed to dry on the bank in the June sun. A cottonwood was found that yielded a nice, respectable wheel twenty-two inches in diameter. The soft wood made Lewis a little nervous about its ability to endure the tough duty of bearing the weight of the canoes and provisions, but there was not another tree "we could find of the same size perfectly sound within twenty miles of us." Lewis's concerns about the wood were justified. The cottonwood proved to be too soft for the wagon tongues and the white pirogue's mast had to be sacrificed to produce them.

Meanwhile, buffalo steaks sizzled over the campfire near the Missouri, and Sacagawea steadily improved. The camp was along the riverbank, where the Corps watched dead buffalo float past camp while living bison walked down to the river to drink. The young mother chewed the well-salted and -peppered meat with increasing delight, and drank some bison "soup." This recovery of their "interpreter's wife" both cheered and relieved the captains. Once again it would seem that the Corps had dodged a bullet.

The great portage was underway, across the flat filled with low-growing sagebrush, prickly pear, and grass that provided a haven for the innumerable jumping grasshoppers and slithering rattlers that, along with the buffalo, provided a constant circus of animals.

John Colter was surprised by a grizzly on a nearby island and retreated into the river with the bear in hot pursuit. Willard, who had also been chased by the bear, alerted Captain Clark, who formed an assault party and reached the island just in time to shoot at, and drive away, the partially immersed bear. Due to impending darkness, the assault was wisely called off.

Feeling somewhat revived on June 19, Sacagawea went into the plain and collected "a considerable quantity of the white apples of which she eat so heartily in their raw state, together with a considerable quantity of dryed fish without my knowledge that she complained very much and her fever again returned." Lewis rebuked Charbonneau for allowing this and treated her with "broken dozes of diluted nitre untill it produced perspiration and at 10 P.M. 30 drops of laudnum which gave her a tolerable nights rest." The nitre or saltpeter (potassium nitrate) was used in this instance for the express purpose of inducing a sweat that would both cool the fever, and clean out the mysterious "acrimonies" that the captains probably believed were contributing to the problem. The opium and the alcohol, both potent central nervous system depressants with pain-relieving effects, contributed to her "tolerable nights rest."

More latitude readings were taken in the clear summer sky and their position was calculated pretty accurately to be 47° 7' 10.3." I wonder what the captains would have thought of, or would have given, for one of our modern Global Positioning System handheld units. Satellites that send messages to such boxes would have been bigger "medicin" to Lewis and Clark than anything they had ever shown to the Indians.

With the prickly pears being "extreemly troublesome to us sticking our feet through our mockersons" and the summer heat bearing down in unyielding fury, the labor of portaging the canoes was horrendous. The men put double soles on their moccasins to try to protect themselves from the one- to two-inch spines, with little success. At times they stripped naked and pushed, pulled, and struggled with the wagons and material. They had to stop frequently, and varying degrees of heat exhaustion were constant companions. Lewis showed, on June 23, a great deal of insight and compassion for the plight of his men: "…at every halt these poor fellows tumble down and are so much fortiegued that many of them are asleep in an instant; in short their fatiegues are incredible; some are limping from the soreness of their feet, others faint and unable to stand for a few minutes, with heat and fatiegue, yet no one complains, all go with cheerfullness."

I sometimes contemplate the degree of hardship this portage must have involved. The best estimate I can imagine to recreate something akin to their experience would be to crawl several times around your block during a hot summer day, on your hands and knees, with limited water to drink.

The men were now acting solely as team members and not individuals, their evolution into a solid group complete. Their dedication to and perseverance in the task at hand had been summed up by Clark as he staked out the portage route on the 20th: "all appear perfectly to have made up their minds to Succeed in the expedition or perish in the attempt."

There were bears all around the portage route. On the 27th, George Drouillard and Joseph Field saw huge grizzly tracks on the muddy shoreline. Spying a twenty-foot-tall tree, they landed and carefully shinnied up the trunk for a bird's-eye view of the area. The climbing had to be a little tough while holding their fifty-inch rifles with one hand and clutching to the rough bark with the other. Once they reached a sufficient height, Drouilland and Field surveyed the immediate area. There was the bear—all five hundred to six hundred pounds of fur, muscle, and bad attitude—trying to conceal himself in the brush. It would now be predator versus predator, and let the best creature win. With all the intensity they could muster, the two men gave a loud "whoop," and the bear immediately went to the alarm stage, crashing through the brush toward the sound. Arriving at the tree, the bear paused to look nearsightedly around, hoping to find his next easy meal. It was his last mistake. The .54 caliber lead ball, from Drouillard's rifle only feet above, slammed into his skull and put the great beast down for the count. This grizzly was even larger than every specimen so far.

This area seemed filled with the great bears. Seaman was in a constant state of alarm at night as grizzlies prowled around the camp. And then there had been Lewis's experience back on June 14, when a grizzly stalked and chased him into the Missouri. Lewis determined, after Drouillard and Shields' bear yielded a skin as big as an ox's, that no man should go out of the two camps unaccompanied, "particularly where he has to pass through the brush."

The area where they portaged is prime hail country, as they learned on June 29. While some of the men were transporting baggage across the open plain, hail stones, some weighing three ounces and measuring seven inches in circumference, began falling from the sky and striking the ground around the men. The hail became heavier and soon started striking the exposed men. Some scampered under the shelter provided by the canoe they were portaging, while others ducked and covered, trying to make themselves as small a target as possible, hoping that the stones wouldn't hit them. But for twenty minutes it continued coming down. The hailstones hit the ground and bounced into the air to a height of ten to twelve feet. Men grabbed anything they could find to cover their heads and bodies. The hail struck their exposed legs, cutting and bruising them. The storm continued until the ground was covered with ice to a depth of 1.5 inches. As the hail slacked off, the men crawled from their makeshift shelters and headed back to basecamp, leaving the provisions on the plain. Lewis noted that "the men were all nearly naked and no covering on the head were sorely mawled with the hail which was so large and driven with such force by the wind that it nocked many of them down and one particulary as many as three times most of them were bleeding freely and complained of being much bruised." He added, in the month's weather observations (describing the hailstorm inexplicably as an event of June 27), "I am convinced if one of those had struck a man on the neaked head it would have knocked him down, if not fractured his skull."

If you do the physics, a hailstone of three ounces and seven inches in circumference hitting you is very similar to being hit by an eighty- to ninety-mile-per hour baseball. The afternoon on that plain near Great Falls must have been terrifying, to say the least. (For those crawling around their blocks, now add neighborhood children throwing base-balls at you.)

What is one man's poison is another man's food, or ice cubes in this instance. Safely tucked away in a shelter at the time, Lewis and other men marvelled at the hail, collecting and measuring the stones. Joseph Whitehouse even noted in his journal that Captain Lewis "made a small bowl of punch out of one of them."[3]

Meanwhile, the storm nearly took the lives of several of the Corps, including Captain Clark, Sacagawea, Pompey, and Charbonneau. For woodsman Clark, the "rain and hail fell more violent than ever I saw before…"

As the storm moved in, Clark, York, Sacagawea with the baby, and Charbonneau had been walking past the five falls from the lower to the upper camp. When the downpour began, they took shelter under an overhanging rock in a steep ravine.

Clark wrote,

> …the rain fell like one voley of water falling from the heavens and gave us time only to get out of the way of a torrent of water which was Poreing down the hill in the rivin with emence force tareing every thing before it takeing with it large rock & mud…

The group was in the path of a flash food. Clark continues:

...I took my gun & Shot pouch in my left hand, and with the right Scrambled up the hill pushing the Interpreters wife (who had her Child in her arms) before me, the Interpreter himself makeing attempts to pull up his wife by the hand much Scared and nearly without motion—we at length retched the top of the hill Safe where I found my Servent in Serch of us greatly agitated, for our wellfar—.

Pompey's clothes were lost; Clark's worst loss, among other items, was the expedition's large compass. Finding it was worth pulling two men off the portage the next day. They found it at the ravine's mouth, after digging into the sand and mud.

On the Fourth of July, while Lewis and some of the men were becoming ever more frustrated with their attempts to assemble Lewis's portable boat that they had lugged up the Missouri for two thousand miles, Patrick Gass, Hugh McNeal, and several others who had not seen the falls were permitted to walk to the river and view the tumbling and rushing waters. In the evening, with the entire Corps assembled around the campfires and, enjoying their Independence Day picnic of beans, bacon, suet dumpling, and buffalo steaks, the captains poured out the last drops of whiskey. Cruzatte's fiddle serenaded the men, woman, baby, buffalo, bears, and rattlesnakes alike. The men danced until 9 P.M., when a thunderstorm cooled off the party. But the "mirth with songs and festive jokes" continued until "late at night" and the men of the Corps "were extreemly merry."

Over the following ten days the portage was completed, and now the men could once again anticipate pushing the canoes upriver. Behind them were the cuts and bruises from massive hailstones, the brutal exertions of towing the canoes over the plain while dodging prickly pears, abundant grizzlies, and rattlesnakes. Drs. Clark and Lewis could rejoice at their gynecological patient's recovery from her fight with the Grim Reaper.

By noon on July 14, Sergeant Ordway arrived at the upper camp with the last of the portaged canoes, as the group readied for their departure up the Missouri the following morning. Late-afternoon heat produced a light thunder shower while the men made camp and tried to situate themselves comfortably for a night under fabulously bright summer stars. They all must have had throughts of exciting adventures, treacherous weather, and exhausting work experienced during the past few months. They would soon begin to penetrate the Rocky Mountains on the great Missouri as it meandered from the distant peaks that were now illuminated by the setting sun.

I wonder if Meriwether Lewis, while he lay on the ground that night with the ever-present humming of mosquitoes around the netting over his head, ever thought back on those days with the Hidatsas, when they tried to warn him about the grizzly bears. I wonder if he thought of his arrogant note that "the Indians may well fear this anamal equiped as they generally are with their bows and arrows or indifferent fuzees, but in the hands of skillfull riflemen they are by no means as formidable or dangerous as they have been represented." If he did think about it, maybe he laughed to himself—maybe he shook his head is amazement—maybe he had a new sense of respect for the Indians and their bows and arrows.

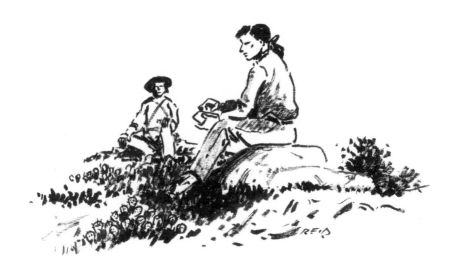

❧ 12 ❧

FROM A TORRENT TO A TRICKLE

To the Headwaters of the Missouri

One never notices what has been done; one can only see what remains to be done...
—*Marie Curie*

The forty or so miles from the city of Great Falls, Montana, to the town of Hardy, have always been one of my favorite drives. On a clear day, the surrounding countryside offers a spectacular view of numerous ecosystems and their diverse scenery. To the west is the front range of the Rocky Mountains, with its dramatic snow-capped peaks. To the southeast is the relatively tame and heavily timbered Little Belt range, home of the "blue-ribbon" trout-filled Smith River, named by the captains after President Jefferson's Secretary of the Navy, Robert Smith. To the north lies flat prairie that seemingly extends all the way to the North Pole and, in winter, feels that way when the frigid winds from Canada blow down into Montana. As you approach Hardy, things change rapidly, with dramatic rock formations rising hundreds of feet, providing pivots for the meandering Missouri. Porcupines, deer, and rattlesnakes frequently make their way across the lanes of Interstate 15 in our modern scene, some luckier than others. Another few miles of interstate and the Dearborn River flows into the Missouri from the west—named by the captains for Henry Dearborn, then Secretary of War. Even with the intrusion of blacktop and cement, this is a scene of spectacular and unique beauty, and it is the area where the Corps of Discovery found themselves moving south, upstream, in July of 1805, minus the blacktop and cement.

Meriwether Lewis wrote, "in some places both banks of the river are formed for a short distance of nearly perpendicular rocks of a dark black grannite of great hight; the river has the appearance of having cut it's passage in the course of time through this solid rock."

Fearing that the united Corps would startle any Shoshones who may have been in the area, the captains decided to split up the group on July 18. Lewis and the majority remained on the river, and William Clark, John Potts, York, and Joseph Field (who may have been along serving as a bear expert), struck out ahead on land, in hopes of making contact with the Shoshone. As usual, the mosquitoes were "verry troublesom," and frequent encounters with prickly pears left their feet wounded, sore, and barely able at times to support them while walking. One night while sitting around the campfire, Clark pulled out seventeen of these inch long spears from the soles of his beaten and weary feet.

On the 19th of July, Lewis and the river party, making their way upstream through the stifling heat of midsummer, entered "much the most remarkable clifts that we have yet seen. these clifts rise from the waters edge on either side perpendicularly to the hight of 1200 feet. every object here wears a dark and gloomy aspect. the tow[e]ring and projecting rocks in many places seem ready to tumble on us." This splendid and breath-taking canyon, five and three-quarters miles long, cut over the millennia by the Missouri, can still be visited today north of Helena, Montana. Lewis wrote, "from the singular appearance of this place I called it the *gates of the rocky mountains.*"

William Clark walked through the present-day Prickly Pear Valley east of Helena on July 19, and named a rambling creek for Sergeant Nathaniel Pryor. Its waters flowed through the valley, making their way from the west and the peaks of the present-day Elkhorn Range. Perversely, Clark's naming failed and it became Prickly Pear Creek for the cactus "so abundant that we could scarcely find room to lye." (A little more than a hundred years later, a young man from Slovenia and his Austrian wife would work a farm on the Prickly Pear's banks, and raise my mother, aunts, and uncle.)

The peaks of the mountain ranges on both sides of the valley, rising from 7,000 to nearly 9,000 feet, still held snow on July 21, but on the water at less than 4,000 feet elevation, the mosquitoes were fierce. Lewis noted the benefit of the mosquito nets, stating, "the men are all fortunately supplyed with musquetoe biers otherwise it would be impossible for them to exist under the fatiegues which they daily encounter without their natural rest which they could not obtain for those tormenting insects if divested of their biers." Three days later he added a description of biblical proportions: "our trio of pests still invade and obstruct us on all occasions, these are the Musquetoes eye knats and prickley pears, equal to any three curses that ever poor Egypt laiboured under..." At least the cooler evening temperatures "some hours" after sunset in the mountain valleys provided the group with mosquito free nights.

While the men toiled, Seaman with his never-ending canine enthusiasm, was busy catching geese along the river, proudly adding some fowl to the men's diet.

The men who continued to row and tow were approaching the limit of their day-in, day-out work schedule. Clark's group hunted on shore, and then the captain encamped to await the boats. Reunited late on the 22nd, the Corps camped on present-day Canyon Ferry Lake, a Missouri River reservoir. Clark "opened the bruses & blisters of my feet which caused them to be painfull." His rationale in "opening up" his blisters is unclear but, based on modern medical thinking, it was not a wise idea. Intact blisters protect the underlying raw skin, giving it time to generate more surface cells that will protect yet deeper layers. Clark's self-treatment rendered the blisters into open wounds. In an era of no antiseptics and, in the field in dirty conditions, he set himself up for acquiring infections on his feet. At the very least he succeeded in making his feet more painful than they needed to be. These raw wounds would take at least a week to heal sufficiently for him to walk without considerable pain. But Captain Clark didn't have a week. He would push onward.

The following morning Clark left camp with a new party of the Field brothers, Frazer, and Charbonneau in hopes of finding the Shoshones. The hiking would have been brutal on his raw and painful feet. By 10 A.M. they had located Drouillard, who had spent the night upriver alone, having been unable to find camp the night before.

Lewis's party brought up the rear in the canoes, utilizing ropes and poles to move upstream. The river bed was slippery, so Lewis had the men attach clumps of brush with wire to the bases of the poles. The traction eased the men's efforts, but they still were exhausted. Lewis joined in and did some poling of his own.

On occasion the men still stumbled upon a grizzly bear, but the great bears seemed "to be more shy here than on the Missouri below the mountains." Lewis's party were eating well without bear meat, though. Geese were numerous but small, and Lewis ordered the men to ignore them; the scrawny bodies did not provide sufficient food to justify using up ball and powder, or time. There were plenty of purple and black currants, and Lewis wrote they were "ripe and Superior to any I ever tasted particularly the yellow & purple kind." Gooseberries, serviceberries and chokecherries all helped balance the diet and add to their bodily stores of vitamin C and other nutrients. There were still some deer, elk, and pronghorns, but the buffalo had disappeared.

The river party now had first-hand information from Sacagawea that they were approaching lands her tribe frequented. She assured Captain Lewis that the river had no further falls, something that Lewis feared was not true, due to the rugged and mountainous country. He noted that the mountains "still continue high and seem to rise in some places like an amphatheater one rang above another as they receede from the river untill the most distant and lofty have their tops clad with snow." As the men neared the head of the Missouri, the clear mountain waters were full of beavers and otters.

On the morning of July 25, Clark and his advance party reached a landmark location where a trio of rivers fed from the distant peaks and mountain ranges join to form the mighty Missouri River. After pausing for a breakfast of deer ribs, Clark sat down in the hot July sun and wrote a note to Lewis, attached it to a pole by the side of the river and set out. He hiked another twenty miles up the westernmost branch and was forced to camp due to his extremely painful foot wounds and Charbonneau's failing ankles. They were, for the first time in fifteen months, off the Missouri.

As the canoes with Captain Lewis passed numerous creeks flowing into the Missouri from the surrounding mountains. He named them after the men of the expedition: Gass's Creek (now Crow Creek), Reubin Field's Valley Creek (North Boulder Creek), Frazer's River (South Boulder Creek), Ordway's Creek (Little Prickly Pear Creek), Howard's Creek (Sixteenmile Creek).[1] The days were the hottest that the Corps had experienced yet this year, and the river's current had become rapid. On the 27th, Lewis wrote that "...the men are in a continual state of their utmost exertion to get on, and they begin to weaken fast from this continual state of violent exertion."

Muscular energy is provided from the food that we eat, the glucose in our blood streams and stored glucose in the form of glycogen in our livers. In spite of their high protein diet, the men's bodies were able to take the protein building-blocks called amino acids and change them into glucose that their muscle cells could in turn burn for energy to push the poles. Prolonged severe muscular exertion can deplete the body's stores of glycogen, and result in the muscles' having little fuel to burn. Muscular exertion also produces lactic acid, which causes muscle fatigue and soreness. Their bodily engines were trying to run without any gas. In addition, the days were hot, and some degree of heat exhaustion was probably present. This is a perfect picture of both glycogen exhaustion and heat-related illness.

But they pressed on, reaching the Three Forks of the Missouri River on July 27. Ordway wrote that Sacagawea recognized this area as the place where she had been taken captive by the Hidatsas four years earlier. She spoke calmly through Charbonneau, and related how her small group had been attacked and had retreated up the western river to hide in the forest. The Hidatsas pursued them, killed four men, four women and a number of boys, and took the surviving females and four boys as prisoners. As she told the story, she seemed to show no emotion at being back in her own neighborhood. Lewis, perhaps showing his occasional lack of sensitivity, observed that "if she has enough to eat and a few trinkets to wear I believe she would be perfectly content anywhere." Even if Sacagawea didn't seem to be excited about their location, her bit of news undoubtedly provided the men with some much needed encouragement. As they listened to the Indian girl, the men's tailoring abilities now were put to use as they busily sewed together some rough buckskin clothing. The two separate parties had reunited but there were still no Shoshones in sight.

On July 27, suffering from constipation for several days, Clark wrote "I was verry unwell all last night with a high fever & akeing in all my bones. My fever & c. continus." Lewis suggested some of Rush's pills and a leg soak in some warm water. Obviously thinking that if a little is good, more is better, Clark took a whopping dose of five of Rush's pills, a dose that contained a potentially fatal dose of nearly 50 to 75 grains, or 3 to 4 grams, of calomel. The presence of the jalap probably produced such a potent and quick bowel movement that some of that calomel exited Clark before it had time to be optimally absorbed. This type of mercury is also poorly absorbed through the intestinal wall, with only about 15 percent entering the blood. Lewis wrote, "My friend Capt. Clark was very sick all last night but feels himself somewhat better this morning since his medicine has opperated." In addition to his thorough bowel "cleansing," Clark must have experienced another effect of the mercury in the calomel—he probably urinated like a racehorse. Whitehouse attributed Clark's illness to fatigue. But as the next several days passed, it seemed to be more than just a bad case of fatigue or constipation. On the 28th, Clark was sick again, and the next day Lewis wrote "Capt. Clark is much better today, is perfectly clear of fever but still very languid and complains of a general soarness in all his limbs. I prevailed on him to take the barks which he has done and eate tolerably freely of our good venison." On the 30th, Lewis reported "Capt. Clark being much better this morning."

As with everything medical that involved the Corps, particularly in our trying to interpret the journal entries about the symptoms and signs described, we venture into the land of presumption and speculation. However, I believe that there are some interesting possibilities that we may consider in Clark's symptoms. Besides possible cases of run-of-the-mill viral illnesses, or wound infection from his blisters, Clark probably to some degree had poisoned himself with calomel.

Clark could also have been suffering from a viral illness we call Colorado tick fever, transmitted by the bite of a tick. The disease is endemic in the Three Forks region, and the symptoms Clark had could certainly have been caused by this organism. Tick fever is the result of an infection of an RNA-containing virus.[2] (Viruses contain either DNA or RNA, not both). This virus is passed along from the bite of the tick *Dermacentor andersoni* and possibly other tick species. The virus is generally passed back and forth between the tick and the rodents on which they feed. The virus does not seem to cause disease in the rodents, and humans are incidental and "dead-end" hosts.[3]

Usually within three to six days after infection, a fever will occur abruptly, followed by severe headaches, muscle aches, and fatigue. Other symptoms such as severe ocular light sensitivity, eye pain, nausea, vomiting and abdominal pain can occur. A distinctive feature of this illness is its "bi-phasic" fever pattern that occurs in about 50 percent of victims. The victim will be febrile for two to three days, recover and feel better for a day or two, only to have the fever return for an additional two to three days.[4]

The tick fever virus enters the body, replicates and circulates in the blood, producing a state we call viremia, or viruses in the blood stream. Once inside the blood, the viruses travel to the bone marrow and infect developing red blood cells. There they hide safely inside cell membranes, protected from the increasing amount of antibodies circulating outside the cells. These antibodies are specifically directed against the invading viruses by the victim's immune system. The symptoms will usually clear up within a week, but the virus's presence in the red blood cells can persist for a month or longer. Rare complications involving the heart, liver, and lungs have been reported.[5]

Another possible medical explanation for Clark's illness could be tularemia, obtained via contact with either an infected game animal in cleaning, or via the bite of a tick or deer fly. This disease has various forms and manifestations, and Clark could have had a less-virulent case.

Another possible tick-borne illness is Rocky Mountain spotted fever. Probably only about 1 percent of ticks in present-day Montana hold the infecting bacterium, known as a *Rickettsia*.[6] The wood tick, *Dermacentor andersoni*, is the chief culprit in the transmission of the disease, which peaks during late spring and early summer. Still another tick-borne bacterium, *Borrelia*, could have been the culprit. Both of these diseases have the potential for fatal outcomes, particularly if untreated by antibiotics, which of course did not exist in 1805.

Symptoms of many of the tick-borne diseases vary from being mild, with fever and muscle aches, to more severe illness including fever, rash, headache, abdominal pain, vomiting, diarrhea, confusion, heart involvement, seizures, coma, vascular collapse, and death. This is an illness to take very seriously and can be cured with modern antibiotics. Clark could have had a mild case of this disease.

On Sunday, July 28, Lewis and Clark named the three rivers that formed the Missouri. The right-hand or western most river, the branch that they would soon ascend, was named the Jefferson, "in honor of that illustrious personage" and "the author of our enterprise." The middle fork was named after the Secretary of State, James Madison, and the left fork after the Secretary of the Treasury, Albert Gallatin.

After two days of rest at the forks, the Corps set out up the Jefferson and, nearly five miles up the rapid current, Sacagawea identified the exact site where she had been taken prisoner. Some of the invalids suffering from their sore feet rode in the canoes as Lewis hiked along the bank. Lewis found himself alone that evening and spent it on an island on the Jefferson, cooking a duck he had shot, and battling the mosquitoes. A large fire kept him company throughout the night. The weather continued hot, with an occasional afternoon or early evening thundershower providing a delightfully cooler evening.

The following evening, without any fresh meat and lamenting the group's inability to conserve food, Drouillard and Lewis tried to surround a grizzly in a thicket and prepared to kill the beast. But the bear gave them the slip.

Lewis's list of disabled read like a modern-day National Football League injury list: Gass with a bruised back from falling in a canoe, Pryor had again dislocated his shoulder, another man with a bad stone bruise, and two with bad boils. There was still no sign of Shoshones, and Lewis was appropriately concerned.

The following day, with a plan born of desperation, Lewis, Gass, and interpreters Drouillard and Charbonneau, planned on ascending the Jefferson to its source and proceeding onward until they made contact with the Shoshones. Summer was rapidly disappearing, and with an unknown portion of the Rocky Mountains to cross, they needed to make good progress so they could get out of the mountains before winter set in. Clark and the rest of the group would continue upstream on the Jefferson River, waiting for Lewis's return and hoping for good news.

On the morning of August 1, Lewis's party set out. The heat of the day was brutal. With no timber to shade their advance, the direct summer sun made everything more miserable. They even took a wrong path that put them several miles away from their desired location. By 2 P.M., they returned to the Jefferson, exhausted by the eleven-mile hike and suffering from the heat. Lewis wrote that "we then hurried to the river and allayed our thirst." He had the added discomfort of loose bowels, produced from his previous evening's dose of Glauber's salts that he took in hopes of curtailing the diarrhea he had been suffering for several days. Revived by the water, Drouillard and Lewis went out to hunt and, fortunately, killed two elk. A fire was struck and some fresh steaks soon started to sizzle. Refreshed from their rest, the group added another six miles before they set up camp somewhere near the present town of Cardwell, Montana. Early morning temperatures of around 50 degrees F. added some incentive to get moving, as the two blankets each man covered himself with provided barely enough warmth to provide a refreshing sleep.

The following morning, wading the Jefferson for the first time, Lewis's group inched across the waist-deep and rapid current. From the opposite shore, they moved across a valley paralleled by two great mountain ranges (the Tobacco Roots and Highlands peaks are in the 7,000- to 10,000-foot range). Although the surrounding peaks still had snow, the valley temperatures were stifling, leading Lewis to comment that they "were nearly suffocated with the intense heat of the midday sun…" Along the way the men "feasted suptuously on our wild fruit particularly the yellow courant and the deep purple servicebury which I found to be excellent." They covered twenty-three miles.

Meanwhile Clark was suffering from a painful sore on the inside on his ankle that was, in his medical opinion, the result of the bite of "Some poisonous insect." His command continued to struggle up the Jefferson.

On August 4, the Lewis party passed a tributary that converged with the Jefferson and named it the "Wisdom" (present Big Hole River). In a few miles, they came to the head of the Jefferson: today's Ruby River ("Philanthropy" to the Corps) and the Beaverhead (continuation of the Jefferson to them). Lewis's men moved onto the Beaverhead, leaving a note instructing Clark to follow them up that "fork." For the next two days they searched for Shoshones without luck.

Lewis's men returned on the 6th to the site where they had left their note. When Lewis sent Drouillard out hunting, he bumped into Clark's party ascending the Big Hole River and told them they'd taken the wrong fork, and to turn back. Clark had not seen the note. It was decided that the green pole where Lewis had placed the note had fallen victim to a beaver.

More problems arose. Clark's ankle abscess finally burst open, discharging a "considerable quantity of matter," but the sore's pain and swelling continued. Shannon was on the Big Hole River alone, sent out by Clark to hunt when his party was on that stream. Drouillard took off in pursuit, signaling shots were fired, but there was still no Shannon. Camp was pitched and the group waited for Shannon to reappear. He didn't show up until August 9, but the time had to be used to dry out the provisions as well as rest the Corps. Along with everything else that was going wrong, on the 6th a canoe had capsized and everything, including the medicine, was wet.

Setting out as usual at sunrise on August 6, Clark's party had been slowly making their way up the rapid Big Hole River, alternately traveling through wooded streamsides and rather brushy plains. They had stopped for breakfast at 8 A.M. Drouillard found them and explained that they had taken the wrong river fork and would have to descend and move up a different fork. As the canoes started bobbing and floating downstream at the whim of the rapid current, near-disaster struck. Private Whitehouse's canoe was upset, and he jumped from his seat in the stern into shallow water hoping to avoid having the boat capsize. The current then caught the craft and quickly turned it, hitting Whitehouse's leg and then trapping it under the hull, pinned to the river bottom. The force on the leg was powerful, and by Whitehouse's report, "was near breaking my leg."[7] His shot pouch, powder, and moccasins were all lost to the stream as the canoe passed over him, pressing him forcefully into the riverbed. Fortunately, the water was deep enough to displace some of the canoe's remarkable weight. As Lewis noted, "had the water been two inches shallower [the canoe] must inevitably have crushed him to death." Whitehouse luckily escaped with some bruises, an unplanned bath, and a harrowing story.

Some great news had come by way of Sacagawea, who recognized the large Beaverhead Rock as being in the vicinity of her tribe's summer home. With the men's food supplies running thin, sickness and injuries occurring with increased frequency, and the brutally hot summer days taking their toll, Sacagawea's news probably provided a much needed boost of morale.

Lewis took off the following morning with Shields, Drouillard, and McNeal. They hiked up the Beaverhead to its beginning, then up its tributary, Horse Prairie Creek, for nearly fifty-five more miles. On the afternoon of August 11, they spied a lone Indian horseback rider descending toward them from the mountains. Lewis tried to signal that he desired to talk by throwing a blanket in the air and allowing it to float to the ground. The rider seemed unimpressed and kept his distance, staring at Lewis and McNeal, while Shields and Drouillard, seemingly oblivious to Lewis's actions, continued to walk towards the Indian. Lewis took out a mirror, some beads and other trinkets, but the Indian still kept his distance. Leaving his rifle with McNeal, Lewis walked toward the mounted Indian. Reaching to within a hundred yards, Lewis stopped and shouted repeatedly the Shoshone word that he thought meant "white man." Apparently having seen quite enough, the young Indian reeled his horse and galloped away. Lewis was furious. Along with the Indian went the Corps' immediate hopes of obtaining horses. Lewis wrote "I now felt quite as much mortification and disappointment as I had pleasure and expectation at the first sight of this indian." Blaming especially Shields for the failure to make contact, Lewis "could not forbare abraiding them a little for their want of attention and imprudence on this occasin."

Continuing upstream on August 12, the Lewis advance party reached Horse Prairie Creek's headwaters, one of the ultimate sources of the Missouri. Lewis wrote that "McNeal had exultingly stood with a foot on each side of this little rivulet and thanked his god that he had lived to bestride the mighty & heretofore deemed endless Missouri." They ascended to the Continental Divide and peered to the west, the land of the Columbia River. Every drop of rain water and every snowflake that fell on this area they now surveyed ran to the Pacific. Their satisfaction must have been great to have finally reached the very source of the great river that they had fought for more than 2,500 miles. But their elation at the ridge on the present day Montana-Idaho border was tempered with the fact that they weren't looking at an easy river ride to the Pacific. They were looking at more ranges of snow-capped peaks.

If the Lewis party was satisfied with their accomplishment, Clark's party on the 12th was discouraged and exhausted. They had had enough of towing the canoes and of wading in the shallow river, and wanted to pack up their gear and hike ahead. Rather than coming down with stern orders, Clark showed his great ability as a leader and wrote simply, "I passify them."

Paydirt was struck on August 13, 1805. Lewis and his group of three had continued down the first miles of the western slope of the Rockies, and within hours happened upon two Shoshone women, a man, and some dogs. Again Lewis tried to approach with friendly gestures, but the Indians ran off. Lewis continued another mile down the dry and steep mountainside, and surprised three females. One ran, but an elderly woman and a young girl froze in submission. Lewis laid down his rifle and approached them. The pair "appeared much allarmed but saw that we were to near for them to escape by flight they therefore seated themselves on the ground, holding down their heads as if reconciled to die which they expected no doubt would be their fate." Lewis took the elderly woman's hand and pulled her to her feet, repeating the "white man" term, and showing her the untanned portion of his arm. The women's fear vanished when Lewis presented them with moccasin awls, pewter mirrors, and colored beads. Using Drouillard and his sign language as his interpreter, Lewis convinced the old lady to call back the young woman, who returned. Lewis in turn painted the women's faces with some vermillion, "which with this nation is emblematic of peace." Drouillard signed Lewis's request that the group take them to the main body of Shoshones. The women graciously started the little parade back to their village.

Tensions accelerated two miles down the road, when about sixty warriors "mounted on excellent horses" came galloping up and stopped a short distance away. Lewis again dropped his rifle and unfurled the American flag, and walked toward the small army of Shoshone warriors. He stopped. The chief and two other men slowly stepped out from the main band and spoke with the women. The Indian women "informed them who we were and exultingly shewed the presents which had been given them." With obvious pleasure and to Lewis's great relief, the chief and his men "advanced and embraced me very affectionately in their way which is by puting their left arm over you wright sholder clasping your back, while they apply their left cheek to yours and frequently vociforate the word 'ah-hi-e, ah-hi-e', that is, I am much pleased, I am much rejoiced. bothe parties now advanced and we wer all carresed and besmeared with their grease and paint till I was heartily tired of the national hug." Taking off their moccasins as a sign of sincerity, the Indians sat in a circle. Tobacco was smoked, and friendships and diplomatic relations were put on their first tenuous footings. The main chief, a man named Cameahwait, conducted the group back to the Shoshone village several miles away. Sitting on green boughs of pine branches and antelope skins, Lewis tried to communicate, through Drouillard's hand signs, the purpose of their trip. The Shoshones' only food was some dried berry cakes, but they generously shared what little they had with the famished party of white men.

The next day, Cameahwait drew in the dirt, showing the Lemhi River branching nearby and flowing into another river that was ten miles below, near present-day Salmon, Idaho. Cameahwait signed that the river was treacherous and flowed through mountains inaccessible to either man or horse. Cameahwait further told Lewis that the Nez Perce Indians, who lived a twenty-day march farther west, had told him that the river flowed toward "the seting sun and finally lost itself in a great lake of water which was illy taisted, and where the white men lived." He was describing the Pacific Ocean.

Lewis and his men camped with the Shoshones, admiring their herd of about four hundred horses and eating salmon provided by the chief. The presence of salmon "convinced me that we were on the waters of the Pacific Ocean," Lewis wrote.

Cameahwait described to Lewis a possible route toward the "stinking lake," or Pacific Ocean, that involved several weeks of travel through hot and arid lands to the southwest. Lewis expressed his desire to go another way if possible. The chief described a more northerly route, one with a treacherous and rocky path through mountains that had no game and were so covered with timber that the Nez Perce "could scarcely pass." Hearing this, Lewis wrote "my rout was instantly settled in my own mind," adding that "if the Indians could pass these mountains with their women and Children, that we could also pass them…"

Lewis now asked the Shoshones to accompany him back to the forks of the Beaverhead River, where, he told them "another Chief and a large party of whitemen" waited. Lewis solicited the help of the Indians and their horses in transporting the Corps' baggage across the Continental Divide. Then, he said, the Corps would trade with them for horses. Cameahwait agreed and gave "a lengthey harrangue to his village." After several delays that apparently arose from the Shoshones' fear that these white men might be leading them to a Blackfeet ambush, on the 15th of August about twenty tribe members began the return trip with Lewis, McNeal, Drouillard, and Shields.

A rather amazing event transpired during that trip to meet Clark. Drouillard had been sent ahead to hunt and had killed a deer. An Indian brought back word of the kill and the race was on. All the famished Shoshones raced to the site, finding that Drouillard had already gutted the animal. They descended on the gut pile, "dismounted and ran in tumbling over each other like a parcel of famished dogs each seizing and tearing away a part of the intestens which had been previously thrown out by Drewyer…" Some gobbled up the raw liver and spleen, leaving blood flowing out the corners of their mouths. One man took about nine feet of the small intestine and chewed on one end while he squeezed the contents out of the other end with his hands! The people even ate the "soft parts of the hoofs." The possibilities they had of ingesting numerous parasites in the raw muscle and organ meats are obvious.

Lewis noted, "I really did not untill now think that human nature ever presented itself in a shape so nearly allyed to the brute creation. I viewed these poor starved divils with pity and compassion." Lewis kept a hindquarter for himself and his men and gave the balance to Cameahwait and his people. Stephen Ambrose's astute reflection on this situation in *Undaunted Courage* is worthy of note: "However heartfelt, his pity and compassion did not extend far enough for him to note that, if the Indians appeared savage with the blood running down their cheeks, they had taken only the parts of the deer Drouillard had thrown away when he dressed the kill. They had not touched the meat."[8]

Lewis and the Shoshones made contact with the Clark party on the morning of August 17. Advance scouting parties of Shoshones reported the presence of the white men coming up the Beaverhead. Both Lewis and Cameahwait were relieved and joyous. Members of the Clark party, including Sacagawea and Charbonneau walking ahead, came to greet the natives. Captain Clark saw that Sacagawea "danced for the joyful Sight, and She made signs to me that they were her nation," whose clothing she recognized. The two groups met and a joyful reunion was underway. Sacagawea recognized a Shoshone girl taken captive with her four years earlier, who had escaped and returned to her own people. The old friends had an emotional reunion.

But the emotional fireworks weren't over yet. As the captains started negotiations with Cameahwait for horses, Sacagawea was called to be a link in the chain of interpretation that went from English to French to Hidatsa to Shoshone and back to English. According to the Biddle edition of the journals, Sacagawea came and "sat down, and was beginning to interpret, when in the person of Cameahwait she recognised her brother; she instantly jumped up, and ran and embraced him, throwing over him her blanket and weeping profusely; the chief was himself moved, though not in the same degree."[9] In his daily entry, Lewis simply said that "the meeting of those people was really affecting, particularly between Sah cah-gar-we-ah and an Indian woman."

Presents of paint, moccasins, awls, knives, beads, and mirrors went to the Indians. In addition, the explorers provided the Shoshones with a culinary novelty with a delicious taste—corn from the Mandans. Cameahwait sampled some squash from Mandan gardens and pronounced it the best tasting food, except for some sugar his sister had shared, that he had ever eaten. York made his usual big hit with the Indians, and everything about the band of white men and their supplies fascinated the Indians. Seaman and his friendly intelligence captivated the Shoshones, and a shot from the airgun astonished them.

But it was now into the waning days of August and time was of the essence. The Corps would make a quick reconnaissance of the immediate rivers and determine if there was any hope of floating down the western slope. If a water route proved possible, valuable time and energy could be saved. If a water route didn't pan out, it would mean a trip over the mountain range. The Corps needed to get out of the high mountains as soon as they could, as horses and men in moccasins don't move any too fast over steep, rocky, and soon to be snowy, mountain passes.

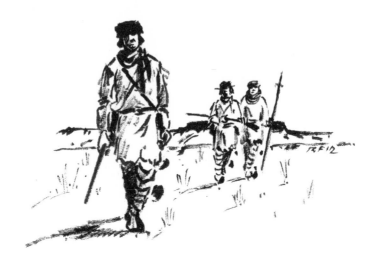

⚞ 13 ⚟

NO PLACE FOR MOCKERSINS

Over the Bitterroots

Let us determine to die here, and we will conquer.
—Barnard Elliot Bee, during the Civil War

Captain William Clark looked disappointedly from atop his horse at the raging and foaming torrent that splashed and roared its way through the canyon of dramatically steep cliffs that shot skyward from the rock-strewn trail on the present-day Salmon River in Idaho. The Shoshones had been right that the river was well beyond any reasonable thought of serving as an exit from the mountains. The maelstrom would not allow an empty canoe to traverse its rapids intact, let alone a loaded one. The banks of the torrent were only dry versions of the river, nearly impassible—large and rugged rocks that made a shoreline portage equally impractical. There would be no easy descent of the western slope of the Rockies and no easy float down to the Pacific.

Thomas Jefferson had hoped for an all-water route to the western ocean, and the captains had hoped for an easy path. Both had proved to be pipe dreams. It was August 23, 1805.

Clark, the Shoshone guide he called Old Toby, and the few men of his advance party began their trek back toward Lewis and the main camp with the unpleasant news. Because Lewis was negotiating for horses at that very time, Captain Clark scribbled a note about the Salmon, gave it to John Colter, and told him to head quickly back over the divide and deliver the news to Captain Lewis. The note described the raging nature of the river and discussed three options for proceeding across the mountains. He also suggested that Lewis buy horses, one for each man if possible. Clark would hire Old Toby and the Corps could either traverse the mountains together, or divide up with one contingent going by the Salmon River with the cargo, and the other crossing the mountains and hunting for their own food. The third option was to return to the Missouri River via a newly learned short-cut, collect provisions from the caches at the Great Falls, and proceed west up present-day Sun River. The Shoshones had told them about this overland route, and noted that they could reach the Great Falls from here in only four days that way.

Clark made camp and, nursing a badly bruised leg he suffered from a fall, ate some chokecherries and hawthorn berries (*Crataegus columbiana*) that made him sick. As we have seen, the seeds of chokecherries are potentially poisonous. I doubt that Clark ate the seeds, but the meat can be very bitter if not fully ripe. Boiling them made them somewhat more palatable. Hawthorn, a member of the Rose family of plants, may contain some chemicals that induce hypotension (lowered blood pressure)[1] that could have combined with the chokecherries to produce Clark's sickness. In addition to his painful leg and sick stomach, Clark endured a night of exposure with heavy dew and wet bedding, the result of his close encounter on horseback with the raging Salmon River.

Thirty-five air miles to Clark's southeast, Captain Meriwether Lewis was busy obtaining horses and a mule to use as pack animals to transport their baggage over the Continental Divide. The Shoshones initially expressed muted interest in trading for horses, but when

Lewis pulled out the beautiful battle-axes that the blacksmiths had made the previous winter at Fort Mandan, their interest showed an obvious upturn. A horse was obtained in trade for the combination of a battle-ax, handkerchief, knife, and some paint. A highly regarded mule traded at nearly twice the price, with an additional knife, handkerchief and pair of leggings thrown in. Lewis provided Charbonneau with some items to trade to ensure that Sacagawea had her own horse. The horses were packed and the twenty-some-mile ascent to the Divide was underway.

No sooner was the main contingent underway, than a Shoshone rode up to Lewis and informed him that one of his men was sick farther back. Lewis ordered the group to halt and, taking along some medicine, he rode two miles back down Horse Prairie Creek to find Private Peter Weiser sick "with a fit of the cholic." Sending Ordway, who had been attending Weiser, to the river for water, Dr. Lewis administered some peppermint and laudanum. Within thirty minutes Weiser felt well enough to climb on board Lewis's horse. Lewis walked back keeping an eye on his patient, and in a short time the men rejoined the rest of the party.

Peppermint oils such as those used on Private Weiser are obtained from the leaves of plants belonging to the genus *Mentha*. Peppermint contains 30 to 50 percent menthol and between 15 and 32 percent of the ketone menthone. These carbon compounds have been used for years as carminatives, or drugs that produce a feeling of comfort in the stomach and relieve the formation of gas in the intestines.[2] Our old friend laudanum, the tincture of opium, would sedate, relieve pain, and slow the actions of Weiser's gut. Weiser's specific problem with his GI tract is unknown, but could have been anything from food poisoning, to any of the ingested parasitic infections that we have already discussed. Abdominal pain, or "cholic" as Lewis saw it, has an extensive list of possible causes. Apparently Weiser recovered well, so it was probably one of the more benign etiologies.

The emergency took up much of the daylight, and the Corps made only six miles in their progress toward the summit, which was still about fifteen miles up the gradually sloping mountains of southwestern Montana.

At camp that night Lewis learned of some interesting Shoshone cultural attitudes and the method by which the Indians name themselves and establish their leadership in the tribe. Lewis noted that Cameah-wait's name meant "one who never walks." He was also called by another name, meaning "black gun." Let's let Lewis tell us about it:

> these people have many names in the course of their lives, particular-ly if they become distinguished characters. for it seems that every important event by which they happen to distinguish themselves inti-tles them to claim another name which is generally scelected by them-selves and confirmed by the nation. those distinguishing acts are the killing and scalping an enemy, the killing a white bear, leading a party to war who happen to be successfull either in destroying their enemies or robing them of their horses, or individually stealing the horses of an enemy. these are considered acts of equal heroism among them, and that of killing an enemy without scalping him is consid-ered of no importance; in fact the whole honour seems to be founded in the act of scalping, for if a man happens to slay a dozen of his ene-mies in action and others get the scalps or first lay their hand on the dead person the honor is lost to him who killed them and devolves on those who scalp or first touch them.

Bravery was the primary virtue among the Shoshone and other tribes, and tribal chiefs were selected based on their feats of bravery in battle. If the tribes were at peace, as Lewis and Clark continually encouraged, this raised an interesting sociological question. Lewis recalled that a Mandan warrior had had the following question the previous winter, after the captain had finished talking up the delights of living at peace with other tribes:

> a young fellow under the full impression of the Idea I have just sug-gested asked me if they were in a state of peace with all their neigh-bours what the nation would do for Cheifs? taking as granted that there could be no other mode devised for making Cheifs but that which custom had established through the medium of warlike acievements.

On August 26, Lewis crossed westward over the Divide (for the second time) and started heading north toward the Shoshone camp, down the steep hillsides toward the valley below. Lewis noted,

> one of the women who had been assisting in the transportation of the baggage halted at a little run about a mile behind us, and sent on the two pack horses which she had been conducting by one of her female friends. I enquired of Cameahwait the cause of her detention, and was informed by him in an unconcerned manner that she had halted to bring fourth a child and would soon overtake us; in about an hour the woman arrived with her newborn babe and passed us on her way to the camp apparently as well as she ever was.

Lewis then noted the apparent ease with which most Indian women gave birth. He noted that some believed it was due to their practice of carrying heavy packs on their backs during pregnancy. But Lewis believed that it was a "gift of nature," noting that the Shoshones' horses had eased the burdens of these women compared to those of other tribes. Lewis also noted the idea that had been expressed to him that Indian women who have become pregnant from white men had more difficult deliveries. He thought that folklore supported his "gift of nature" theory.

John Colter and the Lewis party made contact at 6 P.M. at the main Shoshone campsite near present-day Tendoy, Idaho. Colter presented Lewis with Clark's note, and Lewis immediately began negotiating with Cameahwait for more horses. Cameahwait told Lewis that he was certain that Old Toby knew the way across the mountains better than any other Shoshone, and that he would guide the Corps across to the west. At least that issue was settled. They would soon be underway and with any luck the passage wouldn't prove to be too demanding. They would even have a guide. Lewis wrote,

> matters being thus far arranged I directed the fiddle to be played and the party danced very merily much to the amusement and gratification of the natives, though I must confess that the state of my own mind at this moment did not well accord with the prevailing mirth as I somewhat feared that the caprice of the indians might suddenly induce them to withhold their horses from us without which my hopes

of prosicuting my voyage to advantage was lost; however I determined
to keep the indians in a good humour if possible, and to loose no time
in obtaining the necessary number of horses.

Clark and his scouting party, in the meantime, were limping back toward the Shoshone camp. Game was incredibly scarce, but Clark did note wild hares, "numerous black grasshoppers," and "ground lizards." Clark enjoyed "not one mouthfull to eate untill night as our hunters could kill nothing and I could See & catch no fish except a few Small ones." The Indians he stayed with supplied them with two salmon, and one of the hunters used a novel approach and shot a salmon in the river. Clark noted the generosity of the Shoshones, stating, "...I believe if they had a Sufficency to eate themselves and any to Spare they would be liberal of it."

Awakening the following morning with frost covering their bedrolls, Clark again sent out the hunters. He noted the difference in attitudes toward the current hardships between his men and the Indians.

Those Pore people are here depending on what fish They Can Catch,
without anything else to depend on; and appere Contented, my party
hourly Complaining of their retched Situation and [contemplating?]
doubts of Starveing in a Countrey where no game of any kind except
a fiew fish can be found...

It would seem that all of the physical and mental stress on the Corps of the past few weeks had started to mature into open dissatisfaction and impatience about getting over the mountains—attitudes we did not observe even during the cruel labors of ascending the Missouri or portaging the canoes over the sun-baked plains around the Great Falls. After being given two salmon and purchasing two more, Clark traded three small fishhooks for some salmon eggs to add to their diet. He noted that the salmon were tasty, but that his strength and weight had begun to wither. The hunters came back to camp; once again, they were empty handed.

Clark reached the Shoshone village and a reunion with Captain Lewis on August 29. The captains tried to obtain enough horses to carry their baggage and some extra mounts that the men could take

No Place for Mockersins

turns riding. But the Shoshones, probably sensing that they had a captive market, started to raise their prices. Negotiations centered around assurances from the captains that it was to the Shoshones' advantage to help them cross the mountains, so that the Corps could accompany them on next year's return trip to the plains for buffalo hunting.

Every morning there was now a hard frost, a gentle reminder of the onset of autumn in the mountains. The Corps would pay what they needed to pay. Clark paid dearly for one horse with his pistol, one hundred lead balls, gunpowder, and a knife. Another man traded away one of his rifles in exchange for a horse to ride. Crude packsaddles were put together with boards from provision boxes, and the baggage was lashed onto the horses. Old Toby, his three sons, and the Corps of Discovery with their new herd of twenty-nine horses—with "sore backs," and unaccustomed to packing cargo—departed north along the Lemhi River at 2 P.M. on the afternoon of August 30. As the Corps headed north, the rest of the Shoshone tribe left for the east, the plains and the buffalo.

As the men progressed northward they soon found themselves in treacherous country. Private Joseph Whitehouse noted on September 1 that they had "proceeded on over verry high mountains which was verry bad for our horses to climb up and down…" and "in the afternoon we descended a Mountain nearly as Steep as the roof of a house."[3] Patrick Gass recorded that York's feet became so sore that he was put on horseback.[4]

Whitehouse and John Ordway both recorded that the plentiful "Servis berrys…are verry Sweet and good at this time."[5] The hunters finally met with some success and killed a deer, but only wounded two bears. In the showers and intermittent hail, the men gathered and boiled some chokecherries which, according to Ordway, "eat verry well…"[6] On September 2, Clark wrote that they

> proceeded…without a roade proceded on thro' thickets in which we were obliged to Cut a road, over rockey hill Sides where our horses were in…danger of Slipping to Ther certain distruction & up & Down Steep hills, where Several horses fell, Some turned over, and others Sliped down Steep hill Sides…

They barely made five miles for the day. That day and the next, the group struggled over the rocky and treacherous, snow-covered mountainsides of Lost Trail Pass and back into present-day Montana. The morning of the 4th, the men awoke to snow covering the ground and moccasins that had frozen stiff. They thawed out around a fire and descended the mountainside into the beautiful Bitterroot Valley.

In the afternoon, the Corps encountered another friendly Indian tribe, the Salish. They spoke what Ordway described as "the most curious language of any we have Seen before. They talk as though they lisped or have a bur on their tongue."[7] The camp was in sight of four hundred to five hundred horses grazing on the valley floor. Whitehouse noted that "These Indians received us as friends, & appeared to be glad to see us," adding that they were a "well made, handsome, light coloured sett of people, the most part of them were well cloathed"[8] with robes of mountain sheep and other animal skins. The next day, Whitehouse concluded that "they are the likelyest and honestst Savages we have ever yet Seen."[9] While the Salish were friendly, their dogs were pests, and so hungry that at night they stole and ate several of the Corps' moccasins.

The following day, the captains "informed them who we were, where we Came from, where bound and for what purpose &c. &c.," as Clark recorded, and started negotiating for some of their "ellegant horses." This parley went through five languages. A Shoshone boy who lived with the Salish spoke with Sacagawea in Shoshone, which was in turn translated into Hidatsa, French, and finally English. The captains obtained eleven new horses and exchanged seven of the "sore backed" Shoshone horses for a "fiew articles of merchendize." They now had forty good packhorses and three colts that were bought as candidates for meals should provisions run short. The Salish were on their way eastward, to the Missouri River country to hunt buffalo with their allies, the Shoshone, and the Corps was on their way to the west and their rendezvous with the Bitterroot Mountains. The visit was short, and on September 6, the Corps continued north on the valley floor. To their left was a preview of coming attractions, the spectacular 9,000-foot, snow-covered rocky peaks of the Bitterroot range of the Rocky Mountains.

These mountains certainly didn't look anything like the Appalachi-

No Place for Mockersins

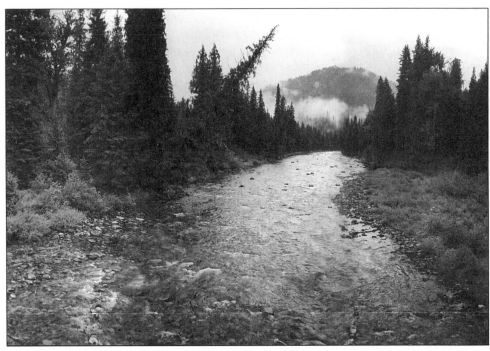

Colt Killed Creek, Lolo Trail. DAVID J. PECK

ans that many of the men had grown up around. Their spectacular rocky and well cut peaks shot into the sky from the flat valley floor. They seemed to rise quickly and forever. The thought of crossing them likely provided a constant stream of apprehension and dread in the weary, hungry, and cold men of the Corps. Clark wrote on September 8, "we are all Cold and wet." Whitehouse said that the peaks were covered with pitch pine and that the tops "are covered with Snow & the snow appears to lay thick in many places."[10] The game situation was again meager. When a hunter had killed two deer on the day before, according to Patrick Gass it was cause "of much joy and congratulation."[11] Venison was augmented with a few ducks and geese, and numerous wild berries making their last stand of the season.

On September 9, the Corps came to rest at a wide plain, near a creek that flowed out of the mountains to the west. They pitched camp and sent out the hunters in a last attempt to bolster the provisions for the upcoming crossing. Latitude and longitude readings were taken. Old Toby now pointed out the passage of four days across the mountains that would land the men about thirty miles above the "gates of the rocky mountain." I wonder if any of the men longed to be heading east, instead of up and over those huge and snowy mountains to the west. They sat in camp, made moccasins, and pondered the inevitable trip up that deceptively mellow canyon. The captains named their oasis "Travelers' Rest."

George Drouillard, John Colter and two of the other "best hunters," sent up to scout for game, returned with a report that "no game is to be found on our rout for a long ways," which likely brought groans from the men. At 3 P.M. on September 11, in a very warm sun, the Corps began its ascent of the Rocky Mountains. They covered seven relatively easy miles.

On September 12, their road took them through heavily timbered country for nine miles. Their path continued over numerous creeks and dead fallen timber that repeatedly retarded their progress. They continued upward, and finally made camp by a creek on a hillside in what Gass described as "a very inconvenient place,"[12] twenty-three miles from their last camp. The Indians peeled bark from the ponderosa pines and chewed it. The mountains had begun to take their weary toll. Clark wrote, "Party and horses much fatigued." The hunters killed only one grouse.

The next morning Lewis discovered that his horse and another had disappeared; he and four men stayed behind to find the animals. Two miles up the canyon, the main party reached a natural hot springs (present-day Lolo Hot Springs), and Old Toby got sidetracked and took a wrong path that led Clark and the men three miles over an "intolerable rout." Once the error was realized and the route corrected, another five miles was put under foot before the Corps stopped on a mountainside to let the horses graze and wait for Captain Lewis. Upon his arrival, the Corps continued down Pack Creek and camped, making seventeen very difficult miles for the day.

On September 14, the going got rougher. Several steep mountains had to be traversed, with snow falling near the peaks. In the valleys, rain and hail fell—making, in Gass's account, for "disagreeable travelling." The hunters took only two or three grouse and, as Gass noted, "without a miracle it was impossible to feed 30 hungry men and

No Place for Mockersins

upwards, besides some Indians."[13] Lewis broke out the portable soup, a nearly unanimously unpopular dish among the men. One of the colts was sacrificed to the Corps' hunger. In honor of the colt, the men named their campsite "Colt Killed Creek."

The morning of September 15, the men ate horsemeat for breakfast. Once again on their way, they descended the Clearwater River for three miles, at which point they struck up a steep mountainside, following a trail Clark described as "winding in every direction" through immense stands of dead timber. Several horses tumbled down the steep cliffs, with one requiring the aid of eight men to right it. The horse carrying Captain Clark's lap desk fell forty yards down a cliff, breaking the desk to pieces but amazingly escaping injury.

In every direction, as far as the eye could see there were more snowy mountains.

The Corps ascended to the top of a peak, and finding the hour somewhat late, camped near a three-foot-deep snowbank left over from the previous winter. Since there was no running water, the men melted the snow and ice. They huddled around their crackling campfires and eagerly boiled more of their colt meat and made warm soup. As they chewed on their horsemeat and sipped the soup for its warmth, the surrounding skies were cold, cloudy, and rather starkly unfriendly. Probably more than one man wondered, "What have we got ourselves into now?" As we read these passages in our positions of comfort, it is enlightening to consider the degree of discomfort these friends of ours withstood, huddled and shaking around campfires, eating meat and drinking soup that we would find thoroughly disgusting.

If the 15th had been bad, the 16th of September got worse. Shortly after midnight it started to snow, and by morning the campsite and the Corps were under two to four inches of snow. The snow continued falling until 3 o'clock that afternoon, providing an accumulation of six to eight inches, enough to obliterate any evidence of the trail. Gass wrote, "the day was so dark, that a person could not see to a distance of 200 yards."[14] They proceeded onward.

A man utterly used to environmental hardship, Clark wrote, "...I have been wet and as cold in every part as I ever was in my life, indeed I was at one time fearfull my feet would freeze in the thin mockersons which I wore..." His more polished version in the Biddle edition of the

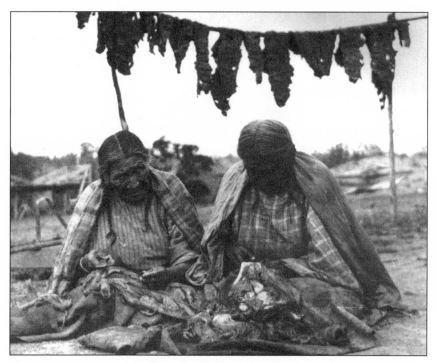

Cheyenne women cutting horse meat for drying. MONTANA HISTORICAL SOCIETY, 955-651

journals notes, "The road was, like that of yesterday, along steep hill sides, obstructed with fallen timber, and a growth of eight different species of pine, so thickly strewed that the snow falls from them as we pass, and keeps us continually wet to the skin, and so cold, that we are anxious lest our feet should be frozen, as we have only thin moccasins to defend them."[15]

Hypothermia and minor frostbite were once again the close companions of the Corps of Discovery. Gass and Ordway noted that men tied rags around their freezing feet in a mostly vain attempt to fend off the cold from their numb extremities.

The miserable crew made camp at dusk, and another colt fell victim to their appetites. Clark noted that "we all Suped hartily on and thought it fine meat." They had conquered fifteen of the toughest miles they would encounter on the entire trip. I think that Patrick Gass summed the situation up well in part of his journal entry of Sep-

No Place for Mockersins

tember 16. He simply recorded that their path that day was through "the most terrible mountains I ever beheld."[16]

In the morning, as the men started preparing to break camp, they discovered that the horses had scattered themselves all over the mountain during the night. Men were sent out to collect the animals, which took until 1 P.M. The wooden packsaddles and baggage were lashed to the ponies, and the rollercoaster ride of up and down the steep mountain slopes began. The walkers' thighs screamed and burned. Some of the slopes were so steep that it made ascending them on horseback impossible. But afternoon found the Corps descending a mountainside, and the weather warming considerably, with bright and clear skies that provided a much-needed shot of encouragement to the dragging crowd. The snow melted in the warm sun and now the moccasined feet were, in places, underwater.

The Corps' bodies were probably in high gear trying to maintain their blood glucose levels for energy. The human body has an amazing ability to regulate the level of energy by providing blood glucose to keep it within a range that will allow an individual to continue to live and function, but the men and woman had by now been in the early stages of starvation for a couple of weeks. The difficult passage through the mountains from the Shoshone camps over a hundred miles away, accompanied by the lean diet of the previous several weeks, had depleted their already very low fat stores. The exhausting passage over the Bitterroots probably used whatever glucose their bodies had stored in their livers and muscles in the form of glycogen. Under well-fed conditions, the liver has only enough glycogen to maintain normal blood sugar levels for twelve to twenty-four hours. As dietary intake dwindles, and glycogen and fat stores are depleted, an interesting physiological phenomenon occurs. The process is under the control of several inter-related hormones including insulin, epinephrine, glucagon, and growth hormone.

For energy sources, the central nervous system (brain and spinal cord) can use only glucose or molecules called ketones that are by-products of fat breakdown. Other bodily cells, such as muscle cells, can utilize molecules called fatty acids that are also obtained from fat breakdown. Once the stored glycogen is depleted in the liver and muscles, the liver is able to take other non-glucose molecules, chemically rearrange them and make more glucose, thereby supplying our cells with energy. Glycerol, another molecule obtained from the breakdown of fat, can be rearranged in the cells of the liver to produce glucose. Amino acids obtained from the breakdown of muscle proteins are the chief source of glucose production in the liver of a starving person. Of course, with muscle breakdown comes muscle wasting and progressive weakness. If starvation continues, the body can also call on the kidneys to produce more glucose from the amino acid glutamine. Unfortunately for the starving person, Paul is robbed in order to pay Peter, and the muscle mass that provides strength for activities like hiking through the Bitterroots begins to decrease, and the victim gets weaker and weaker. By my figuring, the men were starting down the road to starvation and only the relative brevity of their time in the mountains kept them from getting into serious trouble. Their caloric needs must have been remarkable. If it hadn't been for the colts eaten, they would have been in much worse shape than they were.

The best insurance the men had against starvation, the flintlocks, also began to fail them on that same afternoon of September 16. Spying four mule deer coming up the hillside, Clark lay in wait for them. When the deer grazed to within range, Clark got one in his sights and pulled the trigger. "Snap." The gun didn't fire. He once again pulled the cock (hammer) back until it clicked and again pulled the trigger. "Snap," and again, no discharge. He cocked the rifle and pulled the trigger seven times, each time without the rifle firing. His rifle had never misfired in this fashion before and now, when they needed the meat the most, it failed. The piece of flint secured in the cock had come loose, and when the cock fired, the flint did not contact the frizzen to produce a spark that would have allowed the gun to discharge. The deer that would have been dinner bounded untouched into the forest. A second colt was sacrificed that night for dinner.

The 17th of September found the Corps awakening to a cold and cloudy morning. Again, the horses were grazing, scattered all over the mountain. Bringing them all together required several hours of work and energy expenditure. By 1 P.M., in falling snow, the Corps resumed its trek through the forest, frequently hit by packs of snow falling from the pine boughs above. Sacagawea held bundled-up Pompey close to her body to keep the baby warm. They passed over several peaks that Clark described

No Place for Mockersins

as "high ruged Knobs," on an "excessively bad" trail. Snow enveloped the peaks, but the valleys were clear. A few grouse were harvested, but the scrawny birds could hardly provide meat for the crew. Clark added, "a coalt being the most useless part of our Stock he fell a Prey to our appetites." Their total distance for the day was only twelve miles.

The 18th saw a change in plans. The captains noted a distinct attitude of discouragement overtaking the party. Freezing temperatures at night, snow and wetness during the day, little food, and fatigue were all conspiring to defeat the expedition. Rather than all proceeding together for a yet unknown distance, Captain Clark set out ahead along with Drouillard, John Shields, Reubin Field, and three other hunters to attempt to get out of the mountains and obtain some food for the rest. They would hunt and leave meat for the main party. Captain Lewis planned to awaken his contingent early and "determined to force my march as much as the abilities of our horses would permit." They climbed out of their meager bedding in the morning and ate some left-over colt. Willard's horse got lost and delayed the group's departure until 8:30 A.M. Finally, Willard was left to find the horse and catch up. Water was scarce, with only one creek passed during their eighteen-mile hike. Lunch was some of the hated portable soup. By 4 P.M., they encamped on a steep mountain when Willard wandered in, still without his horse. Dinner that night was definitely not from Chez Louis—they mixed portable soup with a combination of some bear oil and twenty pounds of melted candles, probably made of lard.

Meanwhile, the Clark party forged ahead. After twenty more miles of rough passage through the mountains, Clark stood atop a high peak (present-day Sherman Peak, northwest of Grangeville, Idaho[17]) and gazed off in the distance, at a sight that surely lifted his spirits. "I had a view of an emence Plain and leavel Countery to the S W. & West at a great distance." There was finally some hard evidence that this marathon of physical challenge would indeed have an ending. But in between them and the plain were more fallen timber and hardship. They hiked thirty-two miles that day.

They encamped for the night by a beautiful mountain creek. The fullness of the site's beauty was in sharp contrast to the emptiness of their stomachs. They had absolutely nothing to eat that night, though, and named their campsite "Hungery Creek."

On September 19, Lewis and his men set out shortly after sunrise and continued traversing a mountain ridge for about six miles. They witnessed the same sight that had met Clark's eyes the day before, "...when the ridge terminated and we to our inexpressable joy discovered a large tract of Prairie country lying to the S. W. and widening as it apeared to extend to the W. through that plain the Indian informed us that the Columbia river, in which we were in surch run. This plain appeared to be about 60 miles distant, but our guide assured us that we should reach it's borders tomorrow. The appearance of this country, our only hope for subsistance greately revived the sperits of the party already reduced and much weakened for the want of food."

Once again the men were hurting, both physiologically with depletion of their energy stores and thus their physical stamina, as well as psychologically with the effects of their prolonged physical hardships. I believe that this particular day, prior to viewing that distant plain, may have been the toughest one of the entire expedition. They had been on a subsistance diet for weeks while physical exertion was high. The environmental stress was profound on people who had totally inadequate clothing for the snow and cold. The psychological effects of being in an unknown land, on the outbound portion of their journey, with an approaching winter that would force them into an as yet unknown home for several months, were a constant source of stress. There was no possibility of a return trip to their homes and families for the year of 1805. Their collective endurance and commitment was the cohesive force that provided the will and energy to keep putting one foot in front of the other along that Bitterroot ridge. What a boost to their morale this distant plain must have been!

Lewis and the main party continued through another six miles of up and down mountaineering through dead and fallen timber, and reached Hungery Creek, which they followed for another six miles. The trail was hair-raising, to say the least. Lewis wrote, "the road excessively dangerous along this creek being a narrow rockey path generally on the side of steep precipice, from which in many places if ether man or horse were precipitated they would inevitably be dashed in pieces. Frazer's horse fell from this road in the evening, and roled with his load near a hundred yards into the Creek. We all expected that the horse was killed but to our astonishment when the load was taken off him he arose to his feet & appeared to be but little injured, in 20 minutes he proceeded with his load. This was the most wonderfull escape I ever witnessed, the hill down which he roled was almost perpendicular and broken by large irregular and broken rocks." The leftover colt was now gone and the men partook of some portable soup and lay down on the ground and slept.

Lewis also noted that "several of the men are unwell of the disentary," adding that skin problems of "brakings out or irruptions of the Skin" were adding to their mountain nightmares.

Some of the gastrointestinal problems may have been related to eating portable soup. The soup had been made for the expedition in Philadelphia and was probably a paste-like substance produced from boiling and dehydrating boiled meat products. The pasty substance was to be rehydrated with water, and vegetables could be mixed in.[18] It was something to eat when you were starving. Since they had opened the lead canisters that the soup had been stored in, it is entirely possible that the soup mixture had become wet during the past weeks, and thus made a comfortable medium of bacterial growth. This could have produced the diarrhea noted in the journals. Other parasites (*Giardia*) could have been ingested in the mountain water.

The canisters that had held the soup for the past two years was an obvious source of lead ingestion that the Corps didn't want or need. Fortunately, lead poisoning is the result of prolonged ingestion of that heavy metal, and acute lead poisoning does not occur—in contrast to the heavy metal acute poisoning of mercury that we have discussed in regard to the treatment of syphilis. Nevertheless, there is no indication that Lewis knew anything about the less than optimal storage of his portable soup.

On September 19, Clark and his men found a wandering horse and promptly bagged it. After enjoying their breakfast they hung the leftovers in a tree for the trailing main party, who found it the next day. Lewis discovered that the packhorse carrying all his winter clothing was missing, and immediately sent Private Jean Baptiste Lepage, who was supposed to have been watching the horse, back to find it. Lepage returned at 3 P.M. without the horse, and two of the best woodsmen were sent back to find the wandering equine.

While Lewis worried about his winter clothes wandering through the mountains on the back of the lost horse, Clark's advance party finally struggled out of the mountains and down into pine-covered foothills. There they discovered many lodges of the Nez Perce tribe. Soon several Indian boys were encountered, and "ran and hid themselves." Clark dismounted, gave his gun to one of the men, found the boys and gave them pieces of ribbon to take to their nearby village. Soon a grown man appeared and with "great Caution" brought the party into the Nez Perce camp. Women surrounded the party with "much apparent Signs of fear." The Indians fed the men dried salmon, berries, and camas-root bread, of which they ate heartily. By that evening, Clark had started to get sick "from eateing the fish & roots too freely."

Lewis's group was now two days behind. Collecting the horses on the morning of the 21st was a problem, and the trail continued to be nearly impassible, littered with stands of fallen trees through which they plodded for five miles. In the afternoon they passed Clark's campground of the 19th and continued on until they found a grassy area where the horses coud graze. The animals' legs were hobbled to prevent them from wandering too far during the night. An interesting dinner of a "prairie wolf" (coyote), the horse that Clark left, and crayfish from Lolo Creek provided dinner. Lewis wrote, "I find myself growing weak for the want of food and most of the men complain of a similar deficiency and have fallen off very much." Lewis, already anticipating the upcoming river travel, noticed stands of trees that would make "eligant perogues of at least 45 feet in length."

The group's killing and eating a coyote brings up another interesting medical point. The parasitic tapeworm species *Echinococcus*, with its species *granulosa* and *multilocularis*, is present in modern-day western coyotes, foxes, and wolves.[19] These canines pass their infected feces, and herbivorous animals such as mice and other rodents, or deer, moose, etc., eat the plants or drink the water contaminated with the wild canine feces. The herbivores thus become the intermediate hosts to the parasite. The cycle is then completed when the coyote or wolf catches the infected herbivore and consume it.[20]

Disease from the organism *Echinococcus* is caused in humans by ingesting the egg stage of this parasitic worm, from plants or water. The *Echinococcus granulosus* produces lesions predominantly in the liver and lungs, with the species *multilocularis* causing lesions usually in the liver, where they can grow over decades, destroying liver tissue. The infections generally do not cause death, but can produce symptoms in the lung such as cough, coughing up blood (hemoptysis), and chest pain. Liver involvement can produce abdominal pain. The parasites may grow and rupture into the chest or abdominal cavity, causing serious complications in bones, heart, kidneys, gallbladder, brain, and spinal cord. Severe disease is treated in modern times by surgical removal of cysts or with antiparasitic medication.[21]

While Lewis enjoyed his barbecued coyote miles away, Clark was gaining information from the Nez Perce. They drew the captain a diagram of the Columbia and its falls, and told him that white traders came to the falls from downriver and furnished the Indians with beads and cloth.

The hunters sent out returned with nothing. The men's diets now revolved around the Indians' dried salmon, and camas-root bread. Clark obtained a horse-load of camas roots and three salmon, and sent Reubin Field back to meet Captain Lewis and his party.

Camas roots are odorless and tasteless in their raw state. The Nez Perce went through an elaborate method of cooking them in the ground for ten to twelve hours. They were then eaten or dried in the sun, and dried camas could be pounded into dough and recooked. It was pure and wild carbohydrate. The other staple of Nez Perce cuisine was salmon, caught in the spring and fall runs, and then sun-dried for storage.

Arising from their exhausted sleep on September 22, Lewis found to his distress that one of the men had not hobbled his horse and it had wandered off. This man claimed ignorance of the order but nevertheless the mistake delayed their departure until after 11 A.M. After only two and a half miles, the straggling party met Reubin Field and began to gorge themselves on the fish and roots.

With food in their bellies and resting on relatively flat land, Lewis described his feelings of relief: "the pleasure I now felt in having tryumphed over the rocky Mountains and decending one more to a level and fertile country where there was every rational hope of finding a comfortable subsistence for myself and party can be more readily conceived than expressed, nor was the flattering prospect of the final

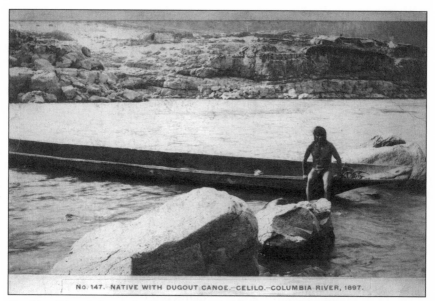

Possibly a Wasco Indian with a high-prowed Columbia River–style dugout canoe.
LIBRARY OF CONGRESS, LC-USZ62-101331

success of the expedition less pleasing." That afternoon the main party wandered into the Nez Perce village. They ate more salmon and camas roots. They would soon regret it.

The next week, from September 23 to October 1, would prove to be a long one indeed. Captain Lewis and all the men started getting very sick with diarrhea and abdominal cramping. Each day's entry by Dr. Clark contains comments about the men's severe complaints of "heaviness at the Stomach" and running of their bowels. Clark noted the severity of the symptoms: "Capt Lewis Scercely able to ride on a jentle horse which was furnished by the Chief, Several men So unwell that they were Compelled to lie on the Side of the road for Some time others obliged to be put on horses."

The men were obviously miserable. They were also probably getting significantly dehydrated. If these men had visited an emergency room in our day, they would have been administered intravenous fluids to rehydrate them, and provided with medication to lessen their probable nausea. But Dr. Clark had a different approach. He used some of Dr. Rush's Bilious Pills. The mercury and jalap in the pills put the already suffering men's bowels into a heightened state of irritation and action. The next day he administered some more cathartic "salts" and some tartar emetic (an antimony-potassium compound used to produce vomiting). Dr. Clark took an already suffering population and made them suffer more. He took already dehydrated patients and made them more dehydrated. Their misery must have been profound! After a couple of days of this therapy, it would be unclear as to whether the men were more sick from their diet or from the medical treatment.

What was going on in the Corps' gastrointestinal tracts could have been from a combination of factors. Drying fish in the sun could have provided a good growth medium for toxin-producing *Staphylococcus* bacteria that would produce food poisoning manifested by the symptoms Clark described. The change to the relatively oily and rich salmon, on which they gorged themselves, could have produced some of the diarrhea. A subsequent expedition into the area in the 1830s suffered similar complaints and also blamed it on the change in diet. It certainly could have been either or both.

Eating sun-dried salmon introduces another problem with potential parasites. The fish tapeworm *Diphyllobothrium latum* is present in salmon and other freshwater fish species. This tapeworm's lifecycle normally alternates between crustaceans (crabs, crayfish, snails) and crustacean-eating salmon. When a salmon eats an infected crustacean, the tapeworm larvae migrate through the fish's intestinal wall and lodge in the muscle, where they continue to develop. After a human ingests raw or poorly cooked infected fish, the tapeworm attaches to the intestinal wall of the human and develops into an adult that can reach lengths of ten meters. A stage of development in this tapeworm, called a plerocercoid, can migrate to various parts of the body, including the muscles and eyes. Many infections can be clinically undetected due to a lack of symptoms, but some infections may produce abdominal pain, nausea, vomiting, weight loss, and vitamin B12 deficiency.[22] A single dose of the appropriate modern medication can wipe out this parasite from the human intestine. (A temperature of 133 F. for five minutes, or freezing at 0 F, for twenty-four hours will kill the worm.)

Other parasitic worm larvae of the ascaroid species inhabit the flesh of seagoing fishes. Since salmon spend part of the life cycle in the ocean, they eat prey containing these parasites (Anasakid nematodes), which in turn infect them. When humans eat improperly cooked fish (such as sun-dried salmon), the larvae burrow into the gastrointestinal walls and can cause severe illness, including peritonitis.[23]

The men slowly recovered from both their gastroenteritis and the treatment they received from Captain Clark. Lewis was sick for more than a week. While some continued to suffer, those healthy enough to pitch in started handcrafting the canoes they would need to float the waterways down to the Pacific. The friendly Nez Perce showed the men their technique of burning the centers from logs, but even with this trick it took ten days to make the five canoes needed. The horses were branded after the Nez Perce agreed to watch over the herd until the Corps returned the following spring.

On October 7, the Corps of Discovery, along with two Nez Perce chiefs who agreed to accompany the men through the Indian villages that dotted the river system below, shoved away from the shoreline of the Clearwater River and started their final descent, and thus the completion of half their transcontinental trip. The men must have been elated, at least those who felt good enough to smile.

Ten dangerous rapids later and twenty-seven miles downstream, the Corps camped. Water had soaked the contents of the captains' canoe, requiring that everything be removed and dried. The surrounding countryside was radically different from the mountains they had just escaped: plain and rolling hills with little or no timber. The Corps had to trade with the Indians for fire fuels.

Old Toby and his son decided not to continue and took off, without being paid, back toward the mountains and its week-long passage. This Indian man, who perhaps more than any single person, had helped so much now quietly and quickly vanished into the mountains, never to be seen again by the Corps.

Except on Captain Clark's trencher, dogs now replaced the salmon as the men's favorite meal. In a practice that will certainly make modern dog owners cringe, dozens of the beasts were purchased from local tribes and became the food that kept the men and woman of the Corps alive.

Clark made an interesting observation on October 17. The Palouse Indians were "subject to Sore eyes, and maney are blind of one and

No Place for Mockersins

Some of both eyes. This misfortune must be owing to the reflections of the Sun &c. on the waters in which they are continually fishing during the Spring Summer & fall, & the Snows dureing the, winter Seasons, in this open countrey where the eye has no rest."

Many tribes along the Columbia and its tributaries suffered from eye problems. Initially causing only irritation of their eye membranes (conjunctiva) and corneas, exposure to the same ultraviolet rays year after year could result in cataracts in the lenses of elderly eyes. This would in turn result in partial or total blindness, without any pain. Acute effects of excessive UV radiation have been discussed in relation to snowblindness, which causes painful burns of the cornea. Low humidity, wind, and high air temperature could contribute to eye irritation and pain.

Diseases including trachoma, which is caused by the bacteria *Chlamydia trachomatis*, were possibly present among the Indians of the area. This infection results in scarring the inside of the eyelid, which in turn causes chronic irritation of the clear cornea as the scarred lid blinks over it thousands of times daily. Chronic irritation and cornea scarring ultimately cause blindness. Although the disease is rare in present-day America, it is endemic in populations with poor hygiene and crowded living conditions, an accurate description of life in an Indian village along the Columbia and its tributaries in 1805.

I believe that it is highly likely that some of the eye infections and problems from which these Indians suffered were also the result of the plerocercoid stage of *Diphyllobothrium*, or other tapeworm plerocercoids, being lodged within their eyes. Regularly handling raw wild meat might have led to oculoglandular tularemia, from the bacterium *Francisella tularensis*. Finally, syphilis could also have a cause of ocular problems that resulted in blindness, as could gonorrhea and other diseases.

For the next two weeks, the Corps steadily made their way down the Snake River and finally reached the mighty Columbia River on October 22. They passed hundreds of Indians from various tribes, gathered for the fall salmon run. These western-slope Native Americans showed marked societal differences from their cousins in the mountains and on the plains. The horses and buffalo of the plains were replaced with canoes and salmon. Instead of mobile teepees, the people lived in wood plank houses. All the villages had large scaffolds covered with drying salmon.

On occasion, the canoes needed to be portaged around dangerous rapids while on other days, rapids that probably should have been avoided were shot with the dugout canoes, sometimes with Indians waiting to see whether the white men crashed in the swirling white-water, or even throwing rocks at them. Although sometimes a canoe overturned, catastrophic accidents were miraculously avoided. The river was spectacular. Often the men could look down into the transparent waters to a depth of twenty feet or more and see the hundreds of salmon below them swimming upstream. The Columbia was immense. It was hundreds of yards wide, carrying the deep, cold, and clear waters that ran to the Pacific from the vast Rockies to the east.

A dramatic and treacherous series of rapids and falls now presented themselves to the Corps in the last week of October. Mighty rapids at the Great Falls of the Columbia (Celilo Falls) were portaged for 457 yards on a "fine morning" of October 23. The canoes were then put back in the river and lowered with strong elkskin ropes through another length of river too treacherous to risk the men's lives. The waters of the river according to Clark's description "Swels and boils with a most Tremendeous manner."

Clark also noted the presence of vast numbers of what he called "flees" inhabiting the area of an Indian camp where fish skins and straw covered the ground. The insects crawled onto the men as they traversed the area and became so vexing that the men stripped naked and tried to brush themselves free of their tiny tormentors. The Corps tried to buy some salmon from the local Indians, but all they were willing to trade to the Corps were "8 Small fat dogs."

On October 24, the two Nez Perce chiefs told the captains that it was now time for them to return to their homes. They could no longer translate the language of Indians along the river and, in addition, they feared for their safety. The area the Corps would now enter was controlled by Chinookan Indians, enemies of the Nez Perce. The chiefs had not only expressed concern for their own safety should they continue with the Corps, but also they had warned the captains the day before that the local Indians planned on killing the party. The Corps was thus put on high alert throughout the night, guarding against any

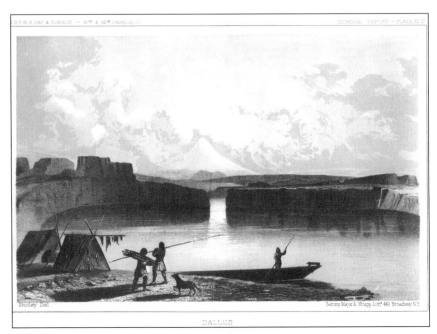

possible attack. Fortunately, nothing became of the rumored threat.

They reached The Dalles on October 24, the Short Narrows of only forty-five yards width, through which all the water of the Columbia was forced, followed by the Long Narrows that was two hundred yards wide. The first fall of this stretch had a drop of twenty feet, "then passing thro' a narrow Chanel for 1 mile to a rapid of about 18 feet below which the water has no poerceptable fall but verry rapid." Clark speculated, after studying the apparent flood plain, that in the spring the high water and its subsequent backup made the level of the river below the nearby falls equal to that at the head. Clark believed that this accounted for salmon being able to pass upstream through the falls. The captains decided to allow the canoes to shoot these rapids, under the leadership of the best sailor in the Corps, Pierre Cruzatte, "notwithstanding the horrid appearance of this agitated gut Swelling, boiling & whorling in every direction..." The guns, journals, and scientific equipment would be portaged around The Dalles, while Cruzatte and some other expert boatmen (and good swimmers) ran the river wild. Apparently the Indians turned out in droves to see this great amusement. Private Whitehouse noted that "Our canoes went with very great rapidity through this place."[24] It would seem that his observation was a little understated.

At the head of the falls lay two Indian villages. The Wishram Indians inhabited the northern shore and the Wascos lived on the southern bank. Here the Corps found a very active center of trade, where thousands of pounds of salmon were drying near a village of twenty large wooden shelters. Numerous tribes came to the area during the fall and traded for food and other items. Indians from the lower river brought goods they had obtained from seafaring white traders on the coast, items such as pots and cloth. Tribes such as the Umatillas, Wishrams, Wanapams, Yakamas, and Walulas came to the great meeting and 19th century trade show every September and October.

While the Corps camped below the falls on the night of October 26, two chiefs and fifteen men from a village came across the river to visit, bringing presents of venison and "Small Cakes of white bread mad of roots." Lewis and Clark in turn presented each chief with a small medal, a red silk handkerchief, arm band, knife, and some paint. The captains' generosity had ulterior motives. Remembering that they would return this way again the coming spring, the captains sought, according to Clark, to "ingratiate our Selves with them, to insure us a kind & friendly reception on our return."

The group gathered around a fire made in honor of the Indians. Cruzatte fiddled, "which pleased those nativs exceedingly," and York danced. Later that evening the hunters returned to camp with five deer, four large grey squirrels and a grouse. One of the guards standing around the river jigged for what Clark called a "Salmon Trout." The captain fried the fish in some bear oil and noted, "I thought one of the most delicious fish I have ever tasted."

The country they were now in was sparsely covered with white oaks and pine. The Indians who inhabited the area practiced the custom of flattening the heads of female children, and some area tribes also flattened the heads of the male babies, both groups limiting the practice to higher classes. This procedure was accomplished by securing boards to provide a nearly constant pressure on the growing skull, forcing it to flatten over a period of months. This produced a sloped

No Place for Mockersins

forehead thought to be a sign of beauty and distinction.[25]

October 31 dawned cloudy and rainy. Clark, Joseph Field, and Cruzatte hiked ahead to inspect the river's upcoming portion. They reached the Cascades of the Columbia, now under Bonneville Dam, the last rapids they faced. To Clark, the "Great Chute" held "great numbers of both large and Small rocks, water passing with great velocity forming & boiling in a most horriable manner." Clark and Field hiked ten miles farther downriver, looking over several vacant Indian villages along the way. At the end of their reconnaissance, they viewed the river running without any rapids, widening westward. An impressive 800-foot-high rock there they named Beacon Rock. On the return hike Clark stopped with several Indian tribes they met and smoked the usual ceremonial pipe.

While visiting with the Indians, Clark witnessed an amazing act. One of his companions had shot a goose that fell into the river and floated into the rapids. An Indian jumped into the river and swam to retrieve the floating goose, 150 feet above the crashing rapids. He returned to shore with his prize. Clark noted, "as this Indian richly earned the goose I Suffered him to keep it…" The man plucked about half of the feathers and, not bothering to gut the fowl, he spitted the bird and began to roast it.

On November 1, the Corps portaged around this last series of rapids. The path was 940 yards "of bad way over rocks & on Slipery hill Sides." Cargo and a small canoe were carried, then the four large canoes lowered over poles "placed across from one rock to another." Three canoes were damaged, but soon repaired.

Clark spotted what he took for sea otters below the falls and attempted to take one with his rifle, but the animal sank into the depths. These "otters" were actually harbor seals that had migrated up the Columbia from the Pacific.

For the first time since they left Fort Mandan, the Corps now entered geography previously described by whites. The lower Columbia had been explored, right after its 1792 discovery, by a British group under the command of George Vancouver, and the captains knew his report. The Cascade Mountains lay within ten miles, directly to the north and south. Mount St. Helens reached its volcanic cone skyward about forty miles to the northwest and Mount Hood lay thirty miles to the southeast. The environment had once again changed dramatically from the dry and barren slopes of eastern Washington and Oregon. Now the surrounding countryside was a dense forest of evergreen trees nourished by rains that blow in from the Gulf of Alaska. The moist and cool air produced frequent fog, at times so thick that the party was forced to wait for it to clear in order to continue their journey to the coast.

Soon the Corps met the Watlala tribe, whose houses—made of split boards covered with bark, with thatch or bark roofs—were nearly fifty feet in length. Their canoes were elegant craft, with painted images of bears and men. The tribe's clothing exhibited a European influence, with many men wearing hats, sailor's jackets, and "overalls." Many men were also armed with excellent weapons obtained from the same European traders. Although the captains and the Corps treated these Indians with "every attention & friendship," they found the Watlalas "assumeing and disagreeable." While the Corps ate dinner, Clark's tomahawk-pipe and a coat were stolen, which prompted the captains' wrath and an impromptu search that finally turned up a capote stuffed under the roots of a nearby tree, but no tomahawk. Sensing their unwelcome status, the visitors left and returned to their village.

The Corps continued down the river that was now a mile and a quarter wide. They paddled for another hour after dark and camped on the northern shore. As the exhausted men lay down to sleep that night of November 4, frustration was added to their already testy state. It had started to rain intermittently. They had camped just opposite of an island inhabited by various species of waterfowl that made such a racket all night that Clark found it impossible to get any sleep at all, describing the birds as "emensely numerous and their noise horrid."

Men who had suffered summer heat and physical exhaustion on their way up the Missouri, endured brutal winter temperatures and frostbite at Fort Mandan, suffered hail storms that left some of them bloody and bruised, who half starved and became significantly hypothermic going over the Bitterroots, now began what Clark described as a period of their greatest testing and physical misery. Winter rains were descending on the Pacific Northwest, and the Corps as yet had established no permanent winter shelter. They were often marooned on small and isolated patches of rocky river shoreline

No Place for Mockersins

with no possibility of moving their location until a break in the weather occurred. They would sit wet, miserable, and cold, with their backs to a forest so thick that it prohibited them from penetrating it for even a short distance to hunt. Their faces were to a stormy and dangerous river estuary, far too dangerous to risk any passage, buffeted by high winds and waves.

But November 7, after traveling thirty-four miles from the previous camp, the view that met their eyes was fantastic indeed. Fantasies of this moment had likely been discussed around campfires and everyone had wondered what the exact moment would prove to be like. The moment of triumph, which for a year and a half had been one of the Corps' key goals, was now nearly a reality. As they paddled down the mighty river, the immense Columbia widened into an estuary several miles across. What was once fresh water below their canoes now tasted salty and smelled of the ocean. Primal joy and excitement reverberated through every man, as well as Sacagawea. Maybe even Pompey, now ten months old, cracked a smile in response to everyone else's happiness. Clark wrote with what can only be described as the utmost satisfaction, "Great joy in camp we are in View of the Ocian, this great Pacific Octean which we have been So long anxious to See. and the roreing or noise made by the waves brakeing on the rockey Shores (as I Suppose) may be heard distictly." What a day that must have been!

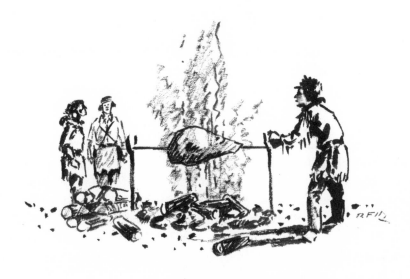

⚶ 14 ⚶

A WINTER OF PORE ELK AND FLEES

The Pacific 1805-1806

He is intrusted with a certain amount of misery
which it is his duty to distribute as fairly as he can.
—Robert Lowe, British Politician

The men and woman must have hoped that the past few weeks would not portend their state of existence for the coming winter, but time would unfortunately prove any pessimism to be fully justified. Although by the second week of December, 1805, Captain Meriwether Lewis had discovered a site on which to build their winter quarters, that was about the only bit of news that was very encouraging. Fleas continued to torment the men at night, crawling on their skin and making a comfortable sleep next to impossible. The rains continued to soak them, and the "great joy" that reverberated through camp on arriving at the Columbia River's estuary had been diminished by a month of brutal rain, wind, difficult hunting, and the anticipation of four months in a relatively warm but very wet forest.

As they had moved down the Columbia, their campsites had been almost continually threatened by the severe weather. Rain and waves crashed and broke on the rocks that served as beds for days in a stretch. The Pacific Ocean coastline, when they saw it, was dramatic with vast beaches dotted with 200-foot-high trees eight feet in diameter. Clark's entry of November 18 noted that the "men appear much Satisfied with their trip beholding with estonishment the high waves dashing against the rocks & this emence ocian." But the beautiful surroundings were veiled by the testy climate, which provided an equal amount of misery.

As they had explored the Columbia's northern shore and lived in constantly wet clothing, Clark had written on November 12 that "It would be distressing to a feeling person to See our Situation at this time all wet and cold with our bedding &c. also wet…robes & leather Clothes are rotten from being Continually wet." Eating dried salmon probably contaminated with *Staphylococcus* bacteria resulted in the familiar complaints of diarrhea and abdominal cramping. On one string of eleven days of continuous rain Clark wrote that this time was "the most disagreeable time I have experienced." Coming from the even-tempered outdoorsman who had endured such extremes of conditions in traveling this far, the statement conveys a remarkable degree of distress. The rain and wind led a discouraged William Clark to scribble a disgusted entry into his journal on November 22: "O! how horriable is the day."

The Corps started splitting trees and erecting their winter fortress south of the Columbia estuary, below the mouth of present-day Lewis and Clark River. On December 11, several members of the team were on the injured reserve list, with problems recorded by Captain Clark as "Sergeant Pryor unwell from a dislocation of his Sholder, Gibson with the disentary, Jo. Fields with biles on his legs, & Werner with a Strained knee." He ended his entry that day with a note about the rain. There was always the rain. Construction of Fort Clatsop proceeded out of necessity during the nearly constant downpours. The men were delighted to discover that the large "balsam pine splits into excellent boards more than two feet in width" that helped them quickly erect the structure and provided effective roof shingles.

The Corps' new neighborhood for the winter was in the vicinity of the Clatsop Indian tribe, who inhabited the country near the Columbia's mouth. These Indians seemed to Captain Clark to be "well disposed" but ruthless traders described as "Close deelers, & Sticle for a verry little, never close a bargin except they think they have the advantage."

Many of the Indians were noted to have skin lesions that the captains believed were evidence of syphilitic infections. Yet the realistic captains handed out pieces of ribbon to some of the men to "bestow on their favorite Lasses, this plan to save the knives & more valueable articles."[1] Either the seriousness of the potential infection or the likelihood of the men contracting it escaped the medical judgment of Lewis and Clark.

The site for the winter fort had been discovered by Captain Lewis during his reconnaissance of the southern bank of the Columbia in an area that the Clatsops had assured him offered abundant elk on which the Corps could survive their winter layover. The coast was about seven miles to the west. The winter quarters would be named "Fort Clatsop" after the local tribe, following the custom established the previous winter with the Mandans. Never fully trusting the Clatsops, who the captains believed to be inherently untrustworthy, they ordered the fort built with defense in mind. It was a square log structure with seven rooms, each with its own fireplace, and a separate smoke room where the game could be preserved as it came in. Gates on either end of the fort would be secured at night, and guards were posted around the clock.

Area Indians made nearly daily trips to the building site, bringing various trade goods such as lynx and otter pelts, and food items of wapato roots and fish. Blue glass beads were the most sought-after item, with white beads, fishhooks, and tobacco also being valued.

The hard working carpenters at Fort Clatsop required food to keep them productive in splitting boards and digging holes. On December 15, Captain Clark and sixteen of the men rowed three miles up a nearby creek and dispersed into the surrounding forests to procure some elk. The hunters found their quarry and began to pack in the meat, quartered for ease of transport. The great coastal elk weighed in at anywhere between three hundred and seven hundred pounds. Part of the group—Ordway, Colter, Collins, Whitehouse, and McNeal—became lost in the thick forest and undergrowth and spent a most disagreeable night in the woods. Whitehouse reported in his journal, "It rained all that night & the wind blew very cold & being without fire, we suffered considerably both from the Rain & wind."[2] As soon as the elk meat made it to the fort, it was placed in the smoke room, where constant fire and smoke was utilized to try to cure it. But the warmth of the Oregon winter caused much of the meat to spoil and become unusable.

By December 22, the men were chinking the fort's logs with homemade material, and several were suffering from boils and bruises. If it didn't rain it snowed. If it didn't snow, it hailed. The wind blew. The men were pelted by the elements nearly every time they walked to the toilet facilities. Inside their fort beginning Christmas Eve, they were at least relatively dry, but once inside, there were fire smoke and the fleas to contend with. It took a stellar effort on the men's part to try to rid their living quarters of the ever-present fleas that infested clothing and bedding.

Fleas are bloodsucking parasites belonging to the class of insects. They obtain food from their hosts, generally mammals and birds. The small wingless insects particularly enjoy living on wild animals, especially rodents. Various flea species usually inhabit their own particular host mammalian or avian species, but they can parasitize other species as well. They thrive in cool and moist environments, hence their abundance along the Oregon coast. They are prodigious jumpers and can easily jump from one host to another. They live and breed in cracks of floors and the dark ground under such places as Fort Clatsop. With a ready food supply their life span involves about a year.

Fleas provide monumental problems for humans, but it would seem that the Corps was able to avoid the most serious: plague and endemic typhus.

Bubonic plague is transmitted from an infected rodent population to humans by the bites of infected fleas or by infected flea feces deposited on the victim's skin and then rubbed into a scratch. Plague is caused by the bacterium *Yersinia pestis* and if untreated is invariably fatal—as evidenced by the millions who died from it during the Middle Ages in Europe.[3]

Various forms of the illness typhus exist, all caused by different species of the intracellular parasite of the genus *Rickettsia*. (One of the *rickettsia* causes Rocky Mountain Spotted Fever.) Epidemic typhus, spread by the body louse, is the more serious form of this disease. Fleas can spread the endemic form caused by the organism *Rickettsia typhi*. Infected fleas can pass this form of the disease to humans with their bites. The fleas obtain the *rickettsia* from feeding on the blood of infected wild mice, rats, and other rodents. Symptoms of endemic typhus include shaking chills, fever, and headache. Fever usually lasts about twelve days, and can be accompanied by pinkish blotches covering the skin of the trunk and spreading to the arms and legs.[4]

It would be highly conjectural to suspect that typhus or plague was part of the Corps' winter of 1805-1806. But even if these two serious results of fleabites were avoided that otherwise miserable winter, the constant torment of the biting, crawling, and bloodsucking insect parasites was most unwelcome.

Christmas Day 1805 was ushered in by the men providing the captains with a salute of firing rifles, followed by an impromptu choir singing a Christmas song. All day was spent inside the huts while the rain poured down. Although the captains noted that "there was nothing in our situation to excite much gaiety," they did their best to celebrate the day "which we have always been accustomed to observe as a day of rejoicing." Clark wrote that after breakfast "we divided our Tobacco which amounted to 12 carrots one half of which we gave to the men of the party who used tobacco, and to those who doe not use it we make a present of a handkerchief." Joseph Field presented the captains with a table and two seats for their room, and Clark with a polished slab of wood to replace his smashed lap desk. Sacagawea gave Captain Clark two dozen white-weasel tails. Clark also received a "small Indian basket" from Goodrich, a pair of "mockersons" from Whitehouse, and a pair of woolen stockings, and a shirt from Captain Lewis. Clark continued, "We would have Spent this day the nativity of Christ in feasting, had we any thing either to raise our Sperits or even gratify our appetites, our Diner concisted of pore Elk, So much Spoiled that we eate it thro' mear necessity, Some Spoiled pounded fish and a fiew roots."

Joseph Whitehouse's entry of Christmas day noted that the men "…are mostly in good health, A blessing, which we esteem more, than all the luxuries this life can afford, and the party are all thankful to the Supreme Being, for his goodness towards us.—"[5] Undoubtedly many stories were shared that day in the smoky rooms of the wooden fort near the blustery coast of Oregon. Stories of past Christmas celebrations, great feasts, families, and warm hearths, with savory stews simmering over the red-hot coals. Stories of Christmases past probably gave way to fantasies of Christmas of 1806.

The game that was brought in daily by the hunters proved to be spoiling entirely too quickly. On December 28, the captains dispatched five men to the coast, seven miles south, with two large kettles to begin to distill sea water. The salt obtained could season and preserve their meat, and serve as a trade item on the return trip. Five of the miles to the coast were through "thick wood vaired with hills, ravines and swamps" and the remaining two miles to the Pacific were through "waving prairies of sandcovered with green grass." Two days later, the sun shone briefly. Blue skies and sun—quite a novelty during an Oregon winter. Hunters returned with fresh elk meat and the captains "had a Sumptious supper of Elk Tongues and marrow bones…" In addition, Fort Clatsop got its last slap of chinking and its last board secured. The Corps of Discovery was now tucked in for the winter.

New Year's Day 1806 must have been a happy occasion. I can nearly hear the men of the Corps slapping each other on the back, and the laughter and anticipation in their voices as they huddled in their huts or wandered between the rooms to visit their comrades. In spite of the rain, wind, and a dinner of "boiled elk and wappatoo" washed down with some tasty "draughts of pure water," the entire Corps realized that, with any luck, this year would see them back to civilization, friends, comfort, wealth, and fame. Lewis wrote that the day "consisted principally in the anticipation of the 1st day of January 1807, when in the bosom of our friends we hope to participate in the mirth and hilarity of the day, and when with the zest given by the recollection of the present, we shall completely, both mentally and corporally, enjoy the repast which the hand of civilization has prepared for us."

On the morning of the 3rd of January, the Clatsops brought berries, roots, and several dogs to trade to the Corps. In addition, they brought another curious substance that caught the captains' interest—whale blubber. This novel food item was obtained from a neighboring nation, who had cut it from the huge carcass of a whale beached near their coastal village.

The Corps' hunters, facing shrinking herds of local game, were now hunting a considerable distance to the east. Harvested animals required longer packs back to the fort. John Colter was out in the bush from January 1 to the 5th, and still returned empty-handed.

At least the salt-making camp found success, and was making between three and four quarts of salt daily. The men found the salt on their daily ration of elk "a great treat."

Captain Clark set out with a dozen others in search of the beached whale on January 6. Sacagawea heard about the planned trip and was upset about not being invited to accompany the group. Lewis wrote that "the Indian woman was very impotunate to be permited to go, and was therefore indulged; she observed that she had traveled a long way with us to see the great waters, and that now that monstrous fish was also to be seen, she thought it very hard she could not be permitted to see either (she had never yet been to the Ocean)."

Once out of the fort and on their way toward the coast, they crossed carefully over a single-log bridge—icy that morning—placed across a creek by the saltmakers. Arriving at the beach, they proceeded to a Clatsop village and paid a man two fishhooks to ferry the party across the wide and deep Necanicum River. Once on the opposite shoreline, they hiked along the beach watching the great winter waves roll and break on the stormy Pacific. Soon, their route became blocked by numerous rocks, requiring the party to climb a steep "mountain" shrouded with clouds, present-day Tillamook Head. The path became so steep that the Corps needed to pull themselves up with the aid of bushes. The upward path took two hours of "labour and fatigue."

At the summit, the fog cleared and Clark wrote, "from the top of which I looked down with estonishment to behold the hight which we had assended" that appeared to be about 1,200 feet and almost perpendicular. At the summit they also met fourteen Indian men and women loaded with oil and whale blubber. They too, had just made the climb, coming up from the opposite direction.

Back at Fort Clatsop, Lewis wrote that the meat was becoming alarmingly scarce. With a third of the Corps gone to the coast, the remaining men shared increased guard duty, which put an added emotional stress on them. Continuing cloudy weather made taking celestial readings impossible for Lewis. The bad weather allowed him time to record his observations about the surrounding Indian tribes being "excessively fond of smoking tobacco," and that both men and women swallowed the smoke and "inhale it in their lungs untill they become surcharged with this vapour when they puff it out to a great distance through their nostils and mouth…" He added that "I have no doubt the smoke of the tobacco in this manner becomes much more intoxicating and that they do possess themselves of all it's virtues in their fullest extent…" If they were hopelessly addicted to smoking, at least they didn't appear to be aware of the use of "sperituous liquors," as they never asked the captains for any alcoholic drinks. Lewis thought this was a great advantage for both the Indians and "for the quiet and safety of thos whites who visit them."

On January 8, after a several-mile hike on the beach and thirty-five miles from Fort Clatsop, the Clark contingent approached a Tillamook Indian village, finding most of the inhabitants busy boiling whale oil with heated stones thrown into blubber contained in wooden troughs. The nearby whale had been reduced to a skeleton, a tribute to the industrious Tillamooks. The Corps traded the goods they had brought along for about three hundred pounds of blubber and a few gallons of oil. Clark complained that the price was astronomical. He was nevertheless thankful for the whale, and noted that he thanked "providence for directing the whale to us; and think him much more kind to us than he was to jonah, having Sent this monster to be *Swallowed by us* in Sted of *Swallowing of us* as jonah's did." After a smoke with the Tillamooks and a night that saw Private McNeal narrowly escape being murdered when a Tillamook woman blew the whistle on a plot to kill him for his clothing, the Corps retraced their steps to Fort Clatsop.

As they had the previous winter, the captains wrote and mapped what they had learned since last spring. The long days of rain allowed naturalist Lewis to describe and draw numerous species of new-to-science flora such as certain maples, Oregon crabapple, Sitka spruce, Douglas-fir, Christmas fern, and fauna such as the condor, white gull, salmon trout (steelhead), Columbian black-tailed deer, Oregon bobcat, and the bottom-dwelling oceanic skate. In addition numerous descriptions and drawings of Indian ethnographic information were added to the knowledge base of the expedition. Cultural information was recorded, such as the technique of head-flattening. Proof of previous Indian contact with English-speaking sailors was recorded by Captain Lewis, noting the Indians' knowledge of such words and phrases as "musquit, powder, shot, nife, file, damned rascal, sun of a bitch &c."

The men of the Corps passed the time in a variety of ways. There were those who participated in the hunting parties, constantly pushing deeper into the surrounding forest in their quest for fresh meat. Skins from the elk were tanned in the frontier method of utilizing the elk's brain as tanning agent. The men then tailored the skins into new garments, and they also became cobblers, cutting, and stitching more than four hundred pairs of moccasins for the return trip.

As Lewis delicately expressed it, "amorous contact" with Indian women had resulted in new contact with "Louis Veneri" and thus the use of mercury to treat the disease. In November, "many of our party" had contracted "the venerial" from a group of Chinook women Lewis said were openly prostituted by their chief and "the old baud his wife."[6] At that time, Clark had recorded that "Those people appear to View Sensuality as a Necessary evel, and do not appear to abhore it as a Crime in the unmarried State."[7] Late in January, Lewis believed that one of the men was cured—at least the visible symptoms had resolved.[8] But, exactly one month later, Lewis wrote again that this man and another were recovering from "the pox."[9]

Lewis wrote in the middle of March that the men had "finally recovered."[10] One must wonder if their teeth were loose and their gums sloughing off after all those weeks of mercury treatment. When the same female group came calling once again at Fort Clatsop on March 15, Lewis "gave the men a particular charge with rispect to them which they promised me to observe." The men who refused the Indian women's sexual offers incited great contempt from area Indians. Clark wrote that the Clatsops, especially the women, seemed "highly disgusted at our refuseing to axcept of their favours…"

Trying to discover what treatment the Clatsops used for syphilis, Lewis was frustrated by the language barrier, but he decided that the Clatsops lacked any such treatment, in that "once this disorder is contracted by them it continues with them during life; but always ends in decipitude, death, or premature old age." He commented that other

Indian tribes, particularly the "Chippeways," used a potion of "simples," lobelia and sumac, that he thought efficacious in treating cases of syphilis.[11]

En route to the coast, Lewis had noticed the relative lack of gonorrhea and syphilis in Upper Columbia Indian population, only two or three cases of the former and "double that number" of the latter; "at least the males who are always sufficiently exposed to the observations or inspection of the phisician" lacked visible symptoms of the venereal diseases.[12] But here around Fort Clatsop, individuals covered in "Sores Scabs & ulsers no doubt the effects of venereal disorder"[13] were often seen, and "Pocks & Venerial is Common amongst them…"[14]

Recurrent dysentery, most likely obtained from both the food and water supplies, added to the the Corps' winter misery. Muscle strains from lifting quartered elk and building the fort, compounded by the cold and damp weather, caused a good deal of musculoskeletal problems for men who had no aspirin, acetaminophen, or ibuprofen to help control their aches and pains.

Frequent respiratory infections were present due to the cramped nature of the men's quarters that easily allowed them to spread among the men. There are at least a hundred different viruses that cause the common cold, in addition to the numerous and more serious influenza viruses that could have accounted for the respiratory infections suffered by the men during the winter of 1805-1806.

That February, Private George Gibson was so sick he was unable to stand, and asked to be brought from the salt works back to the fort. The malaise and fever were from a "violent cold" that Lewis believed he caught by hunting elk in the swamps. Doctor Lewis treated him with doses of the diaphoretic (sweat inducing) medication of "diluted nitre" (saltpeter or potassium nitrate), and laudanum, the same combination he had treated Sacagawea with the previous June at the Great Falls of the Missouri. It was a favorite prescription of Dr. Lewis if his patient had a fever. Gibson would also get some of the Dr. Rush's pills, a treatment without any medical merit that I can determine. Gibson got well in spite of the assault rendered against his body by the era's medicine.

On February 9, while working on the coast and butchering elk he had just killed for Salt Camp, Alexander Willard cut his leg near his knee with his hatchet—"very badly," Lewis recorded. The wound had to be more severe than a scratch to warrant mention in the journals, and the thought of a hachet blade flying through the air and contacting his leg makes us all wince (and me anxious to suture the wound!). Willard's gash was probably dressed with cloth bandaging that held the edges of the wound together and controlled the hemorrhage.

In early February, one of the "nine young men from Kentucky," hunter and blacksmith William Bratton, came down with what would prove to be a debilitating ailment, one that appears in my practice every day—back pain. He was working at the saltworks when he suffered the injury, and the news reached Fort Clatsop by way of the wounded Alex Willard, who limped into camp. On February 11, Lewis dispatched Sergeant Pryor and four others to bring back and replace the sick Gibson and Bratton. On February 15, Lewis wrote that Bratton "is verry weak and complains of a pain in the lower part of the back when he moves which I suppose procedes from debility." Dr. Lewis's answer was to administer some of the cure-all "barks." This treatment continued for several days. It is not clear if the barks were applied in the form of a poultice or if they were given orally. This was probably a totally worthless and potentially dangerous treatment, given our knowledge of the quinine and other alkaloids present in the bark of the cinchona tree. There is mention of Bratton having a cough, but no mention of fever. It would seem on face value of the journal's description of symptoms that Bratton was suffering from a musculoskeletal problem.

There are numerous structures in the human back and spine that can become injured and thus able to generate pain. Muscles can be strained, and ligaments stretched or torn. Discs that normally separate vertebrae can be damaged and at times rupture, allowing the jelly-like contents to push against spinal nerves that exit the spinal cord between the vertebrae, causing severe back pain, leg pain, and leg weakness and, in its most severe form, a neurologic emergency. When the spinal cord becomes compressed by the ruptured disc material, the patient loses neurologic control below the level of spinal injury. Vertebrae in the spine form joints with adjacent vertebrae, in part on small bony projections called facets. Various injuries caused by improper lifting or twisting can injure these facet joints, causing a good deal of muscular spasm and back pain. The spines of every man in the Corps had probably taken terrific beatings from the difficult labor they had performed during their brief lifespans. Some of them undoubtedly had some arthritis in their vertebral joints, and their intervertebral discs were shrinking and dehydrating with age, even though many were still only in their twenties. From the description of Bratton's pain, it is a good bet that this may have been part of his problem. The root cause of back pain is sometimes a difficult problem to diagnose. Back pain can be severe and debilitating and may last for months as it, unfortunately, did for William Bratton.

Many of the men were now frequently sick. Their poorly balanced diets did nothing to help their immune systems resist the ubiquitous viral respiratory infections. After months of elk steak, elk roasts, elk tongue and elk jerky, roots, whale blubber, and fish, they were poorly nourished in every food group except protein. The bright side was that they had three meals a day.

In addition to the scarcity of local game, their once numerous stores of colored beads, knives, and trinkets used for trade items with the Indians had been steadily whittled away. The treasure chest that made itself westward with the Corps now contained one scarlet robe and six blue ones, a United States Army coat and hat, five robes made from their large American flag, and a few ribbon-trimmed pieces of clothing. In other words, the Corps of Discovery that had letters of credit signed by the President of the United States and had all the power of the nation's treasury backing them were nearly destitute of supplies. With nearly four thousand miles between them and a place where they could replenish their reserves, the prospects for business transactions were dwindling rapidly. Fortunately they still had their guns and sufficient lead ball and gunpowder to secure food on the hoof. Although April 1 was the scheduled day of departure from Fort Clatsop, the scarcity of food, their serious state of poverty, and the climate pushed the date up a week. By the third week of March all were ready to leave their water-logged and muddy winter home and start back up the Columbia, to the high plains and western slope of the Rockies and the friendly Nez Perce. From there it would be over the challenging Bitterroots and back to the plains of the Missouri where the problem was not a lack of game, but one of deciding how many elk or buffalo to shoot, and which cut of meat to eat.

Except for Willard and Bratton, who remained on the injured list, the Corps was enjoying reasonably good health by the third week of March. Willard had contracted a bad case of what Lewis thought to be influenza on February 20, suffering from symptoms of a high fever and headache. The journals report him being treated with some of "Scott's pills," which were also administered to several others with comments that "they did not work him," or "they did not operate," or "they opperated very well," leading me to believe that they were another form of cathartic. That Willard was still ill and weak suggests that his case of influenza may have been influenza pneumonia rather than an uncomplicated case of flu. He may also have contracted some other form of bacterial pneumonia, or even pneumonic tularemia, the serious bacterial illness discussed earlier, from cleaning infected wild game. Whatever its cause, pneumonia could certainly result in several weeks of profound malaise. Bratton continued to suffer from his back problem to such a degree that Lewis expressed concern over his recovery in his entry of March 21.

Dr. Clark noted on March 22 that the "Clatsops inform us that Several of their nation has the Sore throat, one of which has lately died with this disorder." They could have been sticken by the pharyngeal form of tularemia, or the life-threatening bacterial sore throat, diphtheria. Their illness also could have been caused by a particular species of *Streptococcus* bacteria (Group A), but many other strep species can also produce serious disease states for humans. This unlucky fellow could have developed complications from his strep throat such as throat abscess, systemic infection spread via the blood, meningitis, endocarditis (heart infection), liver abscesses or other nasty complications too numerous to list. Too bad that the penicillin that could have cured him was more than a century from discovery.

Still, with any luck, the worst was now over. The past four months probably had seemed like an eternity for the men waiting for spring and the return to the United States that it promised. The beat of the pounding raindrops on the roof that barely protected the Corps from the weather was accented by the frequent coughing and sneezing going on all night around them as they tried to sleep. Pompey and Sacagawea had been healthy. The food had been lousy. The salt had helped ease the boredom of their meager diet. Their interactions with the surrounding Indians had not been as enjoyable as they had experienced the previous winter with the Mandans and Hidatsas. The hard bargains area Indians insisted upon during their trading sessions, and the propensity of some to steal various items that belonged to the Corps left a sour taste in the mouths of the captains. The perceived prostitution of the females and the men's resulting cases of syphilis left the captains irritated at both the men and the Indian women. The captains, who had frankly described the attractiveness of other Indian women along the trip, found area women's clothing immodest, but held a higher opinion of Clatsop women than of the Chinooks. The latter were "lude and Carry on Sport publickly," but the former "appear deffidend, and reserved."[15]

On the 22nd of March, in appreciation of his kindness and hospitality, the Clatsop Chief Coboway was presented with the fort and its furniture, as well as a certificate attesting to his kindness. A paper with a map of the connection between the upper branches of the Missouri and Columbia rivers with the proposed route of return to civilization was posted on the wall of Fort Clatsop. A message was written on the papers that read:

> *The object of this list, is, that through the medium of some civilized person who may see the same, it may be made known to the informed world, that the party consisting of the persons whose names are hereunto annexed, and who were sent out by the government of the U'States in May 1804 to explore the interior of the Continent of North America, did penetrate the same by way of the Missouri and Columbia Rivers, to the discharge of the latter into the Pacific Ocean, where they arrived on the 14th day of November 1805, and departed the [blank] day of March 1806, on their return to the United States, by the same rout they had come out.*[16]

The excitement must have been palpable on the rainy morning of March 23, 1806, as the Corps of Discovery rolled up their tattered and damp bedrolls inside the tiny log-walled rooms of Fort Clatsop and the captains secured their precious journals (augmented by numerous newly scribed pages of observations). Sacagawea wrapped up thirteen-month-old Pompey inside the room that had served as their sleeping quarters during the winter, and readied herself to join her husband

Charbonneau on their walk to the canoes. Today was the longed-for day of departure and the beginning of the homeward journey. The wind and rain continued as the Corps made its way down to the river and the waiting canoes. The weather provided by Mother Nature was something less than optimal, but the hunters had already been sent up the Columbia to prepare the way for the trailing Corps. At 1 P.M. the last member stepped into his canoe and pushed it away from the riverbank, and once again the Corps of Discovery was on the move. By Clark's figuring, they were 2,534 miles away from Fort Mandan, and 4,134 miles from St. Louis.[17] This time, however, their departure was in the direction of home, family and, they hoped for the short term, something warm, fresh, and good to eat.

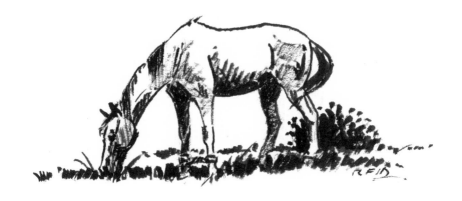

A CLASH OF CULTURES

March-April, 1806

Anger makes us all stupid.
—*Johanna Spyri, author of* Heidi

Once on the Columbia, every stroke of the paddles took them a little closer to home and farther away from Fort Clatsop and its four
months of nearly constant rain, wind, and boredom. The relief the men
felt was tempered with the reality that they were once again paddling
upstream, and soon would be battling a tough westward current. The
riverbanks were densely timbered, with immense stands of trees in
spots reaching the limits of the tidal water, where numerous pieces of
driftwood floated by the advancing canoes. Except for the daily tidal
changes, this estuary seemed more like a stormy lake than the river torrent they had fought on the Missouri River, but the promise of more
rapid waters ahead and those treacherous falls on the Columbia that

would need to be portaged may have challenged their spirits just a bit. By camptime in the evening on that first day out, they had managed to row sixteen miles and reached a campsite somewhere past Point William where they met George Drouillard, and Reubin and Joseph Field. The advance hunters had taken two elk, but the meat was still a mile and a half upstream. It was too far away to be of use today.

The southern side of the river was exceedingly shallow to an amazing distance of four miles from the shoreline. The canoes diverted their path to the northern part of the river where there was "a channel sufficient for canoes." In the early afternoon they halted at a Cathlamet Indian village where they traded for a dog and some seal meat that became dinner for the sick men. The captains noted that the men had been healthier when they had been eating more dog meat, and therefore decided that Willard and Bratton might benefit from a dinner of canine steaks.

The early spring weather continued to be rough, with high winds and cold nighttime temperatures. The 26th of March dawned with winds so strong that the planned early departure was postponed until 8 A.M. A sturgeon was obtained from a grateful Cathlamet chief who had been given a medal, an honor that delighted him. Fortunately, the medal produced some food that ordinarily tobacco would have been necessary to procure. Showing their unrestrained enthusiasm for the weed, two Indian men had followed the Corps for an entire day, trying to sell two dogs in exchange for some tobacco. The supply of tobacco was nearly exhausted and the men who smoked were now forced into a "cold-turkey" quit-smoking program in order to preserve the few twists that remained. Lewis wrote, "Our men who are now obliged to deny the uce of this article appear to suffer much for the want of it." The smokers then substituted saccacommis, as the Frenchmen called a mixture of leaves from the bearberry (*Arctostaphylos uva-ursi*) and the inner bark of the red osier dogwood tree. The tobacco chewers went with their own substitute, the bitter bark of the wild crabapple (*Malus diversifolia*), which the men assured the captains was a good substitute.

By the end of March, the party had worked its way up the Columbia and explored a sizeable river they named the Multnomah, today's Willamette River. Here they camped for a week. Willard was much stronger and Bratton's back seemed to be less painful. The river current

A Clash of Cultures

was noticeably strong, and large pieces of floating logs made the Corps' slow progress upstream fraught with danger. The scenery was stunning when the clouds cleared long enough for a view. To the south, Mount Hood, and to the north conical Mount St. Helens, served as seeming gateposts to the exit from the coast as they jutted above the surrounding timbered mountains.

On April 1, the captains were faced with a discouraging reality. The Corps encountered numerous Indian canoes making their way downriver. The Indians told the captains that their food stores for the winter were nearly exhausted, salmon were not expected on the river until May, and they were coming downriver for food. Between the villages of these Indians and those of the Nez Perce, there were several hundred miles that afforded "no deer, antelope, nor elk on which we can rely for susistence." The Nez Perce had boarded the Corps' horses over the winter, but the captains were concerned that by the first of May the Nez Perce might have crossed the Bitterroots to hunt buffalo. If they took the horses with them, that left the Corps stranded on the west side of the mountain range. Lewis and Clark decided to camp and collect as much meat as was possible and then push on to the Nez Perce. Hunting parties were sent out on both sides of the Columbia, but numerous animals killed proved to be so skinny that they were not even transported back to camp to cook.

On April 5, as the base camp made desperate attempts at building fires and drying the incoming meat, the hunting team of Patrick Gass, Richard Windsor, and John Collins brought back three live black bear cubs. Some visiting Indians were so pleased at the prospect of having them as pets that the Corps traded them in exchange for wapato roots. Lewis, the botanist, was in high gear describing the numerous trees and bushes in the area, cottonwood, ash, willow and huckleberry, to name but a few.

Seemingly friendly Indians came around the campsite the next night, occasionally helping themselves to small items left unattended or unwatched. The Indians seemed to irritate Captain Lewis: "these people are constantly hanging about us."

Irritating problems arose. Clark's small rifle had needed attention on the 8th. John Shields answered the call, repaired the rifle, and earned the captain's written praise of "the party ows much to the injenuity of this man, by whome their guns are repared when they get out of order which is very often." Shields, the oldest enlisted man and a near mutineer against Sergeant Ordway back at Camp Dubois, had endeared himself to, at least, Captain Clark.

On the 9th, with the canoes packed with "dryed meat secured in skins we took breakfast and departed at 9 A.M." Lewis noted that the Columbia was about twelve feet higher than it had been the previous fall, and was at this point about a mile and a half wide. They passed the landmark Beacon Rock, which stood by itself now only seven hundred feet above the current of the mighty Columbia.

The rapid river current made paddling upstream impossible and the towropes made of elk skins were now brought out from storage. Clark commanded the necessary portages, and everyone available helped. Bratton, with his painful back, and three others who were "lamed by accidents" served as cooks for the workers. Three men were needed to guard the goods as they sat on the riverbank and the local Indians crowded around the camp.

Relations with various Lower Columbian tribes took a rapid and progressive downhill course over the next several weeks due to the frequent thievery and hard bargaining by locals, coupled with the Corps' growing impatience and frustration, beginning at the Cascades of the Columbia on the 11th. After Shields bought a dog from them, two Indians attempted to steal it back. He defended himself, drew his large knife, and scared the would-be attackers into the forest. Later that day three men of the same tribe, the Wah-clel-lahs, did the unthinkable and stole Seaman. Learning of the theft, Lewis immediately dispatched three men with orders to track down the thieves and retrieve the dog. Lewis's orders were plain: If the thieves resisted, they should be shot. The men took off after the kidnappers and tracked them for two miles. Discovering the white men coming, the Indians let Seaman loose and fled into the countryside. Meanwhile back at camp the thievery continued. Lewis finally ordered the Indians to be kept out of camp "and informed them by signs that if they made any further attempts to steal our property or insulted our men we should put them to instant death." This was a low point in Indian-white relations. Not only was stealing a capital crime, but any verbal or other insult was considered worthy of a death sentence. Lewis also expressed the growing anger among the

A Clash of Cultures

men, stating that they were "well disposed to kill a few of them." A chief of the tribe apologized and blamed the trouble on "two very bad men" of his tribe, and assured the captains of his personal good will. In a gesture of trust and pacification, Clark and Lewis gave the chief a small medal. Tempers cooled, but the Corps remained vigilantly on guard.

Portaging the Cascades took two days, and then the last boat hawsered over the rapids was ripped away downstream. On April 12, Lewis wrote: "in hawling the perogue arround this point [of rock] the bow unfortunately took the current at too great a distance from the rock, she turned her side to the stream and the utmost exertions of all the party were unable to resist the forse with which she was driven by the current, they were compelled to let loose the cord and of course both perogue and cord went a drift with the stream." The loss now required that all of its cargo be distributed among the remaining four canoes, making them nearly unmanageable in the water. Lewis was forced to give some of their few remaining trade items for two additional canoes. It required three days for the men to inch their way only seven miles upstream on this explosive and violent stretch of river. Along with the canoes, Lewis got four paddles and three dogs, stating that "with most of the party has become a favorite food, by no means disagreeable to me, I prefer it to lean venison or Elk and is very far superior to the horse in any state."

By April 16, the Corps arrived at the beginning of open plains, which extended past the horizon—all the way to the Nez Perce and the foothills of the Rockies. Clark, Sacagawea, Drouillard, Charbonneau, and nine other men took "a good part of our stock of merchandize" and struck out ahead on the Columbia's north side toward the Watlala and Wishram-Wasco Indians. Clark's party camped near the Long Narrows and invited the natives to a horse-trading session. Many Indians showed up with numerous horses, but they wanted half of the merchandise for one horse. Clark wrote, "this price I could not think of giving."

The Watlalas assured Clark that, if he came to their village upstream, they would trade with him. At the village, as the sun sank over the western horizon, Pierre Cruzatte played a few tunes and some men of the Corps danced. Clark traded all the next day, obtaining only four horses.

The air was now noticeably drier and purer. Another novelty—dry earth—was underfoot, and the plains that lay in view were carpeted with what Lewis wrote was "a rich virdure of grass and herbs from four to nine inches high and exhibits a beautifull seen particularly pleasing after having been so long imprisoned in mountains and those almost impenetrably thick forrests of the seacoast."

All able-bodied men of the main party loaded cargo and canoes on their backs on the morning of April 18, and portaged around the Long Narrows of The Dalles. By the time they reached Clark and his group late that day, only two more horses had been added to the Corps' herd. This next day the captains bought five more, for "emence" prices. Both captains were infuriated by the region's "deciptfull" bargaining style, and the many small thefts. At the campsite, Lewis directed the horses to be hobbled and guarded while they grazed. Poor Alexander Willard was among those assigned the task of horse guard duty. He was probably still regaining some of the strength lost during his battle with pneumonia a month earlier. Now, as he slept, daydreamed, or talked with a friend, one of the precious and expensive horses wandered off and could not be found when Lewis ordered the horses picketed for the night. Lewis, with frustration that we can feel, wrote, "this in addition to the other difficulties under which I laboured was truly provoking. I repremanded him more severely for this piece of negligence than had been usual with me."

The next day brought the theft of six tomahawks, and another horse, while Lewis was able to purchase only two new horses. On the 21st, another horse was gone in the morning and another tomahawk stolen. By now the Corps could fit their cargo on the horses and into two canoes, and had cut up two others for firewood. In a taunting act of disgust aimed directly at these tribes, Lewis ordered that "all the spare poles, paddles and the balance of our canoe put on the fire as the morning was cold and also that not a particle should be left for the benefit of the indians." Not even a *particle*. Apparently an Indian came in and was taking an iron socket from the fire. Lewis snapped. Lewis "gave him several severe blows and mad the men kick him out of camp." If that wasn't enough, Lewis now "informed the indians that I would shoot the first of them that attempted to steal an article from us. that we were not affraid to fight them, that I had it in my power at that moment to kill

A Clash of Cultures

them all and set fire to their houses, but it was not my wish to treat them with severity provided they would let my property alone." As the flames of the burning canoes turned into embers, the Corps packed their, by now, nine horses. Bratton, still unable to walk, mounted one, and all left the village that had been a smoldering powder keg of Corps–Indian diplomacy.

Charbonneau's horse spooked on April 22, threw its load and ran downhill to an Indian village. The horse's saddle and blanket were immediately appropriated by the Indians. Charbonneau was able to retrieve the saddle but all the Indians feigned ignorance of the blanket. Lewis would have none of it. He sent an order ahead to Clark to send men back to his aid. Lewis was "determined either to make the indians deliver the robe or birn their houses." The repeated acts of thievery, broken trade deals and what he interpreted as bad hospitality "have vexed me in such a manner that I am quite disposed to treat them with every severyty, their defenseless state pleads," sparing only their lives in return. Private Francois Labiche hurried from dwelling to dwelling until he found the blanket.

For the price of a blanket, Lewis had been ready to torch an entire village and allow the country he represented to suffer the negative consequence. Clark had experienced similar actions at the hands of Indians, but never expressed the level of outrage that Lewis did. Steven Ambrose stated it well: "The resulting conflagration would have been a gross overreaction, unpardonably unjust, and a permanent blot on his honor."[1] For our story, it gives a fascinating insight into Lewis's personality and temper.

As the angry Lewis and his men caught up with Clark, on top of a hill that overlooked the Deschutes River's mouth and a vast expanse of incredible country, the Corps of Discovery achieved another milestone.[2] They had departed from river travel (except for Colter and Potts in one canoe) and their journey through the thick primeval evergreen forest of coastal North America. Now they entered into the relatively dry inland territory that lay in the rain shadow of the Cascade Mountains. Snow-covered 11,000-foot Mount Hood was still clearly discernable to the southwest, with Mount Jefferson to its south.

The meager merchandise stores they possessed a month earlier had decreased still further. What would they do in exchange for food if they were unable to kill enough to keep them going? Would they themselves have to resort to stealing, or would the friendly Nez Perce help them out? They didn't realize it, but in the immediate future, their skills as frontier physicians and their little supply of medicines would be the answer to many of their problems.

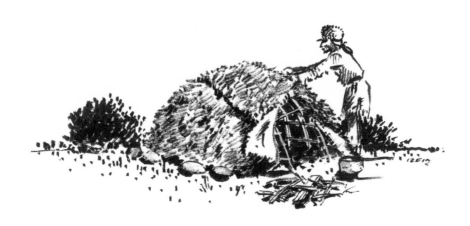

🌿 16 🌿

FRONTIER DOCTOR
AND MEDICAL DIPLOMATS

Great Challenges in Idaho

Natural forces are the healers of disease.
—Hippocrates

The string of men and loaded pack horses now plodded their way like
a giant snake toward the east, through the "rugged" country border-
ing the upper Columbia. At midday on April 23, they reached a Tenino
village and a warm welcome. Dogs and bread made from pounded roots
were purchased for dinner, and a Nez Perce guide they had picked up
downriver suggested they stay for the night, as no wood was to be had
for quite some distance ahead. The day's fourteen-mile hike had been
with what Lewis described as "the greatest exirtion" through the sandy
and rocky riverbank above the Columbia Gorge.

The next day was just as tough. Clark practiced some good anti-
inflammatory physical therapy and soaked his aching feet and legs in

cold water "from which I experienced Considerable relief." As frigid winds blew from the west, poles were sunk in the ground and the thirteen horses that were serving as their pack animals were tied up for the night. Very sore ankles and feet were rested. As usual, a guard stood watch over the growing herd of horses and the sleeping men.

When the group awakened in the morning on plains that extended outward for miles from the abrupt cliffs overlooking the Columbia, they awoke to a novel situation. There was absolutely no dew covering them and the earth was completely dry. It must have been a welcome change. Low-growing grasses provided the horses, some of which Lewis described being "as fat as seals," with good grazing. There were now enough horses to provide two "nags" for Lewis and Clark to ride. Rattlesnakes made their reappearance on the dry landscape, forcing the men to increase their attention on the ground.

Indian relations improved further when the Corps reached the Walula village of Chief Yellepit, about twelve miles below the confluence of the Snake with the Columbia. There they stayed from April 27 to the 30th. The captains viewed Yellepit as a true gentleman, who personally delivered cooked fish and fuel in the form of dried bushes from the treeless prairie. The Corps also learned from Yellepit about an overland shortcut to the mouth of the Clearwater River at present-day Lewiston, Idaho. The trail would save eighty miles of hiking, and Yellepit assured the captains there were plenty of grass, pronghorns, and deer for the taking. A Shoshone woman, living as a prisoner with the Walulas, made the old translation chain of Sacagawea, Charbonneau, Labiche, and Lewis, possible again. Lewis noted that, after several hours of conversation and questions with the Indians about the trip, "they were much pleased."

On April 28, an occasion occurred that led to the most remarkable period of frontier medical practice that took place during the entire course of the expedition.

The Walulas brought "several diseased persons to us for whom they requested some medical aid. one had his knee contracted by the rheumatism, another with a broken arm &c to all of which we administered much to the gratification of those poor wretches."

The most popular and valuable item the Corps possessed was now pulled out of the medicine chest—eyewash. The "eye-water," as Captain Lewis called it, offered an astringent and a mild antiseptic that, Clark wrote, "I believe will render them more esential Sirvece than any other article in the Medical way which we had it in our power to bestow on them…"

The Indian with the broken forearm came to the clinic with his arm supported only in a piece of leather. The deformity of the wrist fracture must have been apparent to the gaze of even an untrained eye. Falling on an outstretched arm probably produced the injury. Captain Clark now became a frontier orthopedist, and splinted the arm with "broad Sticks to keep it in place, put in a Sling and furnished him with Some lint bandages &c. to Dress it in future." This was pretty good first aid. If the bones were not excessively crooked, the arm would probably would have healed well in about six weeks. If the bones were displaced, and the arm had not been manipulated so that the bones were straightened, it would probably have healed but might have been visibly deformed. Clark's reputation for doctoring spread rapidly among the local tribes.

The next day, Clark noted that a man brought "his wife…who was verry unwell [from] the effects of violent Coalds…" Clark wasn't too impressed with the severity of the case, and apparently administered some of Dr. Rush's pills if we can interpret his comments about the medicine being, "as would keep her body open," as referring to the action of some laxative. He also wrapped her up in some flannel, the softness of which no Walula had probably ever experienced. The presumed action of the cathartics and the unusual feel of the cloth probably resulted in the woman's believing that remarkably effective treatment was being given to her by this strange white magician.

The opening day of the Lewis and Clark Clinic had ended with fiddle tunes from Cruzatte while the men of the Corps danced, followed by a Walula—and invited neighboring Yakama—line of 350 men, women, and children who "sung and danced at the same time," jumping up and down to the tempo. A "Medesene man" who "Could foretell things," and who had foretold the Corps' visit, now went to consulting "his God the moon," to see if what the white men said were true.

The benefit the Corps received from the medical treatment rendered by Captain Clark cannot be overemphasized. According to James Ronda, while the Corps had wintered with the Mandans, "the captains had the reputation as powerful spirit beings, some Indians believed that white medical techniques might be especially effective in serious cases."[1] John Ordway mentioned in his entry of that day for April 28, 1806, that the "chief called all his people and told them of the meddicine &c. which was a great wonder among them & they were much pleased &c."[2] These simple acts of compassion, and the administration of the probably not very effective "eye-water," the likely helpful arm splint, and the treatment for the cold were a monumental occurrence for these Indians. The profound good will created by Clark's practice of his brand of medicine would continue farther up the river. Even if the men of the Corps were down to cutting the buttons off their clothes to trade for food, the Corps had stumbled upon what now became their meal ticket over the Rockies—Clark and his travelling medical clinic.

With twenty-three good horses for transport and twelve dogs coming along as future menu items, the men departed the Walulas, on whom Lewis bestowed his great compliment as "friendly honest people." At 11 A.M. on April 30, the Corps struck out across the plains toward the Snake and Clearwater rivers confluence.

By May 3, the Corps had traversed both plains and rugged timbered canyons on their way to the main Nez Perce villages in present-day Idaho. In the afternoon they met one of their Nez Perce friends from the previous fall, a chief named Apah Wyakaikt, whom they called "the bighorn Cheif from the circumstance of his always wearing a horn of that animal suspended by a cord to [his] left arm." The Bighorn Chief had brought along ten "of his young men" who had come "a considerable distance to meet us." The entire party continued up the hillsides through a mixture of rain, hail, and snow to a yet higher plain and camped east of present-day Pataha City in a grove of cottonwoods that offered some slight protection from the cold storm blowing in from the southwest. The Corps ate the last of their dried meat and nearly all of the remaining dogs. The nearby Blue Mountains in present-day Washington were covered with snow "nearly to their bases." This could not have been an encouraging sight for men who were anxious to cross the Bitterroots.

May 4 saw the Corps' arrival at the village of a band of Nez Perce led by the Chief Tetoharsky, who had been helpful to them the previous fall. The village was situated along the Snake River, and the explorers found through the interpreters that if they crossed the Snake at this point, they could pass to the Clearwater River and up to today's Lochsa River in Idaho. There was the home of Chief Twisted Hair and the Corps' herd of horses he had kept over the winter. At 7 P.M., the Corps, with the aid of three Indian canoes, crossed to the north bank of the Snake River and drove onward.

Lewis made an interesting entry in the log on that day, describing the Nez Perce custom of isolating a woman in a small hut during the time of her menses. Menstruating Nez Perce women were not allowed to associate with their families, nor to eat anything, and any item they required people would bring to a distance of "50 or 60 paces and throw it toward them." The similarity between Jewish and Nez Perce cultures, separated by thousands of miles and having taken independent courses, was remarkable to the captains.

The next day, near the confluence of the Clearwater River and its north fork, with his reputation as a physician preceding him, Captain Clark was asked for a vial of his eye-water from a Nez Perce man who had presented him with a " very eligant gray mare." Clark knew his reputation had been built on his treatment of a Nez Perce man the previous fall who suffered from "knee and thye pain." As Lewis now wrote, Clark had "with much seremony washed & rubd" the sore leg of his patient with some "volitile linniment" that apparently cured his problem. The man "soon after recovered and has never ceased to extol the virtues of our medecines and the skill of my friend Capt C. as a phisician."

The reappearance of Dr. Clark and his medicine brought the Nez Perce in droves. With the food stores "now reduced to a mere handfull," the Lewis and Clark Clinic opened for service. Lewis wrote that "in our present situation I think it pardonable to continue this deseption for they will not give us any provision without compensation in merchandize," adding that "we take care to give them no article which can possibly injure them." Considering that Captain Clark took a potentially fatal dose of calomel contained in the five Rush's pills that he swallowed near the Three Forks of the Missouri the previous summer, I think that the captains, at least at times, did not know what was harmless and what was not.

When the hungry and tired Corps prepared their remaining dogs for dinner, the sight was met with laughter from some of the Nez Perce.

One man, as Lewis described, "verry impertinently threw a poor half starved puppy nearly into my plait by way of deresion for our eating dogs and laughed very heartily at his own impertinence..." Of all the men of the Corps this guy could have picked on, he chose the worst target for his jesting. "I was so provoked at his insolence," Lewis wrote, "that I caught the puppy and thew it with great violence at him and struk him in the breast and face, siezed my tomahawk and shewed him by signs if he repeated his insolence I would tommahawk him..." Undoubtedly sensing that he had made a big mistake, the Indian "...withdrew apparently much mortifyed and I continued my repast *on dog* without further molestation."

After that the Corps ascended another four miles up the Clearwater and camped near a Nez Perce village just below the mouth of the Potlatch River, "extreemly hungry and much fatiegued." The Indians proved to be tough traders and refused to trade anything except some roots. But one of the chiefs had brought an ill wife, who was suffering from an abscess on her lower back. The captains' clinic was open and Clark wanted payment for services rendered.

Following a procedure still performed today, he incised the abscess, drained the pus, and put some cloth packing into the cavity. Clark also applied some topical basilicon. Some doses of flowers of sulphur and cream of tartar were given for ingesting later. The cloth packing allowed the wound to stay open and drain, as well as heal without closing up prematurely—prior to resolution of the infection—and forming another festering sore. The basilicon was a mixture of resin, yellow wax, and lard,[3] probably thought to draw out the poison from the tissues. The flowers of sulfur was sometimes used in ointments or salves[4] and sometimes combined with cream of tartar (potassium bitartrate) and administered orally as a cathartic in treatment of skin diseases.[5] The surgical incision and drainage, with packing the wound, was the treatment of choice for abscesses. The rest of the treatment, including administering a cathartic, was worthless. There is no doubt at all that this procedure was very painful to the woman, but no note is made of using any laudanum or opium for pain relief. The payment they received for the surgical services of Dr. Clark was food on the hoof in the form of a horse that was delivered the next morning. It was immediately killed, butchered, cooked, and eaten.

The next morning, surgeon Clark changed the packing material of his patient's abscess. With the sore's inflammation decreased, the woman reported sleeping better than she had since the problem started. More evidence of Clark's greatness to the Indians.

A little girl was brought in with "the rhumatism." She was bathed in warm water that may have provided some momentary relaxation of her muscles and thus some pain relief. Balsam copaiba—an oily, resinous substance obtained from a South American tree (genus *Copaifera*)—was applied topically. Balsams are substances that contain benzoic or cinnamic acids that affect mucous membranes. They have been used through time for treatment of various problems from hemorrhoids and contact dermatitis to urethral irrigation in the treatment of gonorrhea.[6] I do not know what Captain Clark was trying to accomplish in this case, but it seems consistent with his thinking that putting something harmless on the skin was better than doing nothing, particularly in terms of getting some food in return. For several hours Captain Clark dropped his mysterious eyewash into the red and sore eyes of numerous Nez Perce. A second horse was delivered, and the men "obtained a plentifull meal, much to the comfort of all the party."

On the 7th, the Corps moved on and approached timbered hillsides, the first view of "the Spurs of the rocky Mountains which were in view from the high plain today…" Lewis also noted that they were "perfectly covered with snow" and that the Indians reported that it would be at least the first of June before they would be able to cross the range. The disappointment at this news can be felt in Lewis's entry of "this unwelcom inteligence to men confined to a diet of horsebeef and roots, and who are as anxious as we are to return to the fat plains of the Missouri and thence to our native homes."

On May 8, the Corps reached the lodge of their friend Twisted Hair, who had been engaged to care for their horses over the winter. Instead of finding their herd, they walked into the middle of a political fight between Twisted Hair and two other Nez Perce chiefs, Cutnose and Broken Arm. The latter two had been absent the previous fall and, on their return to their village, found that the Corps had come through and left their horses with Twisted Hair. Their jealousy of Twisted Hair's new status led to an ongoing argument, and Cutnose now claimed the horses had been neglected. The next day, with a reminder of two guns and powder as a reward, the Nez Perce began rounding up the twenty-one horses. Late that evening some of the horses were brought into camp while the Corps sat miserably in their exposed campsite, suffering a cold wind that "blew violently," accompanied by rain, hail, and then an all-night snowfall. They all had thought the winter was over!

Hiking onward to Chief Broken Arm's village through eight inches of snow on the 10th, the Corps accepted that they had left the coast too soon. The captains took advantage of a three-day layover while awaiting their horses' delivery. They began with a diplomatic meeting with the combined leaders of the Nez Perce nation, encouraging peace among the tribes of both sides of the Rockies. The Nez Perce countered that they needed guns to protect themselves from the warlike Blackfeet, or at least the presence of American army forts on the east side of the mountains. With negotiations going back and forth through English, French, Hidatsa, Shoshone, and Nez Perce, some of the essence of the discussion must have been lost. At the end of the summit meeting, the captains further influenced their hosts and "amused ouselves with shewing them the power of magnetism, the spye glass, compass, watch, air-gun and sundry other articles equally novel and incomprehensible to them."

As word spread among the Nez Perce of the white visitor's healing powers, Clark's practice as a physician continued to grow. Lewis noted that "many of the natives apply to us for medical aid which we gave them cheerfully so far as our skill and store of medicine would enable us." The captains agreed that Clark, being the Indians' preferred physician, would hold clinic while Lewis worked as a diplomat.

One of the problems listed as being common among the Indians was scrofula, or the infectious involvement of the body's lymph nodes with the tuberculosis bacterium, of the genus *Mycobacterium*. This disease produces enlarged lymph nodes that can drain cheesy material through broken down skin overlying the nodes. The disease is generally painless, and the victim may not have clinical evidence of tuberculosis elsewhere in the body. There was nothing the captains had in their pharmacy that would have been effective in treating this disease. Nothing—except their perceived magical treatments. Tularemia, caused by the bacterium *Francisella tularemia*, transmitted from handling raw game, could have been showing its cutaneous manifestation among these patients, confusing the captains.

Ulcers, various rheumatic complaints, inflamed eyes and "loss of the uce of their limbs are the most common" complaints from the Nez Perce. Lewis thought that a diet of roots may have contributed to the majority of the Indians' health problems, all those except the sore eyes and rheumatism. His reasoning was likely based on the common 18th century medical thought that the body's humors could be imbalanced by the diet.

Clark met a difficult and interesting case of "loss of uce of their limbs," an "extraordinary complaint" in which "a Chief of Considerable note…has been in the Situation I see him for 5 years. this man is incapable of moveing a single limb but lies like a corps in whatever position he is placed, yet he eats hartily, dejests his food perfectly, enjoys his under standing, his pulse are good, and has retained his flesh almost perfectly; in Short were it not that he appears a little pale from having been So long in the Shade, he might well be taken for a man in good health." Clark later recorded that he prescribed cold baths, and left a few doses of cream of tartar and flowers of sulphur as a cathartic, to be given every three days. Dr. Clark also recommended that the man eat more meat and fewer plants.

On the 13th and 14th, the Corps moved to campsite near present-day Kamiah, Idaho, where they would stay for the third-longest time of the whole trek, until June 10. Seven weeks of travel time had not been sufficient to allow for spring to do her work: there was still too much snow on the peaks to pass over the Bitterroots back to the plains of the Missouri. The men passed time with various activities aside from the constant action of the hunters and cooks. Games played included foot races between the men of the Corps and the Nez Perce. Shooting matches were held, and Lewis baffled the Indians, whose bows and arrows had a range of probably thirty yards, with his marksmanship and the power of his flintlock and its range of more than two hundred yards. The Nez Perce displayed their fabulous talents at horsemanship. Team games, including one called Prison Base, an 1806 version of Capture the Flag, cut some of the layover's tedium, and provided the men with some fun as well as the conditioning they would soon need to conquer the Bitterroots. Cruzatte played his fiddle on occasion and both the men of the Corps as well as the Indians danced for each other's entertainment.

Dr. Clark continued to offer his clinic. Two weeks after the paralytic chief came to the captains' attention, Private William Bratton was still suffering with his back problem that had begun at Fort Clatsop. Lewis noted that "he eats heartily digests his food well, and his recovererd his flesh almost perfectly yet is so weak in the loins that he is scarcely able to walk four or five steps, nor can he set upwright but with the greatest pain." John Shields now came up with an idea. He had seen men with similar complaints cured by sweating in a hot house. Bratton was game for anything after months of pain and asked for the procedure. Shields dug a hole four feet deep and three feet in diameter. A large fire was built inside the hole and removed once the earth was heated. The patient was placed on a seat inside the hole and an awning of blankets over willow poles was erected to cover the pit. Bratton was stripped naked, given some water to sprinkle inside to produce "as much steam or vapor as he could possibly bear," and left inside for about twenty minutes. Then he was taken out of the hole and put into icy water not once, but twice. He was then returned to the sweat hole for another round of forty-five minutes. After that he was wrapped in blankets and allowed to cool gradually while drinking "copious draughts of a strong tea" of horse-nettle.

By the following day, Bratton was amazingly "walking about today and says he is nearly free from pain." As Gary E. Moulton notes, various explanations have been offered to account for Bratton's lengthy back problem.[7] Some have suggested an abdominal infection but, given the history and remarkable recovery, I don't know what these theorists could be thinking about. Bratton simply didn't have any evidence that anything was wrong with his abdomen. The possibility of a herniated disc in his spine should be considered given the lengthy period of pain. Over the two-month period, it is possible that the disc material healed but some muscular spasms continued, which could have been relieved by the hot/cold treatments. From my personal experience with back pain, my vote goes to the possibility that Bratton never did rupture a disc, and simply was suffering from a bad case of degenerative disc disease and the arthritis that accompanied it. Or on a less likely note, he was malingering and simply decided that after the sweating it was time to stop faking his pain. Whatever the reason for Bratton's problem, he started feeling remarkably better after his treatments of frontier physical therapy.

That same day of Bratton's improvement, the Nez Perce arrived bearing the mysteriously paralyzed chief. Lewis observed that "this poor wretch thinks that he feels himself of somewhat better but to me there appears to be no visible alteration. we are at a loss what to do for this unfortunate man." So, they comforted him with a little laudanum—for who knows what reason—and some of the rancid portable soup.

By the next day, Clark had an idea. If it worked for Bratton, maybe it would work for the chief. On the 25th of May, they lowered the chief into the sweat hole. But the captains' inability to secure the chief led to the therapy's being cut short when the patient was unable to sit up. Two days later (after a day given to serious hunting and food-trading), the hole was enlarged and the man's father went in with him to support him during treatment. After the sweating, the chief was in considerable pain, a problem relieved with thirty drops of laudanum. On the 28th, Lewis noted an amazing discovery. "The sick Cheif was much better this morning he can use his hands and arms and sems much pleased with the prospect of recovering, he says he feels much better than he has for a great number of months." The following day the man "washed his face himself today which he has been unable to do previously for more than twelvemonths." On the 30th, after another treatment, the chief "could move one of his legs and thyes and work his toes pretty well, the other leg he can move a little; his fingers and arms seem to be almost entirely restored."

What could have accounted for this illness and its apparent remarkable recovery by nothing more than the sweating treatments? The possibility that there was something truly wrong with the man's bodily functions, that he was paralyzed or so weak he could not move, and yet responded so remarkably to the sweating treatments, in my mind is zero. Paralysis-producing diseases to consider in this case could include a ruptured disc in his neck, putting pressure on his spinal cord and resulting in a near-total body paralysis. If this were the case, he would need immediate spinal surgery to solve the problem and he would not have gotten well with sweating. Various other abnormalities of the brain or spinal cord could produce such pathology, but again would not respond to sweating. The mysterious Guillain-Barre syndrome can produce profound muscle weakness without a wasting of muscle mass in the involved limbs. This disease can be preceded by mild respiratory or gastrointestinal infection, followed by progressive bodily weakness. It can also be associated with infectious mononucleosis, hepatitis, or diphtheria. At times the syndrome can be fatal, but total recovery is seen in up to 75 percent of victims. The recovery usually occurs in a few weeks or month, but may take as long as six to eighteen months.[8] Although some factors of the chief's illness may fit, the entire picture does not, and it does not make sense to diagnose the man with Guillain-Barre syndrome.

Another possible explanation goes down the path of psychiatry. It is possible that the chief was suffering a mental disorder manifesting itself in an apparent bodily disease. A person suffering from this problem may not have voluntary control over physical symptoms. In an illness termed Somatization Disorder, the victim has symptoms suggestive of physical illness without any known physiological cause. It is believed that psychological conflicts or unfulfilled needs may result in this problem. We can't do a physical exam and lab tests on the Nez Perce chief, but we do know that he recovered his functional health by way of a treatment that would not heal any known physical cause of his symptoms. We also can't conduct an interview with him to assess his mental state. Could there have been something in his psychological past that could have resulted in his problem? It seems more likely to assign his problem to this cause than any of the other organic problems we have discussed. His recovery after being treated by a white man who was believed to have great medical powers—and possessed such fantastic items as compasses, magnifying lenses, and magnets—may have been a psychological cure of a grand scale.

Showing his up-to-the-minute medical knowledge, Lewis had expressed his wish that he had some electricity available to treat the chief's problem. The study of medical applications of electricity in the early 1800s was in its infancy. As a result of the discovery by Galvani and Volta in the latter 1700s that nerve and muscle function was dependent on electrical principles, numerous electrical treatment fads had developed. One was Englishman James Graham's "Temple of Health," where patients underwent mild electrical stimulation while they watched dancing girls.[9] Benjamin Franklin had experimented with electricity in treatment of some paralytics brought to him in hopes of achieving a cure from their disease by being "electrised," in Franklin's term. Franklin was apparently able to temporarily help some of those he treated who had unclear neurologic/muscular problems, but did not achieve any permanent successes. Electricity, by the time of Lewis's 1803 training, had developed a following among the medical and scientific community in hopes that it might be a cure-all for many mysterious ailments.

Clark's psychiatry skills were put to the test again with a woman who suffered from what Lewis thought hysteria and Clark called hypochondria. She was "much dejected." Clark gave her "30 drops of Laudanum" that depressed her a little more for a few hours. But for these few hours she probably felt much more euphoric. Other visitors to the camp clinic suffering from limb pains were treated with topical liniments, and some patients received one of the many cathartics in the medicine chest. There were always those who wanted the eye-water.

While all this was going on, Clark also was treating a patient dear to his heart. Pompey had taken seriously ill with a high fever and a swollen neck and throat on May 22. He had been cutting teeth and, with some diarrhea for several days, had not been feeling too well. But the swelling on the neck prompted some doses of Clark's favored remedy of "creem of tartar and flour of sulpher," meant to loosen up his bowels a bit, and a "poltice of boiled onions" applied hot and directly on his swollen neck. The next morning the cathartic medicine had "operated several times on the child in the course of the last night," but the neck was still swollen. Three onion poultices were applied to the little boy's neck during the day of the 23rd. The baby fussed all that night, and the swelling increased during the next two days. On May 25, Pompey was given more cathartics, and since they didn't "operate," the captains displayed their unmistakable preoccupation with suspected poisons in the child's colon by prescribing an enema! The next day, Lewis wrote triumphantly "the clyster given the Child last evening operated very well." The swelling was noted to be resolving "without coming to a head" although Clark feared on the 27th that "the Swelling on the Side of his neck I believe will termonate in an ugly imposthume a little below the ear." (Imposthume is the old-fashioned word for abscess.) More onion poultices and cathartics followed. On the 28th, Lewis noted that the child's fever was gone and the "imposthume is not so large but seems to be advancing to maturity." By June 3, Lewis was able to write, "the imposthume on his neck has in a great measure subsided and left a hard lump underneath his left ear; we still continue the application of the onion poltice." Two days later the poultices were discontinued and a plaster of salve made from pine resin, bee's wax, and bear oil was applied. What good that might have done, I am not aware of, but Clark thought it made the inflammation subside completely.

By June 8, some great results had come from the medical diplomacy of Dr. Clark. Lewis noted "The sick Cheif is fast on the recovery, he can bear his weight on his legs, and has acquired a considerable portion of strength." Pompey was "nearly well," and "Bratton has so far recovered that we cannot well consider him an invalid any longer..." Adding some praise for Bratton, Lewis wrote that "he has had a tedious illness which he boar with much fortitude and firmness." All three of their patients with the most challenging illnesses had recovered. The mystery illness of the Indian chief was handled with compassion and concern by Clark, and the bottom line was that the patient improved, resulting in probable elevation to very great status for Captain Clark in the eyes of the Nez Perce. Pompey's abscess had been wisely treated with common sense applications of heat and avoidance of surgery, although with the continuing ignorant adherence to cathartics. Bratton was the lucky patient of some good early American physical therapy that helped bring his two months of debilitating pain to an end.

They moved east to Weippe Prairie and began final preparations for the Bitterroots crossing. Summer was fast approaching, but two giant roadblocks stood in the way of Captains Lewis and Clark, Sacagawea, Pompey, and the men of the expedition—roadblocks that promised one last shot of misery and fatigue. The first was the ninety-seven miles of Rocky Mountain ridges and cliffs of the Nez Perce trail as it wound through the Bitterroots, and the second was the snow that covered it. They knew about the first, but were uncertain about the second. Would the snow be sufficiently melted to let them pass? They certainly hoped that would be so as they packed up their horses on June 15, 1806.

Their interlude with the Nez Perce provides a fascinating look into some of the medical practices and creative thinking of the Corps of Discovery. Their Nez Perce hosts had been friendly enough, certainly in stark contrast to the relations the men had had with the Chinookan natives of the lower Columbia. Now the men yearned to be homeward bound. The warm weather was here once again and the lengthening days of June and its warm sunlight on the vast snowfields of the Rockies steadily cleared them.

The line of packhorses left the Nez Perce villages and headed east into the ever increasing elevations of the western slope of the Rockies, toward what they believed to be their last big challenge. Perhaps the men by this time knew that recrossing the Bitterroots wouldn't be quite as easy as they hoped.

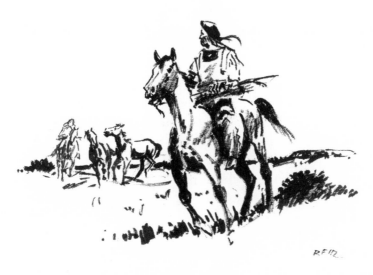

🌿 17 🌿

WILD TIMES IN OLD MONTANA

Act Three: June-August 1806

Maybe one day we shall be glad to remember even these hardships.
—Aeneid, Book 1

The packed horses traveled steadily in rain and mud throughout the day of June 15, 1806. As the Corps of Discovery and their horses went up the muddy slopes, several horses fell, but they struggled on for twenty-two miles through central Idaho. At least the game and grazing were sufficient. All around them Lewis noted the blooming springtime growth of the dogtooth violet, the honeysuckle and white maples.

But the 16th and 17th brought them again to snowdrifts. As the Corps pushed ahead on the morning of June 17 on sunlit southern slopes, snowdrifts twelve to fifteen feet deep and freezing winds that blew across them left Lewis's "hands and feet...benumbed." George Drouillard, the Corps' best woodsman, was uncertain as to which path to follow, and with five days of travel in front of them under the best circumstances, things started looking bleak. Lewis stated it well: "if we proceeded and should get bewildered in these mountains the certainty was that we should loose all our horses and consequently our baggage instruments perhaps our papers and thus eminently wrisk the loss of the discoveries which we had already made if we should be so fortunate as to escape with life." The choice was bitter but obvious. "Under these circumstances we conceived it madnes in this stage of the expedition to proceed without a guide..." If they waited for the snow to melt enough so that they could see the road to travel, they feared that they might be unable to reach the United States that year. They would need guides who could take them over when the snows had receded a bit more. The entire party was dejected. They had never had to turn back during the entire trip and now on their way home they were forced to do so. As if circumstances weren't discouraging enough, the skies dumped rain on them most of the evening.

The next day, Drouillard and George Shannon were sent back down the mountain. Their orders were to find the Nez Perce guides who had promised to accompany them. If the fee of a rifle wouldn't do it, two pistols and ten horses could be added as further incentive. Adding injury to despair, John Potts cut his leg severely with a knife, and John Colter's horse fell with him at the mouth of Hungery Creek, the current "roleing [them] over each other among the rocks."

The Corps retraced their steps behind Drouillard and Shannon, back to Weippe Prairie, feeling "some mortification," reaching the snow-free area on the 21st. Two days later, Drouillard, Shannon, and Whitehouse (the last sent back to trade for salmon) returned with three young Nez Perce men who had promised to guide the Corps to the Falls of the Missouri.

On June 24, the assault of the mountains began anew. In the evening, the guides lit fire to some tall fir trees in a ceremony meant to ensure good weather for the journey. Lewis noted that "the blaze was almost instantaneous and as the flame mounted to the tops of the highest trees, resembled a splindid display of fire-works." Climbing the ridges once again, two days later the captains noted that in the week since they had descended, the snow had melted about four feet. The Indian guides skillfully led their horses across the snowfields, and "along the steep sides of tremendious mountains entirely covered with snow…" The only bare ground visible was at the bases of trees. The rest of the landscape was never-ending snow. But when they camped on Bald Mountain by a spring, grass was plentiful. The men rested and the horses grazed.

Arising early on the 27th, "we resumed our route over the heights and steep hills of the same great ridge." At ten miles, they stopped at the insistence of the Indians and had a ceremonial smoke at an eight-foot-high pile of stones, capped by a fifteen-foot pole, atop a ridge. "from this elevated spot," Lewis wrote, "we had an extensive view of the stupendous mountains…we were entirely surrounded by those mountains from which to one unacquainted with them it would have seemed impossible ever to have escaped…" Their path was composed of hard-packed snow, where the horses' hooves sank only inches into the firm surface. Their progress was remarkably faster than on the crossing of the previous September. Several more days of travel across snow-covered ridges and slopes, with dinners of boiled roots fried in bear's oil, whet the men's appetites for the near future, when they would eat buffalo steaks and white pudding, celebrating victory in their return bout with the mountains.

By noon of the 29th, the Corps was now on the eastern slope and descending past the snowline. Potts' leg wound had become inflamed and possibly infected, but some relief of his symptoms were credited by the captains to a poultice of wild ginger leaves (*Asarum caudatum*), the leaves of which contain some antibacterial properties and also have been used to brew a tonic tea.[1]

That evening, with what I am sure must have been the utmost satisfaction, some of which I wish the captains had detailed in their writings, the men reached today's Lolo Hot Springs, about thirty-four miles up the slope from the Bitterroot valley floor and Travelers' Rest. The aches and pains of the horseback trip were washed and soaked away in the hot springs, where "both the men and indians amused themselves with the use of a bath this evening. I observed that the indians after remaining in the hot bath as long as they could bear it ran and plunged themselves into the creek the water of which is now as cold as ice can make it; after remaining here a few minutes they returned again to the warm bath, repeating this transision several times but always ending with the warm bath." After crossing 120 miles of snowy mountains, that must have been a most excellent and refreshing soak.

Six days after their departure from the west side of the Bitterroots, the Corps arrived once again at Travelers' Rest and immediately noted the sign and presence of mule and white-tailed deer, bighorn sheep, and elk. They had made the crossing five days more quickly than last year. On June 30, Clark wrote a heart-felt if understated assessment of the mountains that had vexed the entire Corps twice in the last year: "Descended the mountain to Travellers rest leaveing those tremendious mountanes behind us—in passing of which we have experiensed Cold and hunger of which I shall ever remember."

The Corps of Discovery's plan at this point was to separate its forces and strike out in different directions on the way back to civilization. Perhaps feeling invincible or at least a bit overconfident, each captain would take a group and explore different areas. Lewis and his men would head east, across the shortcut through the mountains, descend the eastern slope of the Rockies to the Great Falls and explore up the Marias River. The reconnaissance would determine the river's course and drainage, thus perhaps enlarging the territorial claims of the United States. Clark and his men, along with Sacagawea and Pompey, would head southeast, back to Camp Fortunate, travel down the Beaverhead and Jefferson Rivers to the Three Forks of the Missouri. His group would then split up further, with a group under the command of Sgt. Ordway taking the canoes left there the previous summer down the Missouri, through the Gates of the Rocky Mountains, to the Great Falls. At the falls they would reunite with Lewis and his men. Clark and the rest would hike overland to the Yellowstone River and descend it. Pryor and a few men would split off to herd the horses into Canada and use them to obtain supplies from British traders—an effort that failed when Crow Indians made off with the herd. Everybody would meet at the Missouri and Yellowstone confluence, they hoped, around the first of August.

From there it would be a rapid trip to Fort Mandan for a short lay-over, and then a straight shot downcurrent on the Missouri and at long last…St. Louis and civilization. St. Louis would offer a warm meal of nearly anything a guy could want, and some whiskey that no one had tasted in a year, since they had sipped their last taste on the Fourth of

July, 1805, at the Great Falls. The men looked forward to a warm bath and soft beds, fame, and land grants that President Jefferson had told them he would request from Congress (which were indeed approved). And some city women dressed in gowns. But lest they get too excited about all this, St. Louis was still, by Captain Clark's figures, 3,316 miles away.

On July 2, the captains were forced to write their journal entries inside their mosquito nets due to the tremendous plague of those happy insects enjoying their Montana summer. The men went about their chores, preparing to depart. The Nez Perce guides were paid with rifles that John Shields produced by cutting down the barrels of two that were broken off near the muzzle. Filled bullet pouches and powder horns topped off the payment.

On the 3rd of July, Lewis wrote "All arrangements being now completed for carrying into effect the several scheemes we had planed for execution on our return, we saddled our horses and set out I took leave of my worthy friend and companion Capt. Clark and the party that accompanyed him. I could not avoid feeling much concern on this occasion although I hoped this seperation was only momentary." Lewis's detachment included his beloved George Drouillard, Gass, the Field brothers, Werner, Frazer, Thompson, Goodrich and McNeal. The party wound their way through what is now the city of Missoula, Montana, to the fork of the present-day Blackfoot River/Clark's Fork, and up the picturesque grassy valleys that meander through the surrounding ranges of the pine-covered Rockies.

His Nez Perce companions accompanied the group to the confluence of the two rivers but changed their minds about continuing eastward, citing fear of their enemies the Blackfeet, Atsina, and Gros Ventre tribes.[2] Stories from the young Nez Perce men who had accompanied the Corps over the Bitterroots, as well as numerous earlier reports of Shoshone, Flathead, and Nez Perce fatal encounters with the Blackfeet Confederation had Lewis worried. "The minnetares of Fort de prarie [Gros Ventres] and the blackfoot indians rove through this quarter of the country and as they are a vicious lawless and reather an abandoned set of wretches I wish to avoid an interiew with them if possible," was his blunt opinion, based on hearsay about tribes that controlled the landscape through which he now traveled.

The mosquitoes became so troublesome to the group's horses that Lewis had large fires built at night to help drive the insects off. "these insects tortured them in such manner untill they placed themselves in the smoke of the fires that I realy thought they would become frantic." In an area of possible hostile encounters, one must wonder if building huges fires was a wise act. But the confidence grown from successful past Indian encounters, and the misery of the moment, must have helped spark those huge fires that lit up Montana's summer sky in 1806.

Lewis directed Drouillard and the Fields to kill some game to provide their Indian friends with a good store of provisions for their return westward. With fear for their new white friends, on the 4th "these affectionate people our guides betrayed every emmotion of unfeigned regret at seperating from us; they said that they were confidint that the Pahkees [Blackfeet] would cut us off." What a great encouragement this comment must have been—as the group of fewer than a dozen men started their way on an eighty-mile excursion through an area of obvious danger. Every minute of the next several weeks was spent on guard, watching in the distance for some evidence of the Blackfeet.

Lewis and group continued along the Blackfoot River, found the remains of thirty-two lodges that Lewis assumed were Blackfeet, and camped at Beaver Creek near present-day Lincoln, Montana, on the night of July 6.[3] Deer were now fat and plentiful, and Reubin Field even shot a moose in the forest. The rifle only wounded the nearly equine-sized animal, and an apparent encounter with the moose left Seaman "much worried." July 7 found Drouillard shooting three beavers, with the last one gaining some revenge by biting "his knee very badly" and then making his escape. The group struck northeast on a branch of the Blackfoot, and walked up to the head of today's Alice Creek, past numerous beaver ponds. From here they could follow the old Indian road for about a mile as it led up the side of a steep grassy slope sprinkled with the wildflowers, surrounded by pine-topped and green-carpeted mountains to the north, west, and south. As they reached the summit of the mountain, the expansive plains made their abrupt appearance to the east. Less than a day's hike ahead was the Garden of Eden, with buffalo and elk, flat ground to walk on, and warm weather. Most importantly of all, was the Missouri River, with its now friendly and inviting *eastward* current. They had, in the last four days, through the use of this shortcut to the Great Falls, accomplished what had taken them two and a half months to do by water and land the previous summer.

Meanwhile, Captain Clark, Ordway, Pryor, Bratton, Collins, Colter, Cruzatte, Gibson, Hall, Howard, Labiche, Lepage, Potts, Shannon, Shields, Weiser, Whitehouse, Willard, Windsor, York, Charbonneau, Sacagawea and Pompey had left Travelers' Rest and headed toward the southeast on the morning of July 3. Riding a "hard-trotting" horse through the Bitterroot valley did not agree with John Potts, who was still suffering from the healing leg wound. The all-day, thirty-six-mile horseback ride was too much for Potts, and his pain and misery prompted Clark to "give him a pill of Opium which Soon releve him." I'm sure Potts was feeling no pain whatsoever that night and, at least in his mind, was back in a feather bed in St. Louis.

Potts' wound, a cut from a large knife during the return trip over the Bitterroots on June 18, had been reported to be a severe laceration of the inner aspect of his thigh, a wound that Lewis noted resulted in significant blood loss. Lewis had difficulty stopping the bleeding "untill I applied a tight bandage with a little cushon of wood and tow on the veign below the wound." If Potts was still having this much pain from this wound he had suffered two weeks before, and Lewis had bothered to mention it at all, we can be sure that Potts certainly must have filleted his leg open in a dramatic fashion.

We are left by Lewis to speculate exactly what structure in Pott's leg was cut. If we take Lewis at his word that a vein was cut, it may have been the relatively superficial saphenous vein or one of its branches. The function of veins is to return blood to the heart and lungs, after it has made its way through the arterial and capillary systems and released its oxygen to the cells of working muscles and organs. Although blood pressure in the venous system is lower than that in the arterial system, severing a vein could still result in significant blood loss.

Major arteries, however, when lacerated and untreated, can result in the victim's bleeding to death due to the higher pressures involved in the arterial side of circulation. Smaller branches of arteries can pump blood out like squirt guns, a stream shooting from the wound with every beat of the patient's heart. Potts could have partially lacerated the relatively superficial common femoral artery, if the wound was well up on the inner aspect of his thigh. This type of wound would certainly have produced some rapid and dramatic bleeding. Such a wound could have also damaged surrounding musculature, adding to the severity, pain, and delayed healing. The exact nature of Potts' wound is lost to history, but it makes for interesting speculation.

Clark, unlike his fellow captain, stopped the expedition early on the Fourth of July, "a Day commonly Scelebrated by my Country" and "partook of a Sumptious Dinner of a fat Saddle of Venison and Mush of Cows (roots)." The band crossed numerous rushing creeks, fed from the melting snowpacks of today's Sapphire Mountains. The rapid currents at times flowed over the backs of the fording horses, soaking the supplies they carried. At the end of the valley the next day, Clark crossed to the East Fork of the Bitterroot River and continued along its bank, and into the valley of Ross's Hole, where they had met the Salish the previous September. Poor Shannon discovered he had left his tomahawk behind at the site where he had shot a deer earlier in the day. Clark made him go back and get it and, luckily, Shannon returned by sunset.

The night of July 5 was, according to Clark, "so cold that I could not Sleep." The next day they were assaulted by a freezing rain shower accompanied by violent winds, which forced them to take cover for an hour and a half. When the squall passed, they proceeded down Trail Creek into thirteen-mile-wide Big Hole, a high mountain valley rimmed to the east by ten-thousand-foot peaks of today's Pioneer Mountains. The soaked party halted, built large fires, enjoyed the heat, and "dryed our Selves." Nine of Clark's best horses were nowhere to be found the following morning, possible victims of what Clark called "Some Skulking Shoshones." Clark decided to push southward another twenty miles to Camp Fortunate. There he would raise and dry the canoes that had been hidden underwater in the Beaverhead River for the last eight months. In the meantime, Ordway, Shannon, Gibson, Collins and Labiche did their best to try to locate the missing horses.

On their way south, Clark came upon present-day Jackson Hot Spring, "too hot for a man to endure his hand in it 3 seconds." Clark stopped for a little outdoor fun and had Sergeant Pryor and Private Shields cook small pieces of meat in the hot, sulfur-tinged waters. That afternoon they got through Big Hole Pass, and camped on what Clark named Willard's Creek (now Divide Creek).

On July 8, the group reached their campsite of the previous August 17, a site where a cache of provisions had been left. Knowing that the pit contained tobacco, Clark noted, "most of the Party with me being Chewers of Tobacco become So impatient to be chewing it that they Scercely gave themselves time to take their Saddles off their horses before they were off to the deposit." They joyfully dug up the contents, and Captain Clark awarded each tobacco enthusiast two feet of rolled tobacco. The rest was to be sent down the Missouri with Ordway's group to the men waiting at the Great Falls. The canoes were raised, and all except one were in good shape. Clark reflected on the 164 miles they had traveled from Travelers' Rest, noting that "with only a few trees being cut out of the way would be an excellent waggon road."

At 10 A.M. of July 9, Ordway and his men rejoined Clark with the nine horses that had been lost. Preparations were now underway for Ordway, Collins, Colter, Cruzatte, Howard, Lepage, Potts, Weiser, Whitehouse and Willard to descend the Missouri for approximately 150 miles, from the Three Forks to the Great Falls. Clark would continue with the remainder on horseback down the Yellowstone.

Both parties left Camp Fortunate on the frosty morning of July 10, after Clark had awakened to find three-fourths of an inch of ice on water left overnight in a bowl. Clark's party passed down the Beaverhead Valley, past the immense Beaverhead Rock that Sacagawea had recognized the previous August, then filling their discouraged souls with hope that they would soon find the Shoshones, and horses to cross the Bitterroots. They were all probably greatly relieved that monumental tasks were now just a painful memory. The Beaverhead and Big Hole (Wisdom River) flowed together to form the Jefferson, which Clark's entire group followed to the confluence of the Madison and Gallatin Rivers at the Three Forks. They reached that landmark on July 13.

Ordway and his crew departed down the Missouri, waving farewell to Clark on the afternoon of the 13th, after a hot meal. Their next six days were an uneventful trip to the Great Falls. Uneventful except for the mosquitoes, which Ordway described as being "much worse than they were last year."⁴

By July 13, Lewis's party was once again near the Great Falls, having spent two days at the "white bear islands" where the river bottom "on both sides of the river were crouded with buffaloe." Lewis dug up one of the caches only to find that the Missouri's water had invaded the hole, ruining two grizzly skins and numerous dried plant samples. In an occurrence that would foreshadow events in Lewis's future, the stopper in a vial of laudanum had come out, spilling the narcotic fluid into the rest of the medicines, ruining most of the stock "in such a manner that it was past recovery."

On July 13, Drouillard, who had been sent up the Sun River in search of some lost horses, did not return during the evening. By the afternoon of the 15th, Lewis wrote with a worried tone, "I had already settled it in my mind that a whitebear had killed him and should have set out tomorrow in surch of him…" Lewis worried that if Drouillard had discovered a grizzly "in the plains even he would attack him." If his horse had thrown Drouillard and run off, "in that situation the chances in favour of his being killed would be as 9 to 10." Much to everyone's relief, Drouillard rode into camp that afternoon, minus the horses, which had apparently been stolen by a band of Indians.

July 15 also saw the curtain rise on Act Three of "Wild Times in Old Montana." Lewis dispatched Hugh McNeal to ride across the sixteen-mile portage route to the lower camp of 1805 and check on the cache and the state of the white pirogue. Nearly reaching the lower portage camp, McNeal unknowingly rode his mount to within ten feet of some brush that contained a huge grizzly. The bear came out and, terrified, the horse reared and threw McNeal to the ground—right at the bear's feet. The equally surprised grizzly stood up on his hind legs to see what was going on. McNeal grabbed the barrel of his rifle, scampered to his feet and swung the rifle for all he was worth, clobbering the bear over the head. "…the bear stunned with the stroke fell to the ground and began to scratch his head with his feet; this gave McNeal time to climb a willow tree which was near at hand and thus fortunately made his escape." The bear walked circles around the base of the tree for several hours, and finally wandered off. McNeal, probably with equal amounts of relief and anxiety, climbed down, found his horse two miles away and, along with his broken rifle, rode back to camp, with a story that has impressed everyone for the last two hundred years. Lewis wrote "these bear are a most tremenduous animal; it seems that the hand of providence has been most wonderfully in our favor with rispect to them, or some of us would long since have fallen a sacrifice to their farosity."

On their descent of the Yellowstone, Clark and his overland party were to have their own "wild times" with numerous grizzly encounters and other adventures. Private Gibson suffered a deep puncture wound in the thigh. His pain soon made horseback riding impossible, so Clark sent John Shields to find trees from which they could build canoes to float down the river. During the foray, two bears chased Shields on his horse.

One of my favorite tasks as a physician is to clean and treat wounds such as the one suffered by George Gibson. His wound—and the added dangers of the nonsterile field treament he received—remind me of a time when I spent two hours removing rock and dirt from a bicy-clist's elbow. I painstakingly removed every piece of visible foreign body, thoroughly rinsed and washed the cavity with a disinfecting sponge, and placed the patient on antibiotics. In spite of all this, the wound still got infected. Such wounds are nasty to suffer and difficult to treat.

Gibson had fallen from his horse onto an inch-diameter, broken and burned stick that ripped into the quadriceps musculature of his thigh to a depth of two inches. This wound should have been anaesthetized and surgically explored to remove any dirt, pieces of wood, and dead tis-sue—to minimize the possibility of subsequent infection. There was probably some significant but short-lived bleeding and a good deal of pain. Gibson's wound was dressed by Clark and, luckily, began to visi-bly improve within a couple of days. Gibson fortunately recovered with-out any apparent infection.

Once the canoes were finished and the float began, several grizzly bears appeared along the route. Some were hunted while others were just observed in passing. As the canoe floated at 8 A.M. on August 12, "a Bear of the large vicious Species being on a Sand bar raised himself up on his hind feet and looked at us as we passed down near the middle of the river. he plunged into the water and Swam towards us, either from a disposition to attack't or from the Cent of the meat which was in the Canoes. we Shot him with three balls and he returned to Shore badly wounded."

Both captains witnessed uncountable numbers of buffalo. With mating season at hand, Lewis—nearing White Bear Island—noted that "the bulls keep a tremendious roaring we could hear them for many miles and there are such numbers of them that there is one continual roar." Clark's note describing his experience several hundred miles away stated that on July 25 "emence herds of Buffalow…with those animals the bulls keep Such a grunting nois which is very loud and disagreeable Sound that we are compelled to Scear them away before we can Sleep." Clark had to pull his canoes to the shoreline one day for nearly two hours to allow a continuous flow of the beasts, "as thick as they could Swim" to pass across the river. The days of gut-gnawing hunger were now far behind.

On July 19, the Ordway group reached the shore of White Bear Island. He met Gass's group of five who had come overland with Lewis and, together with the help of four horses, took the canoes and supplies once again across the portage route to below the series of falls. The men assembled the wagons, and with difficulties of broken wheels and wagon tongues, completed the portage on July 26. Weiser managed to cut his leg severely, becoming the newest invalid. Occasional rains made the plains so muddy that the wagon wheels sank several inches into the greasy earth. But the rain was somewhat welcome in relieving men and horses from the ever-present mosquitoes. When it wasn't raining during camptime, the men built fires of dried buffalo dung, which produced clouds of smoky early American insect repellent.

On July 16, Lewis, Drouillard, and the Field brothers left for their much anticipated reconnaissance of the Marias River. Lewis wanted to take more men, but the lack of horses made strengthening the little army impossible. They headed into a plain that "as far as the eye can reach looks like a well shaved bowlinggreen." After stopping for two hours to sketch Rainbow Falls (the middle of the five cascades), they pushed ahead to camp at the "Great Falls," site of today's Ryan Dam. With only four men going into Blackfeet country, Lewis' adventure up the Marias to establish the location of its headwaters and survey its drainage was the most dangerous and reckless undertaking to date for the Corps. Lewis wrote of his belief that should they encounter the Blackfeet in their weakened state, they would likely be robbed of their supplies, guns, and horses. Therefore, he wrote, "I am determined to take every possible precaution to avoid them if possible."

Nothing much went smoothly on that trip. On July 21, one of the packhorses fell into the river and wet the scientific instruments. Lewis dried them and their cases. On Cut Bank Creek, the Marias' north fork, the horses bore the men "between clifts of freestone rocks...the bottom narrow below us," and the rocky trail made the unshod horses' feet "extreemly soar." There was no wood to start fires, so buffalo dung was used. The weather turned "extreemly cold," with periodic wind and rain, and Lewis noted "our situation extreemly unpleasant." Drouillard found recently abandoned Indian camps, and their fear of an unwanted encounter grew. Following Cut Bank Creek upstream kept taking them to the southwest—the wrong direction for extending the Louisiana Purchase's boundary. They stopped at what Lewis named "Camp Disappointment," and he tried for two days to take celestial readings, but cloudy weather wouldn't allow it. Without longitude readings, but with the threat of running into hostile Blackfeet, he decided to call it quits and return to the Missouri.

Drouillard, separated from the trio of Lewis and Joseph and Reubin Field on July 26, soon became an unknowing spectacle for eight Blackfoot warriors who, along with about thirty horses, stood atop a sharp barren ridge watching his every move. The nearby Lewis and Field brothers discovered the Indians, and Lewis immediately pulled out his telescope to survey what he described as "a very unpleasant sight." Believing that he could make the best of the situation, Lewis slowly and cautiously approached the band of young warriors, who initially acted "much allarmed," then approached cautiously. The men dismounted and untrustingly shook hands. Drouillard was retrieved, and through Drouillard's sign language, Lewis conducted an interview with the men, who were Piegan Blackfeet. The Indians seemed "much agitated with our first interview." Lewis tried to curry favor by giving one of their three indicated chiefs a medal, another a handkerchief and the third a flag, "with which they appeared well satisfyed." Reassuring the young men that he was "glad to see them and had a great deel to say," Lewis invited them to camp for the evening. The united band went down a steep bluff and formed a camp on today's Two Medicine River.

With tobacco smoke filling the air around their campfire, conversation with the hands followed for several hours, Drouillard signing back and forth with the Indians. Lewis learned that there was a large band of Piegans within a half-day's march, near the base of the mountains. The Indians told of their trading furs with white men for liquor, guns, and ammunition about six days north on the Saskatchewan River. Lewis gave his standard speech about creating a peace between the Blackfeet and their enemies, the Shoshone, Nez Perce, Crow, and Flathead nations. He talked about future trade with the Americans and assured them that if they would accompany him back to his men at the mouth of the Marias that he would "give them 10 horses and some tobacco." The Indians "made no reply." The parley ended.

Everyone except Meriwether Lewis lay down on buffalo robes to sleep. The captain kept the first watch until 11:30 P.M. and then awoke Reubin Field for his shift. All had been quiet for Reubin when he awoke his brother for his turn at guard duty. Joseph, sitting next to his sleeping brother, twisted around and laid his rifle behind him on the ground. He sat and watched.

At daylight, the Indians gathered around the fire and hatched their plot. One of the warriors quietly walked behind the drowsy Joseph, quickly grabbed both the Fields' rifles, and started running away. Two others simultaneously grabbed Lewis's and Drouillard's rifles. Fully aroused by the action, Joseph hollered to his brother, who "instantly jumped up and pursued the indian," running him down within about twenty yards. Reubin grabbed his knife while he ran and, as he wrested the guns from the young man, plunged the blade into his chest. The warrior staggered about "15 steps and fell dead."

Meanwhile, Drouillard, who had been awake when a Piegan grabbed his gun, cried, "Damn you, let go my gun!" That immediately awoke Lewis. Drouillard wrestled his rifle back. Lewis, undoubtedly in a severe state of mental fogginess, said "What's the matter?" Within seconds it all became crystal clear. Reaching for his rifle and finding it gone, Lewis pulled out his pistol and ran after the Indian fleeing with his rifle. Lewis's shouted command to drop the rifle, with the added incentive provided by the cocked rifles of the Field brothers, led the Indian to comply. Lewis told his men to hold their fire.

The Blackfeets' attention now turned to driving off the horses, and they hazed them up the river. Being unhorsed in this country could be a death sentence. Lewis was in hot pursuit, ordering the other Corps members to fire on the Indians if they persisted in stealing the horses. A young Blackfeet ran the horses up a canyon about a hundred yards away from the campsite. Lewis, speaking English to the non-English–speaking men, shouted that he would "shoot them if they did not give me my horse." He raised his rifle and one of the two jumped behind a rock. The other stopped, and Lewis shot him in the guts. The wounded warrior crumpled first to his knees and then to the ground—but, using his right elbow, raised himself enough to aim at the captain's figure fifty feet away, and squeezed the trigger. The lead ball whizzed by Lewis's uncovered head so closely that he felt "the wind of his bullet very distinctly." The wounded man crawled away to hide behind a rock.

Lewis now "leasurely" walked back to camp. Within seconds, Drouillard and Lewis were saddling and packing horses, and the Field brothers soon returned with several more. Lewis threw the Indians' abandoned belongings, including shields, bows, and quivers of arrows, into the campfire. The young men, in their confusion, had left one of their two guns by the campfire, and it now became property of the Corps of Discovery. Lewis also grabbed the flag that had been given as a present the day before, and then walked over to the body of the dead man. Noticing the medal of peace around his lifeless neck, Lewis left it there, so "that they might be informed who we were," openly advertising that the white men had nothing to fear from the Blackfeet. It was a highly defiant act, much more one of military triumph than of diplomatic initiative.

From a medical standpoint, the young stabbing victim most assuredly died within seconds, as a result of the knife piercing his thoracic cavity and producing massive internal injuries. The stab would have created a pneumothorax, or collapsing of the lung, inside the thoracic cavity. John Ordway's report, as it was relayed to him, was that "he drew but one breath   the wind of his breath followed the knife & he fell dead."[5] From this graphic description, we can hear the sound of outside air rushing into the wound.

But the bleeding involved in a knife-produced pneumothorax would probably not be sufficient to cause such a quick death. The several-inch-long blade probably directly wounded the heart, causing massive internal bleeding, and the heart ceased to function. This could have occurred either through direct trauma to the cardiac muscle, causing its pumping action to fail, or through damage to the pericardium, the sac that surrounds the heart. A wound to the pericardium could have produced bleeding inside the sac, creating pressure that inhibited the filling of the heart's chambers. The condition—known as a cardiac tamponade—could progress to the point that the pericardium was so full of blood that the heart muscle could not function as a pump. But this process would still not have produced a death within fifteen seconds. What probably occurred with the wound Reubin Field inflicted was that the point and blade severed major pulmonary arteries or veins, resulting in rapid internal hemorrhage, a rapid drop in blood pressure, unconsciousness, and a quick death.

Although we do not know if the man shot by Lewis was dead or not, I find it improbable that he survived. At about fifty feet or so away, the .54 caliber rifle ball probably had the muzzle velocity nearly equal to a modern .357 magnum. The diameter of the ball in the .54 is larger, creating an impact roughly equal to that of the modern-caliber projectile. The bullet from the flintlock did not penetrate as far as a modern bullet would have due to its shape. Once it pierced the skin, muscular wall, and omentum, the bullet probably ruptured portions of intestine and perhaps some major arteries in the mesentery, the apron of tissue overlying the intestines. If the bullet partially severed one of these mesenteric arteries, significant bleeding could have continued to the point of causing death. But if one of the mesenteric arteries was totally severed, it could have contracted enough to stop the bleeding. The lead ball could have hit the liver, pancreas, kidneys, or spleen, organs that are highly vascular, and would have produced significant bleeding and death within minutes to hours, depending on the rate of hemorrhage. The quickest death for the unfortunate victim would have occurred if the bullet penetrated and pierced the aorta that runs down the left side of the spine within the chest and abdomen. This would have resulted in death within seconds to minutes. The slowest and most painful scenario would have resulted from the lead ball's piercing the large intestine, spilling the contents into the abdomen, and setting up an infection that could have taken several days to kill the man. A painful way to die, to be sure.

The forensic pathology of the incident is fascinating, but the bottom line was that there was at least one, and probably two, dead young Blackfeet, one with an identifying medal around his neck, given to him by his killers. What were Lewis and his party to do? They were suddenly faced with the very real possibility of being overcome, then possibly becoming victims of their own weapons, or losing their horses more than a hundred miles away from the Missouri. Lewis expected more Piegan warriors to return once they heard of the fight, and also was aware he'd freely said that more of his men waited at the mouth of the Marias. Perhaps they should have never camped with the young Blackfeet, who were obviously prepared for trouble. But Lewis had wanted to give his "peace among the tribes" speech. We can't be certain about the extent of the negative impact this incident had on the future relationship between the two cultures, but it certainly was not positive, and the Blackfeet and whites continued to be major thorns in each other's sides for years to come.

The four horsemen now fled for their lives across the northern Montana plains "and pushed our horses as hard as they would bear." By 3 P.M. and sixty-three miles away from the site of the fight, they reached the Teton River, and took an hour's break to take some food and water and allow the horses to graze. Some late afternoon rain moistened the ground and provided a perfect softened track for the horses. After another seventeen miles they stopped at dark, killed a cow buffalo, cooked dinner, rested for two hours, and remounted. Under a surrealistic night sky, with moonbeams filtering through broken rain clouds and illuminating the flat prairie, they passed through thousands of buffalo dotting the plains. By 2 A.M. on July 28, nearly twenty-four hours after starting their ride from hell, they stopped, turned their horses loose, and lay down on the ground a few miles west of present-day Fort Benton, Montana.[6] Lewis noted that the party was "very much fatiegued as may be readily conceived."

"I was so soar from my ride yesterday that I could scarcely stand" were his words the next morning. Drouillard and the Fields were in similar pain as they struggled to their feet, but "I encourged them by telling them that our own lives as well as those of our friends and fellow travellers depended on our exertions at this moment." Muscles pushed beyond their normal limits, muscles that were already in outstanding condition, ached and groaned with overexertion created by the nearly one-hundred-mile, eighteen-hour ride. Their goal was to reach the Missouri as soon as possible, meet their fellow soldiers and make their stand or escape, whatever should be required. By 9 A.M., the weary quartet began a twenty-mile ride to the Missouri and, with what Lewis described as "unspeakable satisfaction," spied their comrades descending the river in the canoes. They rode the horses to the riverside, the canoes reached the riverbank, they stripped the horses and, with some military humor, Lewis "gave them a final discharge." Lewis and the others hastily arranged their gear and, with shaking limbs, climbed aboard the dugouts.

By 1 P.M., Gass and Willard joined the reunion, having brought the horses downriver from the falls, as Lewis had previously ordered; the animals had been used to hunt and then pack in meat for the enlarged group. Now Lewis's band of four men had grown to twenty. The group paddled to the island to retrieve the red pirogue left there thirteen months earlier, but found the boat needed so much repair that it would not answer its original calling. They cannibalized it, pulling nails and stripping iron for some future use. The white pirogue, along with five small canoes, then embarked from the Marias-Missouri confluence and added another fifteen miles to the distance between Lewis's men and the Blackfeet.

With lightning and thunder crashing overhead, hail and rain pouring down, and his body still unbearably sore, Lewis spent the night lying in the wet canoe. Within hours the group retraced their Missouri trek through the forty-mile stretch of enchanted rock formations of the White Cliffs area, and camped at the same site where they had rested on May 29, 1805. Lewis noted the river's being high and that "every little rivulet now discharges a torrant of water bringing down immece boddies of mud sand and filth from the plains and broken bluffs." He scooped up some of the river to relieve his thirst, "so thick with mud and sand that it is with difficulty I can drink it." I shudder to think what kinds of organisms may have been in his cup of water—and marvel that he drank it at all.

Their goal now was to reach the Yellowstone River and Captain Clark as quickly as they could, although they needed to send hunters ashore. The men now harvested deer, elk, buffalo, and an occasional grizzly in this wildlife-rich area.

With one more swipe of intended disaster, the Missouri River had yet another surprise for the Corps of Discovery. Willard, now fully recovered from his probable springtime pneumonia, and Ordway had been out hunting on August 4. They had killed two deer and a silver-gray grizzly but their hunt had extended into the night. Trying to catch up to the main team and still canoeing at 11 P.M., the men found themselves in a mass of partially submerged trees, a nest of swirling liquid danger. Willard, in the back of the canoe, tried to steer through the mess but was unable to avoid a tree that knocked him overboard into the black river's rapid current. He grabbed the tree and held on for dear life while the current floated Ordway and the canoe a half-mile downriver. Ordway maneuvered the canoe to shore and ran back up the bank to find Willard. Willard, hanging on to the tree trunk, may have shouted his inquiry, "Is everything all right?" But he couldn't hear Ordway's reply due to the current roaring around the sawyers. Willard grabbed a couple of pieces of floating wood, lashed them together, tied his clothes on the float and let go. He maneuvered his way through the danger and floated a mile downriver until he could get back into the canoe. Soaked to the bone, the two men paddled a short distance downstream and joined their comrades around a friendly, warming fire with yet another exciting tale of adventure.

By August 7, 1806, the Lewis party arrived at the mouth of the Yellowstone and found a note from Clark, who abandoned the campsite due to too many mosquitoes and too little game. Lewis in turn left a note for Collins and Colter, thought to be behind hunting, and proceeded down the Missouri into present-day North Dakota. Many of the men were nearly naked, their buckskins rotten with continued use in wet weather. But at least it was summer and there was plenty to eat, and that river current was still flowing in the right direction.

The Missouri River, from the confluence of the Yellowstone, past the Great Falls and the Gates of the Mountains, to the Three Forks and over the great divide, then the trek to the Bitterroot valley and over those great mountains had provided the explorers with many of their greatest adventures and most precarious situations. There had been the grizzly encounters too numerous to mention—any one of which would provide the story of a lifetime for one of us modern-day folks. They'd had hardships of travel and disease, injury from hailstones, a flash flood in a narrow ravine, and a deadly encounter with young Blackfeet. Sacagawea had nearly died the year before at the Great Falls, and many a night the men had sat around campfires pulling prickly pear spines out of their feet. There had been days of blistering heat and mornings of frost-covered blankets. Elation at discovering the Great Falls changed to apprehension at the sight of the jagged, snowy Bitterroots. This had been a land of beauty and danger, celebration and dejection, health and sickness. Willard and his late night swim in the middle of the river was yet another narrowly escaped disaster—and the last act in the Corps of Discovery's "Wild Times in Old Montana."

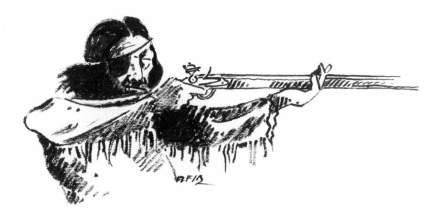

⚜ 18 ⚜

NEAR DISASTER AND THEN...

Back Home: August and September, 1806

*Oh! Weep no more today! We will sing one song for the old
Kentucky Home, For the old Kentucky Home far away.*
—*Stephen Foster*

By the second week of August 1806, there was undoubtedly a high
level of excitement among the men. On August 12, Meriwether
Lewis and his men met two trappers from Illinois who were ascending
the Missouri. The men reported having passed Captain Clark the day
before, on his way downstream. These were the first new faces of civilization the men had seen in nearly two years.

Lewis' ability to ask questions of the trappers was hampered by his
extreme pain, and also due to the fact that he was laid out in the bottom of a canoe, unable to move, with a bullet wound in his back end.

"Damn you! You have shot me!" he had screamed the previous morning.

Lewis and Pierre Cruzatte had pulled their canoe to an island to stalk an elk herd, and as Lewis and Pierre Cruzatte made their way through the brush Lewis spied an animal, raised his rifle to shoot and suddenly felt a lead ball rip into his left buttock, and through his right buttock, lodging itself in his buckskin pant leg. Shouting his fury at Cruzatte but receiving no answer, Lewis feared that Indians were attacking, and ran limping back to the canoe, shouting his warning to the men waiting on the river. While Patrick Gass aided the wounded Lewis, the remaining men assaulted the island but found no Indians. They did find Cruzatte, however, but he seemed to know nothing about the incident.

The lead ball that came from the muzzle of Cruzatte's Harpers Ferry rifle had entered Lewis's "left thye about an inch below my hip joint, missing the bone it passed through the left thye and cut the thickness of the bullet across the hinder part of the right thye; the stroke was very severe..."

It sounds as if the approximately half-inch ball had penetrated the gluteus muscle of the left buttock, passed out the skin of the left buttock and entered the right buttock at a shallower depth, but enough to "cut the thickness of the bullet." Lewis probably had almost no fat at all in the area, so the wound probably damaged the muscle significantly. Only an inch or two deeper lies the main nerve of the entire leg, the sciatic nerve. In spite of the muscle damage, Lewis had made his retreat back to the boat using his gluteus muscles with every step. Within moments they rebelled with pain and stiffness to such a degree that he no longer wanted to move.

Lewis treated and packed his bleeding wounds with some packing cloth but, noting that although in great pain, he wrote with some relief that "I was hapy to find that it had touched neither bone nor artery." In what Lewis described as "infinite pain" when he moved, he lay in the bottom of the dugout for the rest of the day and, in fact, slept in the same position, experiencing "a very uncomfortable night," adding that "the pain I experienced excited a high fever."

It should be noted that in 18th century medical jargon, the "high fever" described by Lewis was probably nothing more than a rapid pulse produced by the extreme pain, and by a very high level of sympathetic nervous system activity the pain produced. The sympathetic nervous system controls our bodily functions that help us escape dangerous situations. If this system goes into high gear, stores of epinephrine are released into our bloodstreams, making our hearts beat faster, and we breathe more quickly through dilated and relaxed airways, a good reaction if you are running for your life.

It is very interesting to consider that if Pierre Cruzatte was fifty yards away from Lewis when he shot him, that as little as one fiftieth of an inch change in his aim would have resulted in the bullet's going an inch deeper and very possibly wounding Lewis's sciatic nerve, leaving him with a worthless left leg and very painful wound. If Cruzatte had been seventy-five yards away, only a one seventy-fifth of an inch change in his muzzle's position could have produced a crippled Captain Lewis. That is less than a twitch in Cruzatte's arms that supported his rifle. I'd rather be lucky than talented. Lewis, at least in this aspect, was incredibly lucky.

As Clark's party awaited the arrival of the rest of the men, George Shannon was up to his old tricks. He had once again lost his tomahawk or left it behind at the previous night's campground. Clark ordered him back to find it. (I am inclined at this point to write Shannon a prescription of Ritalin, which in all honesty would probably have helped him pay a little more attention to his actions. It seems that if he wasn't losing himself, he was losing his tomahawk.)

On August 12, Gass wrote that Captain Lewis was in good spirits, and Lewis himself wrote first about meeting the trappers who brought news of Clark (and then decided to return to the Mandan-Hidatsa villages with Lewis) before adding that "my wounds felt very stiff and soar this morning but gave me no considerable pain." The cure-all poultice of Peruvian bark was applied to the wound.

That same afternoon, John Colter and John Collins canoed into Lewis's camp, having been separated for the last nine days. They had been hunting and believed that Lewis was somewhere behind them. They waited for several days and then, seeing no one, correctly concluded that they were the ones who were behind and played catch-up until that moment. Within hours, the Lewis canoes floated to within sight of Clark's campground.

Clark wrote, "I was alarmed on the landing of the Canoes to be informed that Capt. Lewis was wounded by an accident—. I found him

Near Disaster and Then...

lying in the Perogue, he informed me that his wound was slight and would be well in 20 or 30 days this information relieved me very much. I examined the wound and found it a very bad flesh wound the ball had passed through the fleshey part of his left thy below the hip bone and cut the cheek of the right buttock for 3 inches in length and the debth of the ball." Although Cruzatte got the blame, Clark held no bad feelings towards him, noting that Cruzatte "is near Sighted and has the use of but one eye, he is an attentive industerous man and one whome we both have placed the greatest Confidence in dureing the whole rout." Captain Clark took over as Lewis's personal physician and continued to pack the wound, an experience that on one occasion made Lewis faint from the pain involved.

A lesson learned: I have enjoyed many a hunting trip. My memories of the fun and adventure with friends and family are treasures of my life. But I have never, and will never, go hunting with a near-sighted man wearing no glasses, and having but one eye.

On August the 14th, the fleet of the Corps of Discovery began to see signs of Indian villages along the riverbanks and, with salutes firing from blunderbuss rifles, they triumphantly paddled into the Hidatsa and Mandan villages, where they had wintered in 1804-1805.

Lewis of course arrived laid out in the canoe. Clark enjoyed a happy reunion with the chiefs of the Hidatsa and Mandans and disappointingly learned that the Sioux were still at war and "had killed Several of their men Since we had left them…" Because of these continued hostilities, the chiefs were afraid to accompany the Corps back down the Missouri through the heart of Sioux territory. After much reassurance and promises, only one of the chiefs agreed to go along and visit the great father in Washington.

The group of intrepid explorers had already started to dissolve. Once again back home, Sacagawea and Charbonneau and their eighteen-month-old son Pompey stayed in the Mandan village. Charbonneau received his pay of $500. Clark offered to take Pompey back to civilization and raise him as if he were his own son, but the little boy's parents said they would wait till he was a little older. John Colter, with the captains' blessing, left the group and reascended the Missouri with the two trappers they had met a few days earlier. He would make history as the first white explorer of what is today Yellowstone National Park. Apparently the impending return to civilization did not hold much allure for Colter.

On August 17, the rest of the Corps, full of anticipation but with Lewis still out of commission, departed the village that had provided them with so much comfort against the ravages of the winter on their trip up the river. The boats once again passed by the Arikara villages and floated through channels and past falling riverbanks that offered more welcome views in the downstream direction.

By August 22, Lewis was able to walk a little for the first time since the shooting, and he directed Clark to discontinue packing his wounds. On the 27th, Lewis took a prolonged walk to look at some buffalo. He paid the price for his activity with pain well into the following morning, and took it easy the following week. September 3 saw Lewis able to walk slowly without pain and, on the 9th Clark noted, "My worthy friend Cap Lewis has entirely recovered his wounds are heeled up and he Can walk and even run nearly as well as ever he Could." Clark added that the wounded area was "yet tender &c. &."

Ninety well armed Indian men had appeared on the bank of the Missouri on August 30 and, as Clark noted, with "their hostile appearance we were apprehensive they were Tetons." Clark met a delegation on a sandbar between the Indians and the Corps' location. His translators spoke Omaha and Pawnee to the Indians, neither of which they could understand. It was quickly learned, through a few words of Sioux, that they belonged to the Teton Sioux of Chief Black Buffalo, who had provided the Corps' closest encounter with trouble during the fall of 1804. Wanting nothing to do with the group and refusing seemingly friendly overtures of several young men in the delegation, Clark told the Indians to go back to Black Buffalo and say that "they had treated all the white people who had visited them very badly; robed them of their goods and had wounded one man whome I had Seen [one of the trappers Colter joined]." Adding that the Tetons were "bad people and no more traders would be Suffered to come to them," Clark told them that in the future whites would come up the river "Sufficiently Strong to whip any vilenous party who dare to oppose them," and that they had armed their Mandan and Hidatsa enemies with "a cannon" and "Guns Powder and ball." He then directed the young men to tell Black Buffalo to stay "away from the river or we Should kill every one of them…" After the

Near Disaster and Then...

young men swam back and relayed their message, they shouted at Clark and his men "to come across and they would kill us all." Clark ignored them and the standoff ended.

By the first week of September, the days were once again quickly shortening, with brisk air filling the night skies over South Dakota. Strong winds blew over the river, pelting the exposed camp with sand and rendering "the after part of the night [of September 8] very disagreeable."

In the afternoon the Corps had met a trader with two small vessels full of merchandise coming up river. The captains asked about the latest news. The trader didn't have much news, but said that the British had fired on two American ships in the port of New York. The captains learned of the death of the brilliant Alexander Hamilton at the hands of Aaron Burr in a duel, and that two Indians had been hanged for murder in St. Louis.

The news of home made it seem all the closer, and the men now rowed with the added strength provided by the excitement of nearing their friends and homes. Sixty or seventy miles a day passed under the hulls of the canoes. Various trading vessels were periodically encountered and eager inquiries made about news from the homefront. The men who wanted it were treated to a dram of whiskey from the traders. An old friend of both the captains, Robert McClellan, commanded one of these trading parties. Feeling a little sick to his stomach, Clark tried perhaps a new remedy—some chocolate given by McClellan, "of which I drank about a pint and found great relief."

The banks of the river in Missouri Territory were now filled with sycamores, ash, mulberries, and elms. Buzzards, crows, hawks, and "hooting owls" hovered over the party as they steadily advanced mile by mile, closer to their goal. The men probably started allowing themselves to think about the comforts of civilization more than they had ever done during the previous years of living in the wild. George Shannon continued to periodically not think, and once on the 12th left his powder horn, bullets, and knife behind—and did not even realize it until the next night.

On September 18, John Potts developed a probable case of ultraviolet light burn on his corneas. Shannon experienced similar symptoms. With the men's rapid progress downriver covering great distances, the menu began to suffer, and on the day of Potts' and Shannon's eye problems, the men had nothing to eat except some pawpaws and custard apples. The pawpaw was apparently black haw or *Viburnum prunifolium*. This plant contains natural chemicals (anticholenergic) and its roots and inner bark were used by Indians to brew a tea to treat stomach cramps.

Soon after Shannon and Potts got sick, others suffered inflamed and swollen eyes, "and the lid appears burnt with the Sun," leaving three incapacitated. Clark surmised that it was probably from the sunlight reflected off the water. But why did this hit much of the group suddenly and why in September with the falling incidence of reflected light on the river? Perhaps windborne dust joined the ultraviolet radiation. Dr. Chuinard suggests infectious conjunctivitis,[1] but this condition does not usually produce such painful symptoms that would incapacitate the men, unless they were suffering from ocular tularemia, or their corneas were affected by an herpetic viral infection. Ann Rogers suggests the possibility of contact dermatitis from handling of the pawpaws.[2] But why just on the eyes? If they had touched a substance that gave them an allergic inflammatory reaction, it would have also been present on their hands and anywhere else it touched. This does not seem to me to be a viable explanation. On the 20th, the three men who couldn't even row due to their eye pain were divided among the other canoes. Two canoes were left behind.

On the afternoon of September 20, with the men "being extreemly anxious to get down," a scene occurred that brings a smile to our faces as we imagine it.

I would like to ask you, the reader, when was the last time that the sight of a cow brought you great joy? This is precisely what happened to the bearded and tattered men. As their canoes hit the first outskirts of civilization, they "Saw Some cows on the bank which was a joyfull Sight to the party and Caused a Shout to be raised for joy." Remember this the next time you see a cow in a pasture.

Soon after, the Corps reached the small French village of La Charette, where the men discharged their firearms in celebration. They landed and were treated to a "very agreeable supper." Friendly conversation followed with both the French- and the English-speaking inhabitants. The captains were informed that nearly everyone back in civi-

Near Disaster and Then...

lization by now believed the Corps were dead. The men were invited to various homes for visits with local families and were undoubtedly treated to culinary delights long since forgotten, such as fresh milk, sweets, coffee, and tobacco—as well as human contact that soaked their souls with joy.

The newly energized men departed La Charette on September 21, and passed outposts of civilization new since they had gone up the Missouri. Inhabitants inquired as to who they were, expressing surprise. As John Ordway wrote, they "had heard and believed that we were all dead and were forgotton."[3]

By evening they arrived in St. Charles, once again firing "three rounds" off in celebration. The citizens excitedly gathered around the men, once again in amazement, saying "we were Supposed to have been lost long Since, and were entirely given out by every person &c." as Clark recorded.

Most of the men got some rooms in town, along with what Ordway called "refreshments." The next morning Clark wrote a letter "to my friends in Kentucky" and then they descended another few miles to the year-old U.S. Army Fort Bellefontaine at the mouth of Coldwater Creek.

The morning of the 23rd of September, 1806, dawned and the men immediately prepared for their last day on the river as official members of the Corps of Discovery of North America. The Mandan chief, Sheheke, and his family were taken to the "publick store" and furnished with white men's clothing. We can only imagine what went through his mind as he browsed at the array of gear that was available on that army outpost.

By noon on that rainy and dreary day, that long anticipated return to their friends and countrymen became reality as the canoes were finally paddled into St. Louis. The captains allowed the men to "fire off their pieces as a Salute to the Town." The city folks swarmed down to the riverside to greet the explorers and gave them three cheers. I'm sure much excitement and laughter was evident as well as a tremendous relief and satisfaction born of knowing they had whipped the entire wilderness of North America for two years, four months and fourteen days, and had now returned to tell about it.

The local press immediately sent dispatches to the east, describing the expedition and its course to the Pacific and back, and announcing that "some of the natives and curiosities of the countries through which they passed" had been brought back to St. Louis, and that the expedition had "only lost one man." The article ended with the note that "They have kept an ample journal of their tour; which will be published; and must afford much intelligence."

Captain Lewis quickly scribbled a several-page letter to President Jefferson beginning:

> It is with pleasure that I anounce to you the safe arrival of myself and party at 12 oClk. Today at this place with our papers and baggage. In obedience to your orders we have penitrated the Continent of North America to the Pacific Ocean, and sufficiently explored the interior of the country to affirm with confidence that we have discovered the most practicable rout which dose exist across the continent by means of the navigable branches of the Missouri and Columbia Rivers.[4]

Several more pages followed with information about the fur trade, Indian relations, and activities of British fur traders in the region. The letters were sent with Drouillard to Cahokia to catch up with the mail.

The grunge and some of the beards of twenty-eight months were probably washed away and shaved off in hot baths all around St. Louis. Rotten buckskins that stank from the smoke of hundreds of campfires were exchanged for new cotton shirts and pants. City food was probably the utmost novelty after endless days of bland roots and venison, elk, bear, crayfish, coyote, ground-squirrels, and stuffed buffalo intestine.

St. Louis was in an uproar. Celebrations were held over the next few days. William Clark's old friend, Major William Christy, now a St. Louis tavern keeper, held a party there on the night of September 25. The celebrants raised eighteen toasts, starting with one for President Jefferson, "The friend of science, the polar star of discovery, the philosopher and the patriot." Other St. Louis residents probably pushed into the crowded space to gain a glimpse of the explorers returned from the dead, and to join in the cheers that followed the last toast, to the captains whose "...perilous services endear them to every American heart."

But I think that the supreme satisfaction of having returned home was best expressed by the simple and heartfelt entry made by the highly dependable and trustworthy Sergeant John Ordway. Ordway had written in the beginning of the trip that "I am so happy as to be one of them pick'd men from the armey," and his anticipation of some reward "if we live to Return." Through unbelievable toils and dangers, he had most certainly returned, and probably he expressed the feelings of all of his fellow members of the Corps in his journal's last entry, dated September 23, 1806:

> *all considerable much rejoiced that we have the Expedition Completed and now we look for boarding in Town and wait for our Settlement and then we entend to return to our native homes to See our parents once more as we have been So long from them.—   finis.* [5]

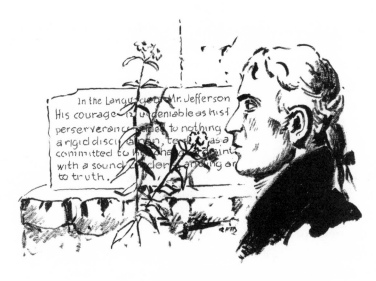

In the Language of Mr. Jefferson
His courage was undeniable as his
perserverance yielded to nothing
a rigid discipline, temperate as a
committed to life on the constraint,
with a sound understanding and
to truth.

☙ 19 ☙

GHOSTS OF EXPLORATIONS PAST

Fates of the Corps of Discovery

"Life's too short for worrying."
"Yes, that's what worries me."
—*Anonymous*

As I wrote in the introduction, in my occasionally romantic imagination and admitted fascination with the story of Lewis and Clark, I fantasize that some day, on one of my outings in western Montana, I will come around a corner on a forest trail or over the top of some windswept ridge and discover the Corps of Discovery sitting round their campfire. I will be hailed by a friendly shout from William Clark and be invited to sit down with them and hear some of their stories and enjoy a bite of the white pudding. As the fire snaps and sparks, I ask the men what it was like to be trapped on the Great Falls plains being pelted with giant hailstones, or how they endured their weeks of grueling labors on the Missouri and in the Bitterroots. It would be great to hear Cruzatte and Charbonneau arguing back and forth in French about the meaning of a word, or to see Sacagawea rocking Pompey to sleep, illuminated by the campfire. Imagine the thrill of hearing Lewis's account of the all-night ride across the prairie of the Marias River, expecting to turn around and find dozens of very angry Blackfeet galloping down on him, or of getting a one-on-one lesson from George Drouillard in sign language.

But as much as I'd like for this event to occur, it undoubtedly will not. Those healthy young men of 1806 are gone. Some got old. Some got sick and died before their fourscore years on this planet had expired. As the good book says, "For what is your life? It is even a vapor that appeareth for a little time, and then vanisheth away."

As our tale of adventure comes to a close, we will stop and look at the last remaining medical aspect of interest. No writing about medicine and the Corps would be complete without a discussion of what happened to some of the key figures of the Corps of Discovery after their return.

Many of the men fell into the same degree of obscurity on their return that they occupied prior to their moments of glory. William Clark tried to account for the men's whereabouts later in his life. Some of what we know is as follows.

Pierre Cruzatte, the fiddling French boatman, and shooter of Captain Lewis, may have joined a later expedition into the Rockies under the command of John McClellan. Clark listed him as "killed" by 1825-28.[1]

Joseph Field, the prodigious hunter whom Lewis trusted enough to make one of only three men he took into the heart of Blackfeet country, was listed as "killed" within a couple of years after his return to St. Louis. The circumstances surrounding his death are not known.[2]

The captains on their return praised Reubin Field with a letter to the Secretary of War recommending him for a commission to the rank of lieutenant in the regular army. But the size of the army was not being increased in 1806 and Reubin, instead of becoming an army officer, got married and settled down as a farmer. He died of unknown causes in 1823.[3]

Nathaniel Pryor, with the frequently dislocated shoulder, remained in the army and was one of the group who returned Mandan Chief Sheheke to his home in present-day North Dakota. He rose to the rank of captain during the War of 1812, left the army and became a trader with the Osage Indians along the Missouri. He married an Osage woman and had several children. He died of unknown causes in 1831. His name lives on, in the town of Pryor, Oklahoma, as well as with the Montana town and mountain range that bear his name.[4]

John Shields, the magnificent gunsmith and originator of the sweat bath that cured both Bratton and the Nez Perce invalid, returned to trap for a year with his apparent relative, Daniel Boone. He died of unknown causes in 1809.[5]

Patrick Gass, the replacement sergeant after the death of Charles Floyd, lived to the ripe old age of ninety-nine, outliving all the other members of the Corps. The skillful carpenter, and writer of the first (and the driest) expedition journal to be published (in 1807), stayed in the army and lost an eye during the War of 1812. A living example that "hope springs eternal," at the age of sixty he married a woman more than forty years younger than he and fathered seven children.[6]

The member of the Corps whose fame most closely approaches that of the captains is the legendary John Colter. Although at the onset of the journey he was not as accomplished a frontiersman as Drouillard, his decision to leave the Corps on the final leg of the journey and reascend the Missouri has led to his renown among American mountain men. After trapping the Upper Missouri for the winter of 1806, Colter descended to the Platte River and there met American fur entrepreneur Manuel Lisa, who lured him into returning to the Yellowstone once again. Colter, with two Indian guides, traveled to the mouth of the Bighorn River in present-day Montana. Encountering hostile Indians, the two guides took off, leaving Colter alone in the middle of a Montana winter. He continued into the eastern part of the Yellowstone, all alone.[7]

In 1808, Colter and fellow Corps member John Potts were trapping together near the Three Forks. While paddling on one of the rivers near the Three Forks, they met with a group of Blackfeet warriors on horseback. The Blackfeet motioned them to shore. Colter got out, but Potts apparently panicked and pushed the canoe into the river. The Indians became threatening and Potts responded by shooting one of them. It was Potts' last mistake and last shot. He was soon riddled with Blackfeet arrows, and Colter became a prisoner.[8]

Ghosts of Explorations Past

The Indians decided to give Colter a sporting chance. They stripped him naked, gave him a head start, and then chased him. Unlike his friendly foot races with the Nez Perce, this race was now for his life. Colter left all but one of the warriors in the distance, and killed the closest one with the man's own spear. He continued running to the Jefferson River, jumped into the water, floated with the current, and hid himself under a log jam. The remaining members of the Blackfeet pursuit party searched for him in vain. Once the Indians departed in frustration, Colter pulled himself out of the river and resumed his journey in the nude across the Gallatin River, into the Yellowstone Valley, and on to Lisa's fur trading post on the Bighorn River,[9] a distance of about 150 miles.

Colter returned to St. Louis in 1810, married and began the life of a farmer. He died in 1813, at the age of thirty-eight a victim of "jaundice," the probable result of a liver problem. It could have been the result of an overwhelming case of viral hepatitis or possibly the result of the invasion of the liver by some malignancy, an infected gallbladder, amoebic obstruction of his gallbladder, some other parasitic manifestation, etc., etc., etc. Our speculation could fill another book.

George Drouillard was another of the great American mountain men. He became a valued member of the team assembled by Manuel Lisa and helped establish the fur trade in today's southwest and central Montana. The master of the Indian sign language, himself half Omaha, chose a life in the wilderness. This great man ran out of luck and died of massive trauma, the victim of Blackfeet arrows while trapping beaver near the Three Forks in 1810.[10]

William Bratton, who had what the captains called "the strictest morals" and also enjoyed some exclusive company by outrunning a grizzly, the man who suffered so long with his painful back, lived a relatively long life in Indiana and Ohio. He married for the first time at the age of forty-one, and fathered eight sons and two daughters. There is no mention of his back problem ever returning, and he died at the age of sixty-three. His headstone reads, "Went with Lewis and Clark in 1804 to the Rocky Mountains."[11]

John Collins, one of the recipients of a court-martial for stealing whiskey early in the trip, was killed in 1823 by Arikara arrows while accompanying William Ashley's trapping adventure.[12]

Silas Goodrich, victim of syphilis and the mercury treatment meant to cure it, was simply listed as "dead" by 1825-28 in Clark's record. One must wonder if the syphilitic *Treponema* didn't escape the mercury and ultimately kill him, or how much of his kidneys may have been damaged by the mercury.[13]

Francois Labiche the interpreter was living in St. Louis in 1825.[14] The cause of his death is not known.

Hugh McNeal who, along with Lewis explored the little creek near the Continental Divide and "exultingly stood with a foot on each side," and who clubbed a grizzly and then spent a couple of hours in a tree while it paced around the trunk near the Great Falls, died prior to 1825 of unknown causes.[15]

John Newman, the mutineer who worked hard to restore his reputation after his court-martial, was sent home with the return party from Fort Mandan in the spring of 1805.[16] The man who was whipped and discharged from the Corps died from Yankton Sioux arrows in 1838.

George Shannon, eighteen in 1804, was the youngest soldier in the Corps and the soldier with the greatest talent at getting lost. He had a leg amputated as a result of complications from a wound suffered while returning Chief Sheheke to North Dakota with Sergeant Pryor's party. In 1810, he assisted Nicholas Biddle in preparing the first edition of the journals. Shannon studied law and practiced in Lexington, Kentucky. He served as a state senator in Missouri and died of unknown causes in 1836, at the age of forty-nine.[17]

York remained Clark's slave until he reached the age of forty-two. During that year of 1811, Clark gave him his freedom. York became a freighter but eventually failed, possibly the victim of some swindlers. He died of the bacterial intestinal disease cholera sometime before 1832.[18]

Alexander Willard, the sleeping sentry who escaped the death penalty only to receive a hundred lashes, suffered probable pneumonia during spring 1806, and spent time in the middle of the Missouri holding on for dear life to a submerged tree, was married in 1807. He was hired by Captain Lewis as a government blacksmith in 1808. He served in the War of 1812, and fathered twelve children. Apparently always the adventurer, he moved to California, shortly after the gold rush of 1849, and died near Sacramento in 1865, aged eighty-eight.[19] Pretty good for

Ghosts of Explorations Past

a guy that narrowly escaped a firing squad. I have had the pleasure of meeting some of his descendants.

Sacagawea and Charbonneau probably lived with the Hidatsa until 1809 or 1810. They then brought four- or five-year-old Pompey to St. Louis and allowed Captain Clark to raise the boy. Sacagawea's death is a matter of debate. Some say she died in the winter of 1812, and others that she lived into old age. Charbonneau lived to be eighty, working as an interpreter for William Clark with the Mandan and Hidatsa tribes.[20]

Jean Baptiste Charbonneau or, as Clark called him, "Pompey," lived an interesting life. In 1824, he met the traveling Prince Paul of Wurttemberg, Germany. As apparently everyone else did, Prince Paul took a liking to Pompey and convinced him to return to Germany. Pompey lived in Europe for six years, learned several languages, and returned to the States. He then lived the life of a mountain man and guide for the army. He settled in California, but left for the gold fields of Montana in 1866. He caught pneumonia, and died along the route at the age of sixty-one. He is buried near Danner, Oregon.[21]

William Clark's return to civilization saw his marriage to the teenaged Judith, whose namesake river still flows into the Missouri in central Montana. He outlived her, then married her cousin. His life as a public servant, as both a Commissioner of Indian Affairs and as Governor of Missouri Territory, met with much more success than the political life of Meriwether Lewis. He was highly respected by the Indian tribes he administered west of the Mississippi. They depended upon him to be their spokesman and advocate with the American government.

Clark's love for his friend inspired him to name his first born son, Meriwether Lewis Clark. The favorite physician of the Nez Perce and a brilliant and personable co-leader of the Corps, William Clark died in 1838, of unknown causes at the age of sixty-eight.[22]

Lewis did not fare as well. Faced with numerous problems upon his return to civilization, including failed courtships, assignment to political positions for which he was ill suited, nefarious land schemes and loss of personal wealth, and suffering from depression greatly worsened by the use of alcohol and opium,[23] Captain Lewis went progressively downhill from the time he reentered society in 1806. In 1809, Lewis died probably by his own hand, in Tennessee en route from St. Louis to Washington, D.C.

If Meriwether Lewis was addicted to opium, he was not the first to experience the hell of this problem. It has caused colossal medical and societal problems with its profound effects on human physiology and behavior since it started to be cultivated by the human race sometime between 4000 and 3000 B.C.

Opium is a milky substance obtained from the immature flower pod of the opium poppy (*Papaver somniferum*). The raw opium in Lewis's pills contained dozens of alkaloids, the most abundant being morphine and codeine. Morphine was identified and isolated from raw opium in 1803, but its spectacular efficacy in relieving pain did not come into general use until the 1830s. Besides relieving pain, morphine causes intense euphoria and tranquility as well as the less desirable side effects of depressing the drive to breathe and producing a whopping case of constipation. Opium and its alkaloid products were included in over-the-counter tonics, elixirs, cough drops and medications to calm down unruly babies in the United States until 1914.

Although Lewis wrote that he was taking opium pills of one gram, it is highly doubtful that those pills actually contained a gram of opium, which would have been a potent dose. When Lewis took his opium— up to three pills at night and another two in the morning if they "did not operate" on his self-diagnosed malarial fevers—he was ingesting an unknown quantity of morphine, codeine, and several dozen other pharymacologically active substances produced within the cells of the magic poppy.

Morphine from raw opium was readily absorbed from Lewis's intestine into his bloodstream, where it then flowed to his liver. That organ inactivated a good deal of the opium before it entered his central nervous system and general circulation. (This is why opiate pain-relieving drugs started being administered with a hypodermic syringe after its invention in 1853, to avoid the "first pass" effect of the liver's inactivating some of the dosage.)

The euphoric effect produced by the morphine would have been present with the first pill taken. Within a period of weeks, Lewis could have become sufficiently addicted to opium to experience symptoms of irritability and aggression should he try to discontinue the medication. Opioid withdrawal produces an intense craving for more of the substance, nausea, cramps, a depressed mood, inability to sleep, increased sensitivity to pain, and increased anxiety.

If Lewis was drinking heavily at that time, which we know he had done on occasion during his life, the alcohol abuse would have produced and magnified the same ugly results just listed. You can start to gain some insight into the tremendous effects that Lewis's drinking and opium use could have produced in bringing him to a point of dispair and ultimately to suicide.

Besides the ease with which he could obtain opium and alcohol, Lewis may have been influenced by incorrect medical theory of the day. John Brown, teacher of Lewis's teacher Dr. Rush, classified a depressed psychological state as being an "aesthenic" disease, the result of insufficient nervous stimulation. Dr. Brown's medical treatment was a bottle of alcoholic drink to solve the problem. The captains even treated a mentally ill Indian woman with some of their opium on the return trip. Unbeknownst to the captains, or any medical professional of their day, alcohol and opium, mixed with depression, are a lethal combination.

There are endless arguments about Lewis's state of mind prior to his death, and within the circles of Lewis and Clark aficionados, controversy still exists as to whether Meriwether Lewis was murdered or died by suicide. The late Dr. E.G. Chuinard wrote a series of articles in 1991, citing evidence that he believed proves that Lewis died as the victim of murder.[24] He wrote in response to the late Dr. Paul Cutright's writings that supported the premise of suicide. As Dr. Chuinard cited his regret at the passing of Dr. Cutright prior to the publication of his articles, I too must express my regrets that I never got the opportunity to met either Dr. Chuinard or Dr. Cutright and discuss the issues surrounding Lewis's death. Both men loved the Corps of Discovery and contributed greatly to the knowledge that the public enjoys of it today. I salute them.

Gilbert Russell, in 1811, wrote a letter to the first superintendent of the U.S. Military Academy describing Lewis's death:

> Some time in the night he got his pistols which he loaded, after everybody had retired in a separate building [at Grinder's Stand on the Natchez Trace near today's Hohenwald, TN] and discharged one against his forehead without much effect—the ball not penetrating the skull but only making a furrow over it. He then discharged the other

against his breast where the ball entered and passing downward thro' his body came out low down near his back bone.[25]

Lewis lingered for some hours.

Dr. Chuinard asserted that, if Lewis had shot himself in "the breast," the slow death "is totally unbelievable!" Chuinard raises the interesting question in his article: "The second shot would be expected to have killed Lewis instantly, or have disabled him," adding "What do the supporters of suicide think that this second shot would have done to the heart, lungs, aorta and/or intestines? Certainly Lewis would have been in dire shock and soon have bled to death or perhaps paralyzed from spinal cord injury."[26]

To Dr. Chuinard's conclusions concerning the implausibility of Lewis's shooting himself and surviving for two hours, I present the following observations.

We may interpret the nonspecific term "breast" as meaning somewhere on the chest. If Lewis held a pistol to his chest, with the muzzle aimed at a slightly downward angle as is suggested by the description of the resulting wound, the bullet probably entered his chest, passed through his lung, penetrated the thin muscular diaphragm, and wounded either his spleen or his liver depending on whether the bullet entered his left or right chest. The lungs, spleen, and liver all have remarkable blood supplies and, if wounded, can bleed to the point of causing death. As the bullet passed into Lewis's chest, it would have created a totally or partially collapsed lung from the introduction of atmospheric pressure into the thoracic cavity. The wound probably resulted in a slow exsanguination (bleeding) into his chest and abdominal cavities. This could have definitely gone on for two hours prior to his death, not causing the "instant death" that Dr. Chuinard believes it would have. I believe that it is less likely, but still possible, that the bullet could also have wounded the heart superficially, resulting in the sac surrounding the heart slowing filling with blood (hemopericardium), and the resulting increase in pressure surrounding the heart (pericardial tamponade), which would ultimately cause it to stop beating.

Any trauma surgeon could tell you stories of talking to gunshot victims who are carrying on conversations and seemingly stable for hours, then suddenly lose consciousness and die, as the result of bleeding in the chest, abdomen, or sac surrounding the heart. People who suffer gunshot wounds do not always die instantly as we have seen on television shows. Mortally wounded victims can continue to function until the effects of their internal wounds compromise the functions of their heart and blood pressure. This would certainly fit the picture of Meriwether Lewis's survival of two hours after he shot himself. With such a gunshot today, it is likely that a surgeon could save the victim's life.

Some authors have suggested that malaria contributed to Meriwether Lewis's mental state and death. Let's take a closer look at the two most common *Plasmodia* that caused malaria in early America: *P. vivax* and *P. falciparum*.[27]

Malaria arises from the parasitic infection of our oxygen-carrying red blood cells (RBCs), and its symptoms from destruction of the RBCs, which the human body continuously produces in bone marrow. As RBCs travel through the blood vessels, they can flatten and change shape, squeezing through the tiny capillaries to give off their life-sustaining oxygen, while the liquid portion of the blood (plasma) nourishes our hungry cells with its energy-rich glucose. These red cells live for several months cruising through blood vessels to every nook and cranny of the body. There are, of course, always younger and older RBCs in our bloodstreams.

As mentioned earlier, the most severe form of malaria is caused by *P. falciparum*. One reason for its severity is that, unlike *P. vivax, falciparum* parasitizes all ages of RBCs, whereas *vivax* infects only young RBCs. Besides thus infecting more cells, *P. falciparum* also alters the cells' membranes, preventing them from changing shape to slip through capillaries. The stiff, rigid RBCs can clog—and thus stop blood circulating into—capillaries supplying the brain, kidneys, and other organs.

Falciparum is the only type of malaria that can result in "cerebral malaria,"[28] which develops as brain capillaries become clogged with parasite-laden RBCs. These "traffic jams" are thought to produce impaired consciousness and coma.[29] Victims of cerebral malaria usually suffer from low blood sugar, anemia, and kidney failure, dying within days. Such victims would have been unable to carry on the travel schedule that Lewis did in the days preceding his death: He had traveled on rough trails via horseback for the previous ten days.

The milder malarias caused by *P. vivax* and *P. ovale* are so similar that they are considered identical.[30] After the initial infection the *vivax* parasites, unlike the *falciparum*, may lie dormant from six to eleven months in the victim's liver. This accounts for symptoms of fever, chills, headaches, etc., even if the victim has not been bitten recently by a mosquito. *Vivax*-caused malaria is common in temperate regions, where cold winter termperatures wipe out entire populations of infected mosquitoes. Every spring, a new batch of uninfected mosquitoes hatches, and again feed on *vivax*-infected humans to begin the cycle again.

Symptoms of malaria include a pattern of chills lasting from fifteen minutes to several hours, followed by a "hot stage" lasting hours (coinciding with the rupture of parasite-laden RBCs). High fevers during this phase can cause brain damage and convulsions. The final stage is typified by profuse sweating, fatigue, and sleep.[31] The men of the Corps, who were probably all victims of either *vivax* or *falciparum* malaria, could have been protected to some degree by their immune systems' responses to previous infections. Some probably lived with few, if any, recurrent malarial symptoms, while others could have suffered repeated bouts, particularly if their malaria was *falciparum*-caused.

Did Lewis have cerebral malaria? Or, could he have been so distraught over a recurrent bout of malaria that he committed suicide? Possibly, but I find it difficult to imagine that symptoms of fever, chills, headache, and nausea he had experienced previously would have caused Lewis to take his own life this time. I think it is more likely that the malaria, added to the effects of opium addiction, alcoholism, and other psychological problems, combined to have this effect.

One medical author has cited his belief that Meriwether Lewis had personality changes caused by neurosyphilis, that Lewis recognized that he was suffering from neurosyphilis and thus committed suicide to avoid the progression of the disease. Neurosyphilis is a tertiary form of syphilis that causes progressive degeneration of the spinal cord and peripheral nerves, affecting both mind and body. This author states that Lewis caught the disease during the Corps' stay with the Shoshones, as evidenced by Lewis's writings of skin eruptions several weeks later on September 19, 1805. The author also stated that a board of "world class epidemiologists" had concluded that neurosyphilis was the most likely explanation of the symptoms Lewis suffered from during his final days.[32]

First of all, Lewis could not have known for certain that he was suf-

The Fatal Gunshot of Meriwether Lewis

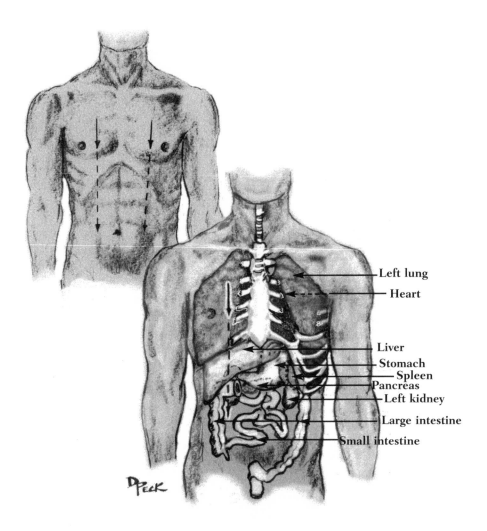

Front (anterior) view of possible bullet routes and the resulting organ damage resulting from such wounds.

Diagramatic Lateral Views
of Possible Bullet Path

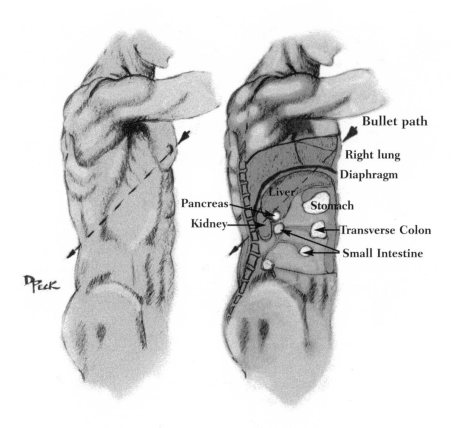

View on right shows bullet path and damage done to lung, liver, pancreas, kidney or spleen depending on whether the bullet entered the left or right side of chest.

fering from neurosyphilis, because the condition was not even described in the world of medicine until 1882, when Bayle described "dementia paralytica," or paretic neurosyphilis. It was the first psychiatric disease for which a specific pathology and cause were found.[33] This fact does not mean that Lewis did not have neurosyphilis, it just means if he did, he didn't know it. His health could have deteriorated, and he may have even suspected syphilis, but I still do not believe these scenarios to be valid.

Although several Indian tribes offered young women to the captains for bed partners, there is no evidence in the journals that they ever took advantage of the opportunities. In fact, the captains wrote about the Indians' irritation at their refusals. So it is very presumptive to assume that Lewis caught syphilis anywhere along the route. Apparently there were others among the Corps who did not sleep with Indian women. William Bratton was specifically mentioned as "having the strictist morals," which suggests that he did not have sex with the Indian women. In addition, few of the men were mentioned as being victims of a "salivation," the mercury treatment for association with "Louis Veneri."

Could Lewis have contracted syphilis after his return to civilization in September of 1806 and subsequently be suffering from the effects of neurosyphilis in 1809? Possibly. However this diagnosis would have to be totally presumptive. Edmund C. Tramont, writing in one of the most respected textbooks of infectious disease, noted that neurosyphilis mimics

> *any degenerative neurologic process, or disorder that cause chronic inflammation (e.g. tuberculosis, fungal or sarcoid meningitis, tumors, subdural hematoma, Alzheimer's disease, multiple sclerosis, chronic alcoholism), or any disorder affecting the vasculature of the central nervous system. The axiom that syphilis can mimic any disease is particularly apropos with regard to the central nervous system.*[34]

So without any confirming laboratory test to establish that Lewis's system had been infected by *Treponema pallidum*, you can take your choice from the above diagnoses, any one of which would produce the same symptoms. Since we know that Lewis was drinking heavily towards the end of his life it would seem much more logical to attribute the psychiatric changes he suffered to the deleterious effects of alcohol.

As noted earlier, the journals' references to "skin eruptions" have been cited as evidence of syphilis. This generic description from the captains could mean any one of several hundred types of skin rashes, sores, or manifestations of myriad infectious diseases other than syphilis. The early stages of syphilis were well known by the captains, so why didn't they refer to these "eruptions" as the "pox" as they did on other occasions? Why didn't Lewis treat himself with mercury if he knew he had contracted syphilis? Or, if he had treated himself with mercury, why didn't any of the other journal keepers write about Lewis's case of the pox when they noted him using mercury on himself for the several weeks that a "salivation" would have required? Did Lewis forbid the reporting of his condition? Did he do everything to hide the treatment? Did the commanding officer let down his guard, knowing of the likely resulting infection and its subsequent horrible treatment?

If we assume for a moment that Lewis did contract syphilis and either did not treat himself, or the treatment he underwent was not effective, what could have been the outcome?

There have been two major studies on the progression of syphilis in untreated victims. These were performed in Oslo, Norway[35] and in the United States in the 20th century.[36] They showed that only about a third of those syphilis victims who were *untreated* progressed to having neurologic involvement. Most people who die of complications of syphilis die from cardiovascular disease, by developing inflammations in their aortas and accompanying complications. The odds get even smaller that Lewis had neurosyphilis, given the probability that if Lewis knew he had contracted syphilis that he would have at least treated himself with mercury, knowing the potential for death in an untreated victim. Given that Lewis's personality seemed rather obsessive/compulsive, it seems totally inconsistent with his character that he would have contracted what he believed to be syphilis and decided not to treat himself.

The author who believes Lewis suffered from neurosyphilis also expresses seeming amazement at the assertion that Lewis would commit suicide "simply because he was psychologically depressed."[37] Hundreds of people across the United States commit suicide every day because they are depressed, even without the compounding problems that alcohol abuse and dependence would bring to an already depressed personality. The *Diagnostic and Statistical Manual of Mental Disorders*, the handbook of psychiatric diagnosis, notes that "Major Depressive Disorder is associated with high mortality. Up to 15 percent of individuals with severe Major Depressive Disorder die by suicide."[38]

Even though I believe in the complete plausibility of Lewis's last days as I have presented them from a medical viewpoint, the certainty of what really happened on that fall day of 1809, somewhere around some dingy log cabins called "Grinder's Stand," deep within the state of Tennessee, is about as clear as the springtime runoff. There are just too many questions within multiple credible scenarios, involving people of probable ill repute, to insist authoritatively that Lewis killed himself.

There was much conflicting testimony given by Mrs. Grinder regarding the facts of the case. She was the supposed "eye-witnesses" to the event and gave different and conflicting versions of what occurred throughout her lifetime. There were numerous people involved in giving their opinions pertinent to this case in the early 1800s—personalities who are utterly unable, 200 years after the fact, to be challenged, probed, or checked for their reliability and honesty. Once again what we are left with is our own ability to reason and take an honest look at the facts as we understand them today. People of high intelligence and good repute often come to differing conclusions regarding the death of Lewis.

Whoever pulled the trigger on the gun that fired the fatal bullet for Meriwether Lewis cannot take away his hallowed place in American history. His accomplishments were many, as were his mistakes and faults. He was undoubtedly a complex man, with much more than his share of talent. The uncertainty of the purveyor of his death, as well as the two centuries that have passed since that October day of long ago, cannot fully eclipse the great element of tragedy involved.

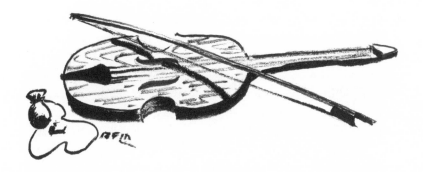

⚓ 20 ⚓

FIDDLES AND FRIENDSHIPS

The Sinews of Success

*It is not so much our friends' help that helps us as
the confident knowledge that they will help us.*
—*Epicurus*

The Corps of Discovery of North America accomplished a fabulous
feat in returning from their exploration of more than eight thousand miles through the western two thirds of the continent. Although
their exploits involved much more than the wilderness adventure and
the medical thought and practice of the day that we have focused on, I
have left the detailed discussion of the politics and other aspects of the
trip to those who have already done it so well. My effort, I hope, adds
another piece to the great puzzle of understanding and appreciating
what these men, woman, and child accomplished.

Not only did the group conquer Mother Nature and her hazards over the twenty-eight months of travel, but also they were able to conquer an even more insidious enemy on their road to success—themselves. How did thirty-one men, a young woman and her infant son, each and every one with a different personality, different likes and dislikes, diverse ethnic backgrounds and languages with their own racial and sociological biases, some with modest educational backgrounds and others illiterate, with various religious and moral backgrounds, form a cohesive team that was able to survive the rigors of their life in the wilderness? How were Sacagawea and Pompey able to make such a journey? Thirty-three different personalities in nearly constant contact with each other for two and a half years. As with any group, some of the members were probably unlikable and abrasive while others were winsome. A few were probably humorous, others dullards. There were probably the shy and the gregarious. Maybe a few were cowardly on their own, but fortified by the courage of their fellows: they rose to the occasion at hand.

The most obvious factor, and also the most important, was the incredibly effective leadership of Lewis and Clark. Meriwether Lewis and William Clark were masterful commanders of the small army. Cool-headed decision-making on numerous occasions avoided disaster, injury and perhaps death to themselves and their men.

Clark's courage and ability to be unintimidated by an entire armed force of Teton Sioux, an act that likely saved the team from a fire fight and possible annihilation during the summer of 1804, is a stellar example of effective leadership. Captain Lewis displayed spectacular calmness when on the slippery mud of northern Montana he saved the life of Private Windsor as he dangled over the edge of a cliff in June 1805. The experience they possessed in the wilderness and their characters of steel, shown by these acts of courage under very threatening circumstances, are blueprints of competence.

Their combination of strict discipline savored with a healthy dose of understanding and compassion kept the men on the straight and narrow. In the early months of the trip, when various men tried to undermine the captains' authority, they were dealt with swiftly, fairly and with a proper degree of severity. By the time the Corps reached Fort Mandan during the fall of 1804, there apparently was absolutely no question in any of the men's minds as to who was in control, and what was expected of them all.

On numerous occasions during the expedition the captains shared the toil of poling, hunting, riding, and starvation along with the men. The captains slept in the rain, suffered diseases along with their men, ate the rotten elk meat, and braved the dangers of potential and real hostilities at the hands of some Indian nations. They generally didn't have it any better than the privates, and the men deeply respected them because of that fact. Private Whitehouse, in the preface to his journal, stated that the captains "claim my utmost gratitude: and the humanity shown at all times by them, to those under their command, on this perilous and important Voyage of discovery…"[1]

As with all successful teams, the Corps had its individual talents that contributed to their successes. There were the men with their fabulous hunting skills that kept the Corps alive. Drouillard, Colter, Reubin and Joseph Field, Shannon and the other hunters were human predators in the finest sense. Drouillard's ability with the sign language and John Shields' ability to repair the intricate mechanisms of the flintlock rifles illustrates two totally different but equally necessary skills. Cruzatte, although half blind and a lousy shot, was a fabulous boatman. The huge shot of morale that his talent with the fiddle around many a campfire supplied to the Corps cannot be overestimated. Labiche and his ability to speak French and English made the translation chains from the captains to various Indian nations possible. Sacagawea was a great mellowing influence on the men, and she and little Pompey provided a touch of gentleness and feeling of home to the otherwise undiluted dose of testosterone on the trek during 1805 and 1806. Sacagawea's presence with the small army also eased many an initially tense situation with native people, and her native language made acquiring horses to cross the Bitterroots much easier. Charbonneau made the most delicious white puddings of buffalo intestine stuffed with kidney suet, then fried in bear's oil. Granted, the American Heart Association will not list this on their approved diet, and none of the fast food chains across the country are likely to feature it, but it put joy in every hungry stomach and weary heart along hundreds of miles of the Missouri River. Patrick Gass was the talented carpenter and Ordway was the stalwart sergeant. York was a steady and trustworthy companion. And then there was Charles Floyd, who reminded all of them just how close their daily paths took them to disaster and death.

Their trip through the unknown is a primer on innovative responses to numerous problems. Guns broke and needed to be fixed. Canoes were built by hand. Horses with sore hooves were shod with leather boots. Animals were killed and skinned, and the leather made into clothing. When they needed fish to eat and had no hooks, they shot them. When they ran out of tobacco they smoked wild herbs. They ate nearly every type of animal they encountered in order to survive.

In their medical practices, both Lewis and Clark enjoyed apparent success with the "simples." Lewis brewed his chokecherry branch tea, and Clark enjoyed spectacular successes with his Indian sweat bath, thanks to the suggestion of gunsmith John Shields. When the barks and laudanum didn't seem to be curing Sacagawea's bout of abdominal pain, Lewis sent a party to a nearby spring in order to obtain some mineral water, hoping it would help.

The vitality of youth and well functioning immune systems allowed them to survive wounds, numerous bacterial and viral infections, near starvation, malaria and other parasitic infections, and weather extremes. The fact that most people will get well without any medical intervention was never so clearly illustrated as during the twenty-eight months the Corps was on the trail. Their endurance and survival in the face of the illnesses they suffered, with the pathetically inadequate medical care available, should haunt me every time I write a prescription for an unneeded antibiotic or whine about my own back pain.

The psychological stresses of being isolated from civilization for so long may not have been an overwhelming burden for many of the men. Frontier people lived in isolated areas, and there were obviously no such things as radio or television. The incident that occurred early in the trip, with the men watching Charles Floyd quickly fail and die, with no hope of any effective medical intervention must have been a blow to their morale. Stephen Ambrose suggested to me that he believes one of the biggest psychological stresses occurred when the smokers ran out of tobacco. Seeing so many smokers on a daily basis who refuse to quit in spite of having pneumonia, chronic bronchitis and emphysema, makes me agree with him. The Corps' knowledge that they were far removed from any help from the civilized world and that they had only themselves to depend upon, must have caused psychological stress for some of the members. The ultimate proofs of my theory are the shouts of joy that went up from the men on seeing *cows* in the fields as they paddled back into civilization.

The psychological stress was also handled by having some good, simple fun. The men danced and sang songs around the campfire. They continued their holiday traditions by doing whatever they could that was in some way festive, to commemorate the days that held special meaning for them. They awoke the captains on Christmas mornings with firing guns and a Christmas carol or two. July Fourth was remembered at the Great Falls with the last few drops of their whiskey supply, dancing and much laughter. They held foot races with the Nez Perce and had shooting contests. They played the game of prison base like a bunch of neighborhood boys on a Saturday afternoon, and the captains played backgammon. The effects of the exhausting travel, the mosquitoes, the heat and the cold, and the limited diet were often offset by their friendships, laughter, a welcome campfire and the fiddle. Joseph Mussulman, writing in the journal of the Lewis and Clark Trail Heritage Foundation, *We Proceeded On*, notes that laughter transcends "all barriers—age, sex, race, nationality, language, and adversity." He also prods us to imagine "the hearty haw-haws that taunted the hapless Private Alexander Willard when he caught up with the rest after dropping his gun in a creek while en route back from retrieving the tomahawk he had left behind at the previous day's camp."[2] York's playful chasing of Indian children who screamed with delight, and the amazement of the native peoples at his black skin must have provided some light-hearted moments. Even the repeated encounters with the massive grizzlies, and their avoidance of any injury at the claws of these beasts, probably provided many a campfire story, laughter and a sense of having cheated the Grim Reaper once again. Lewis's journal note of "I expect these gentlemen [the grizzly bears] will give us some amusement shortly as they soon begin now to coppolate," makes me laugh, two centuries later.

All in all, what a marvelously fine honed team had been together. The camaraderie that can only develop through shared adversity and trust, coupled with times of humor and relaxation, put the Corps of Discovery at the head of the list of effective teams. The men's character and the endeavor they had committed themselves to, created an expedition that lacked modern conveniences and survival gear, but lacked nothing in determination, innovation, and valor. As Lewis wrote on several occasions, the men had committed themselves to the success of the venture and would sooner die than be defeated in their mission.

In 2000, *Outside* magazine published an article on their "super heroes."[3] These adventurers have distinguished themselves by climbing high peaks, snowboarding off sheer snowy cliffs, windsurfing massive waves, exploring Antarctica, etc. All the "super-heroes" were asked about their most harrowing moments during their highly adventurous lives. Some of the answers dealt with topics such as escaping from armed rebels, walking along precarious "knife-edge ridgelines" and nearly being blown off by wind gusts, near drowning in pounding surf, floating on an ever dwindling piece of ice in the middle of the subfreezing ocean, and being trapped under a rock buttress in the French Alps with an avalanche crashing overhead. Each of the these gutsy "award winners" had in their own ways challenged nature, and returned intact to tell us about their adventure and close calls in the bush.

But how would their moments of danger measure up when compared with such events as rowing and poling dugout boats for several thousand miles, surviving subzero weather without any modern clothing in huts built with their own hands, hunting their own food supply for more than two years, surviving encounters with grizzly bears, being pelted with giant hailstones falling at eighty miles per hour, surviving a flash flood, crossing a mountain range for more than a hundred miles in the snow (twice), with rags wrapped around their feet to protect them from the cold, tolerating an insect wonderland with no modern repellents, walking thousands of miles with flimsy homemade leather moccasins, suffering hunger and malnutrition for prolonged periods of time, and being shot in the butt and treated in the bush for three weeks? Not to mention doing this all in the middle of an uncharted wilderness, with no modern navigation, communication or survival equipment, while keeping track of it all with a quill pen.

It is astonishing that the captains lost only one of the crew to death. The men survived everything the outdoors could throw at them and nearly everything that the world of disease could muster against their success. It would seem that many of the treatments rendered by the captains, particularly the frequent purging and occasional blood-lettings could have been forgotten about all together and would have resulted in a healthier and happier Corps.

But there is more to effective medical practice than simply administering the correct medications. Meriwether Lewis and William Clark cared for their patients with compassion and, as Jefferson described it, "fatherly concern." Through myriad physical problems, with little training and few resources, Lewis and Clark did the best job they could as America's first wilderness physicians. The best-trained physician in the nation then, practicing in Philadelphia with all its resources, would not have performed better than the captains did in the wilderness. And, the captains also had phenomenal luck throughout most of their staggering challenge.

Through their trip, much information was gained by white America about the cultures, languages, and politics of the native nations of the Missouri—information that would not always be used with wisdom or much insight by the "great father" in Washington.

They didn't find an all-water route to the Pacific. There simply wasn't one to be discovered. Their attempts at creating peace among the Indian nations were mostly a failure. Hundreds of years of inter-tribal warfare would not be stopped by a few words of friendly exhortation from the captains.

Lewis accurately described hundreds of new-to-science species of North American flora and fauna, even though the *Megalonyx* and Drouillard's snake that gobbled like a turkey were not among them. In a tribute to his pioneering work in botany and zoology, Jefferson nominated Lewis as a member of the prestigious American Philosophical Society in Philadelphia, where his original journals rest today.

The first steps to solidifying American influence in the Louisiana territory as well as reaching the disputed northwest were accomplished. Maps now existed of America's new backyard. Lewis and Clark's moccasins hadn't even had time to dry after their return to St. Louis before more Americans started to ascend the Missouri to its headwaters and trap beaver.

The Corps of Discovery's wilderness exploits are the most wonderful adventure story in American history. The makeup of the expedition team and the adventures they encountered during their epic journey will continue to fascinate future generations of Americans. Yet-unborn

Americans will in future years wander the Missouri, Rockies, and Columbia, experiencing a little of the magic left behind along the trail of Meriwether Lewis, William Clark, George Drouillard, Sacagawea, little Pompey, and the rest.

Unfortunately, reading stories cannot provide the chill of a winter wind in the face, the burning thigh muscles, the mind-numbing hunger, or the elation of seeing the rising Rockies for the first time. But through the captains' writings, their stories of the men and the Missouri, its sawyers and falling banks, the hoards of mosquitoes, the terrifying encounters with the grizzled bear, their diet of wild foods, and the innumerable dangers overcome, the eight thousand miles of trails and river mixed with their curious brand of wilderness medicine will always offer images of adventure and fascination to those who love and cherish American history and wilderness adventure. Proceed on!

APPENDIX ONE

Riddles of Nature: The World's Medical Expedition

A physician is one who pours drugs of which he knows
little into a body of which he knows less.
—Voltaire

Medical thought and practice during the time of Lewis and Clark did not exist in a vacuum. Medicine, as developed through the centuries by creatively thinking men and women, many of them true renegades, was the result of thousands of years of changing thinking. When their turn in the spotlight of history came, these people challenged the accepted thinking of their day. Many were ridiculed by the so-called masters of their times. All of them stirred the pot of stew, adding new spices in the form of theories about medicine and disease. Who were the great thinkers and physicians of old, whose ideas and lives contributed to medical thought as it existed in the early 1800s, and influenced Lewis and Clark?

Embarking on a study of medical history is similar to an exploration of the wilderness in both nature and scope. "Wilderness" has a connotation of the uncharted and unknown, terms that characterize medicine for the entirety of human history. It is equally true that even as modern science and medicine are cracking the code of life in mapping the human genome, we find that the more we learn, the more we realize how much we still do not know. The history of medicine is similar to the wilderness in scope due to the tremendous diversity of theories of disease and of treatments utilized throughout the ages. The more one studies medical history, the more they may feel lost in the center of a dark and mysterious forest, wandering in one direction, only to turn around and wander aimlessly in another. But within the forest are a multitude of fascinating and captivating curiosities. We are able to stop on our trail to observe a few of the numerous theories and practices that constitute the annals of medicine. Many observations will be of comical oddities to a person of the 21st century, and others are curious concepts that will dumbfound the modern mind. But at the end of our historical expedition, we know that trail will lead us out of this dark place, into the "enlightened" medicine of the early 1800s.

It is an arbitrary decision where we decide to enter this vast forest of historical medicine but, more than any other tradition, early Greek medicine was the starting point for the medicine of Lewis and Clark.

Prior to the Greeks, disease was assumed to be the result of the work of supernatural forces. Many diseases were believed to have been sent by gods, as illustrated in the myth of Pandora's opening her notorious box of good and evil.

Supernatural diseases called for supernatural cures such as utilizing spells, amulets, and a forerunner of cardplaying, bone throwing.[1] Lest we modern Americans feel too smug about our state of enlightenment, note that we who live in the 21st century seem to have no shortage of our own crystal gazers, New Age healers, and hitchhikers on mythical flying saucers.

Somewhere during the sixth century B.C., philosophers from the Greek city of Miletus sought to explain natural phenomena such as earthquakes, thunder, and solar and lunar eclipses in natural terms, regarding these as manifestations of natural occurrences, not as supernatural incidents.[2] In addition, Pythagoras, the ancient Greek genius of mathematics (580-489 B.C.) began his teachings of natural explanations of disease at the medical school of Croton, in southern Italy.[3] One of his contemporaries, Alcmaeon of Croton, provided his own philosophical input that stated that diseases could be explained solely in natural terms, and that health was a balance of the powers within the body.[4] This rational approach to explaining natural events previously believed to be cryptic had a direct effect on the medical thought of the day. Epilepsy, for example, with its dramatic manifestations of seizure activity, was now being explained as a result of natural phenomena rather than the supernatural.

A truly monumental theory which in some ways survived for centuries was developed by the young Greek, Empedocles of Agrigentum (504-433 B.C.). He formulated a theory that suggested a unity among the material world. His four elements of the world—air, fire, earth, and water—were created by a combination of the earth's four fundamental qualities: hot, cold, wet, and dry. This system gave rise to an extension into the physiological arena, when the young Greek philosopher theorized that human flesh and blood were composed of equal mixtures of these factors. Disease could now be explained as an imbalance of the four elements.[5]

Hippocrates of Cos (460-379 B.C.) is credited as being the "father of medicine" although very little is actually known about him. His numerous books about the art and practice of medicine are called the *Corpus Hippocraticum*. This Greek physician was thought to be the greatest of the ancient physicians due to his knowledge of anatomy, emphasis on good diet, and his treatment of fractures, wounds, and other medical problems. Hippocrates also stressed the professional and ethical obligations of a physician to his patients. Hippocrates touted observation of the patient, encouraging a practical approach to curing the disease, rather than the abstract theoretical explanations of their origin. He supplied groundbreaking advice in clinical observation of patients, instructing his students to observe the patient's face, skin texture and tone, and numerous other clinical pearls. Palpation of the patient's body, visual inspection, and a good sense of smell helped the Hippocratic physician provide a treatment based on the idea that nature, or *physis*, provided a strong healing force, which was the physician's job to aid, and not overpower.[6]

One of the volumes of the *Corpus Hippocraticum* contains a comprehensive theory of the nature of disease and the function of the human body. This theory detailed the presence of four bodily humors: black and yellow bile, phlegm, and blood, and their correlation to the four elements of earth, fire, water and air. Blood was the dominant humor during the spring, yellow bile was the summer humor, black bile was chief in autumn, and phlegm predominated during the winter. Imbalances of the humors produced disease.

It was during the 3rd century B.C., in the city of Alexandria, that the dissection of the human body was first legalized. Prolific and groundbreaking work on human structure included the first description of the eye, brain, and duodenum (first part of the small intestine), as well as of the male and female genital organs. Separate motor and sensory nerves within the body were noted for the first time. A fascinating theory that broke with Hippocrates' humoral theory was popularized, stating that the external air, called "pneuma," circulated through the arteries, vitalizing the atoms that make up the body's elements. Disease was a problem with the "solids" and not with the "fluid" humors.[7]

As control of much of the western world shifted to Rome during the following centuries, the Greeks continued to lead the way in medical thought, easily outdoing the Romans who were apparently too busy conquering the world and putting on spectacles of blood sport. Greek physicians served the Roman emperors, caring for the medical needs of the Roman legions. In recognition of their great value to the empire, Julius Caesar decreed in 46 B.C. that all foreign physicians in Rome would be granted Roman citizenship. One Greek physician in particular, a bright young fellow named Dioscorides, served as an army surgeon under Nero (54-68 A.D.). This prolific herbal master described several hundred plants and their medicinal uses, laying a groundwork for the materia medica for centuries to come.[8]

One of the most influencial physicians in history was the son of a Greek architect. He was born in Pergamum, in 130 A.D. He is distinguished among even the greats of medicine for his work in anatomy and physiology. His influence on medical thinking is comparable to that of Hippocrates. His name was Claudius Galen.[9]

Galen, well educated for his day, studied at Smyrna, Corinth, and Alexandria. He returned to Pergamum and took up a position akin to being a modern day NFL team physician, except in 155 A.D., the athletes he took care of had rather remarkable occupational risks. As the team physician to the gladiators, Galen had the opportunity to develop skills in surgery and physical therapy. After four years of trying to patch up these human chopping blocks, he had a reputation that allowed him to move to Rome, where he became the personal physician to Emperor Marcus Aurelius. While in the emperor's service Galen wrote extensively on his theories and practice of medicine. He extended discoveries from his anatomical work on pigs and monkeys, often erroneously, onto human structure. But his contribution to understanding the structure and function of the nervous system, showing that nerves did not arise from the heart as had been believed, secures his position as a groundbreaking anatomist. In experimental physiology he tied the ureters (tubes which connect the kidneys to the bladder), and noted that urine backed up, showing that urine was produced in the kidneys and not in the bladder as previously believed. He used the inspection of urine, known as "uroscopy," as well as interpreting the patient's pulse, in diagnosing disease.[10]

Galen is best remembered for his theory of blood flow, which unfortunately was wrong. This theory, however, would be cited by medical experts as the embodiment of truth for the next fifteen hundred years. Galen believed that blood was produced in the liver from digested food that was transported there from the intestines. The liver would utilize the "natural spirits" which came from the magical "pneuma" that entered the body with air breathed into the lungs. Some of this new and vitalized blood flowed via veins to the body's periphery. The remaining blood went to the right ventricle of the heart, in turn sending a small portion to the lungs. The remaining blood passed through "pores" (which do not exist) into the left ventricle. In the heart, another portion of the pneuma, termed the "vital spirit" regulated blood flow and body temperature. The "animal spirit" portion of pneuma was present in the brain, center of sensory and motor function.[11]

Although a pathfinder in many areas, Galen persisted in believing the Hippocratic humoral theory of pathology. If Galen's diagnosis involved "too much black humor in the blood," he would counter that imbalance by administering milk, which is white, practicing the belief that "contraries are cured by contraries." He prescribed and formulated medicines containing dozens of ingredients, and was a great fan of bleeding and intestinal cathartics. He believed that all wounds produced pus as a normal process of healing, not realizing that pus was a sign of infection. This concept of "laudable pus" was so accepted by the medical world, that physicians did not think of pus as undesirable until the 1800s. Imagine the untold millions of infected wounds that occurred during the seventeen hundred years this theory was popular, which were observed and dismissed as normal by physicians of the day.[12]

Galen's vast contributions to medicine lay in his great diagnostic and observational skills as well as contributions from his work with physiology and his experimental nature. He desperately wanted to learn the reasons behind the function of the human body. His interest in diagnosis of a disease and then formulating a prognosis for the patient was an important step in medical thinking. Although Galen was stuck in mental quicksand, thinking that imbalances of black and yellow bile, blood, and phlegm caused disease, he correctly believed that malfunctions of specific organs caused distinct diseases. Galen was a genius of his time and, after he died in 203, the medical world went into a scientific doldrums for more than a thousand years.

During the middle ages (500-1500 A.D.), Greek medicine continued to be the system adopted by the western world. Greek medical texts were translated into Latin, chiefly by the most educated members of society, the Catholic monks. Monasteries became centers of learning, knowledge, and medical education. The monks became, if not medical pioneers, at least the keepers of the flame that had been lit by the Greeks. Medical thought was the result of theories built on the weakest of empirical evidence. Research and justification for a medical theory arose from the research of books filled with erroneous information. A classic case of "don't confuse me with the facts, my mind is made up," can be seen in looking at the state of anatomical dissection during the Middle Ages. While a barber-surgeon would dissect a body, the physician professor would oversee the dissection, reading from Galen's text of anatomy, ignoring the reality in front of his eyes, describing Galen's five-lobed liver and other erroneous anatomical structures. In the words of medical historian Dr. Erwin Ackerknecht, "such was the weight of binding tradition and authority."[13]

The Middle Ages were not devoid of true medical progress. Some incentive for changed thinking about disease came through the great Black Plague of 1348–1361, which resulted in mortality rates near 90 percent for those unlucky enough to contract the disease,[14] and killed about one-fourth of Europe's population during the Middle Ages.[15] The idea of a quarantine was instituted during the Middle Ages in an attempt to control such devastating killers. This disease could not be accounted for by the humoral thinking of Galen.

Deathblows to the medical philosophy of Galen began to occur during the Renaissance. At the dawn of this age, men of spectacular talents lent their work and thoughts to help establish a new lineage in medicine. The science of anatomy made the most outstanding progress during this era, but much was accomplished in the fields of therapeutics, surgery, and disease description. Fabulous anatomical drawings were produced by Leonardo da Vinci (1452-1519), and the diseases of small-pox, measles, plague, and syphilis were described by another gifted Italian, Fracastoro (1484-1553).[16]

The founder of modern anatomy is a title that has been assigned to Andereas Vesalius (1514-1564), a medical professor born in Belgium, educated in France, and based in Italy. Vesalius, whose innovative medical program utilized bedside teaching rather than simply mastering facts from medical texts, taught in Venice. Through his direct examination of the dissected body, Vesalius published the classic human anatomy text, De Humani Corporis Fabrica. Although Vesalius supported the theory of humors, his anatomical work flew in the face of Galenic ideals, and Vesalius consequently encountered terrific criticism from the medical establishment. This ultimately discouraged him to the point that he quit his research career and became court physician to the King of Spain.[17]

In the beautiful cemetery of St. Sebastian's Church in Salzburg, Austria, lies the body of the physician who may have provided the push to the first falling domino that led to the end of medical thought based on Galenic ideals. This Swiss/Austrian (1493-1541) was born Philippus Aureolus Theophrastus Bombastus von Hohenheim. Consistent with his seeming iconoclastic personality, he renamed himself, as Theophrastus Paracelsus.

Paracelsus is reported to have begun his teaching career at the University of Basel by letting everyone know exactly where he stood on certain established medical ideas. His approach was to publicly burn the works of Galen and other current medical authorities. The less than subtle action earned him the lasting hatred of many mainstream physicians of the day. Paracelsus displayed a deep intolerance for popular medical ideas and instead stressed experience and empirical treatments. His observations, for example, noted the relationship between mining and lung disease, a problem he observed in local coal miners.[18]

Paracelsus also practiced alchemy, the 16th century forerunner of modern chemistry, and experimented on the use of lead, sulfur, iron, potassium, and arsenic as medicinals. He replaced the Galenic model of humoral imbalance with his own alchemical theory. Paracelsus believed that the elements of salt, sulphur, and mercury were the source of both disease and healing.[19] He is also credited with being the originator of laudanum, an alcoholic extract of opium, and with using mercury for the treatment of syphilis as our friends Meriwether Lewis and William Clark did extensively.

Paracelsus' somewhat accurate medical thinking was sharply contrasted by his apparent construction of a new system of thought based not on science but on his own philosophies. He held many bizarre alchemical theories, such as the center of the sun being made of gold. He also supported the theory of "signatures," which stated that plants and mineral substances displayed some natural sign indicating a purpose for their medicinal use. For instance, St. John's Wort has red flowers that, because colored like blood, would be of use in treating wounds. The mineral topaz could be used to treat jaundice, due to its yellow coloration. Walnuts, with their rough surface, would help cranial ailments. Spotted lizard skin helped cure malignant tumors, and wart-like toads could treat the wart-like lesions of smallpox, syphilis, and other diseases manifesting themselves in skin papules. In spite of his ridiculous ideas about some things, Paracelsus made some real contributions to medical progress.

At the time that a wooden ship sailed from England to establish the Jamestown colony in the new world, and nearly two hundred years prior to the travels of Lewis and Clark, profound changes started to occur in the scientific world. Icons of physics such as Newton, Galileo, and Kepler did their landmark works in mathematics and astronomy, thus destroying such long held beliefs as that of the earth's being the center of the solar system. Chemists such as Robert Boyle (1627-1691) did fundamental work in proving the presence of oxygen in the atmosphere, and our dependence on it. Boyle's law concerning gases is still studied by every beginning chemistry student in the world. Acids and bases were also discovered. The 17th century was a watershed era in the development of scientific knowledge that would open doors to numerous medical secrets undiscovered since the dawn of time.

Medical science took a profound leap forward with the invention of the compound microscope, built by the Dutch lens maker Anton van Leewenhoek (1632-1723). Little did he know, that first day he peered at the tiny "animalcules" dancing in the drop of water under his glass lenses, that his device would open up the world of microscopic anatomy, pathology, and microbiology, all fundamental sciences of modern medicine.

Great progress was accomplished not only in studying the structure of the human body, but also in understanding its function. Physiology made great strides during the 1600s in understanding workings of organs such as the pancreas and gallbladder. The color change that differentiates venous and arterial blood was discovered to occur in the lungs. Robert Hooke (1635-1703) assured himself a hallowed spot in medical history by doing research into the physics of respiration. His greatest contribution, however, would come in formulation of the cell theory. This bedrock of modern biology basically states that all living organisms are made up of individually functioning cells. The presence of the microscopic blood vessels we call capillaries were first described by Marcello Malpighi (1628-1694). He also described the microscopic structure of lung, kidney, liver, skin, and spleen. The existence of the lymphatic system was described by several different scientists during the middle of the 1600s.

Perhaps the greatest discovery of the 17th century was that of the Englishman William Harvey (1578-1657) on the blood's circulation. Harvey studied the mechanical nature of the heart and its one-way valves, and showed that the blood circulates through the lungs in a one-way direction. With the addition of Malpighi's discovery of the capillaries, the circuit of the blood's course through the body was known. Harvey's discovery, like many throughout history, was met with enthusiastic condemnation by many authorities in the medical world. But his anatomical and qualitative evidence was overwhelming, and thus the ancient concepts that Galen had created concerning the heart and blood flow were finally put to rest.[20]

The 1600s also witnessed advances in the medical clinic. Thomas Sydenham (1624-1689) was touted as the "English Hippocrates." His return to an emphasis on observing the patient and the disease process was of paramount importance in advancing clinical medicine. Such was his stature as a physician that his medical books were still being issued in 1776 to American physicians. He also originated the idea of "morbific matter," the elusive and never-discovered, disease-producing substance.

Sydenham also employed a new medicine that had proven effective in the treatment of some illnesses manifested with fever. This medicine was the bark from the cinchona tree of Peru, first imported to England in the 1630s, and known as "Peruvian bark." The medicine was ground into a powder to be administered. We now know that this bark contains the chemical quinine, which is effective against the organism that causes malaria. Administering a medicine that cured a disease exclusive of other therapies helped disprove the ancient theories of imbalanced humors.

Although great strides occurred during the 1600s in basic medical science and clinical practice, a medical student of the day still was trained in nonscientific disciplines as a basis for developing medical judgment. Rhetoric, reasoning, philosophy, and mastering Latin were believed to be the building blocks of a sound medical mind.

One group of medical practitioners believed that life could not be explained in merely mechanical or chemical terms, and that something else was within living tissues, which made them alive. During the 1600s arguments about the nature of life raged across the continent of Europe. It would seem that these arguments are still occurring in the early 21st century.

Frederick Hoffman (1660-1742) of Germany was a staunch "mechanist," believing that the body consisted of "fibers" that could expand and contract, and were controlled by what he called a "nervous ether" emanating from the brain.[21] The "vitalists" gained new momentum in Germany under the work of Georg Stahl (1660-1734). Stahl believed that "anima" inhabited the living body and their actions prevented its death or "putrefaction." He felt that all living tissue responded to stimuli, which he used to support his vitalistic position.[22] Stahl was open in his disdain of anatomy and physiology, and the apparent mechanistic nature he believed they encouraged.

During the 18th century, the "ivory tower" of medical education was probably at the University of Leyden in Holland, which flourished under the charismatic and eclectic Hermann Boerhaave (1668-1738). In the estimation of many medical historians he was the most influencial physician of the first half of the 18th century. Boerhaave was a master of the arts, music, and literature, and a much beloved teacher. His emphasis on bedside clinical teaching and observation of the patient had a profound effect on medical education. His practical approach to medicine is summed up in his statement, "keep the head cool, the feet warm, and the bowels open."

For most English-speaking medical students in the 18th century, their best professional educational opportunity was to travel to Scotland's University of Edinburgh and study under the famous William Cullen (1710-1790) and John Brown (1735-1788). Although their theories, which reflected their fascination with stimuli and the body's response, should be considered of minor importance in the overall evolution of medical thought, they were on center stage in the 18th century. They would profoundly influence the thinking of a young American physician, Dr. Benjamin Rush, later the medical advisor of Meriwether Lewis.

Dr. William Cullen wrote the text *First Line of Physic* in 1776, which was popular for years in medical education. Cullen was a "vitalist" and proposed that all life existed in the form of what he called "nervous energy." He believed that disease was a disruption of this force. It must be noted that Cullen's view of medicine, although developed during a time of increasing knowledge of basic medical sciences, was still a system of philosophic medical practice. Although new in substance, it was similar in essence to systems concocted for centuries by medical theorists. It was built on a solitary concept of "nervous force" and, due to the immature state of chemistry and other basic sciences, it would go down in history as yet another vain attempt to explain the body and disease.[23]

Cullen's pupil John Brown (1735-1788) is a most interesting character. His theories, in retrospect, did not have much of a positive or lasting influence throughout the world, but his influence in early America was quite important. His theory was a direct extension of Cullen's, and proposed that all life consisted in a state of nervous stimulation, produced by both internal and external forces. The internal forces were emotions, muscular contractions, and sensory information. External forces were those of air temperature, diet, or the state of the air. A state of health depended on a proper balance of these factors, and disease resulted from underexcitation (asthenic diseases), or overexcitation (sthenic diseases) of the body. All disease was considered either "constitutional" or "local." Treatments within Brown's simplistic system were aimed at correcting these imbalances.[24] If a patient was suffering from overstimulation, he should be administered something to calm him. Brown's favorite treatment was opium. If excitation were insufficient, Brown's answer to the problem was to excite the patient a bit with some ethyl alcohol (not knowing that alcohol was a nervous system depressant). Apparently John Brown suffered from an extreme imbalance of stimulation as he died at the age of fifty-three, the result of his alcoholism and opium addiction. He should have taken the old adage to heart: "The physician who treats himself has a fool for a patient."

Additional treatments utilized during the period focused on ridding the diseased body of some illusive disease-causing elements. This was accomplished in a variety of ways. Cathartics and enemas could rid the elements from the intestines. Emetics could rid them from the stomach. Diuretics could increase urination, and diaphoretics could increase sweating. Blistering relieved congestion in the internal organs. Through the utilization of these medicines, both natural (herbs, ground-up beetles) and man-made concoctions of chemicals, it was thought that a proper balance could be achieved within the diseased body, thus producing a state of good health. There was little understanding of the physiology involved, and treatments were employed that supported the erroneous assumptions of the day.

American medicine embarked on its own path through the medical wilderness. Our isolation of three thousand miles from the shores of Europe, and the four-month, perilous journey required to get to American shores, created some unique and interesting situations in North America that led to our own brand of medical thought and practice. But some of our most prominent physicians gained their medical knowledge under the influence of teachings from such men as William Cullen and John Brown.

APPENDIX TWO

Medicines of the Lewis and Clark Expedition

Helpful Pharmacy Terms

Analgesics—drugs that produce pain relief.

Astringents—drugs that harden or contract tissues.

Carminatives—drugs that produce a feeling of comfort in the stomach and intestines and relieve the formation of gas.

Cathartic—acts on the intestines to stimulate bowel movements.

Counterirritants—drugs that act on the skin causing redness. They were believed to relieve inflammation in remote organs or tissues. By acting on the nerve endings in the skin they also relieve pain in remote organs.

Dermatitis—inflammation of the skin.

Diaphoretics—drugs that produce perspiration.

Diuretics—drugs that increase the production of urine in the kidneys.

Emetics—drugs that produce vomiting.

Emollients—drugs that soften and protect the skin.

Lavage—the act of washing a tissue with some solution.

Purgatives—drugs that stimulate bowel movements, same as cathartic.

Poultices—drugs that were applied to the skin to relieve pain or to dilate blood vessels on the skin, functioning as a counterirritant.

Resins—thick, sticky chemicals from the sap of various trees; many were dissolved in alcohol.

Stimulants—drugs that stimulate the patient, causing an increased level of consciousness, activity.

Tinctures—drugs mixed in an alcoholic solution of usually from 10 to 20 percent concentration.

Tonics—drugs that were thought to increase vigor and health.

Lewis & Clark's Medicine Chest

Assafoetic—ill-smelling (similar to garlic) Indian spice, used as a carminative to lessen abdominal distention, abdominal cramping. No documented use during the expedition.

Balsam copaiba—an oily, resinous substance from the South American leguminous tree, genus *Copaifera*, containing benzoic or cinnamic acid. Probably used as a carminative, diuretic, or orally as a treatment for gonorrhea. It is possible that this was also used in solution to lavage the penile urethra with a penile syringe in treatment of gonorrhea. It can also be used to treat contact dermatitis.

Balsamum traumaticum—This substance contains benzoin (a thickened sap from the Peruvian tree *Styrax benzoini*), aloes, and balsam of tolu, from the plant *Myroxylon balsamum* (a sticky reddish substance that dissolves in alcohol but not in water). Likely used to treat respiratory problems by increasing respiratory secretions, and in inflammations of the nose, throat, and bronchi.

Calamine ointment—mixture of zinc oxide and ferric oxide, used as an ointment to reduce skin irritations.

Calomel—mercurous chloride, used principally as a purgative. Increases bile duct secretion producing dark stools; also a diuretic; given orally, has an anti-syphilitic action; ingredient of Dr. Rush's Bilious Pills.

Cream of tartar—Derived from the juice of grapes and deposited in wine casks together with yeast, a purgative.

Dr. Rush's Bilious Pills—a potent combination of calomel and jalap. Used for many ills during the expedition. Lewis bought fifty dozen of them to take along!

Epispastric ointment—used to produce blisters on the skin to act as a counterirritant, which was thought to withdraw fluid from deeper tissue into the blister, thus competing with tissue excitability elsewhere. The active substance is a cantharide, obtained from dried beetles found in various temperate climates, especially in Spain and Italy.

Glauber's salts—Sodium sulfate, a saline cathartic.

Gum camphor—When taken internally it is a stimulant and diaphoretic. Obtained from the camphor tree, *Cinnamomum campho-*

ra, a large evergreen of the laurel family. Also used on skin diseases as a counterirritant, which causes mild skin irritation, a feeling of warmth, and analgesia for aches and pains.

Ipecacuan—From the roots of the Brazilian tree *Cephaelis ipecacua-naha*. A favorite of producing emesis, used sparingly on the expedition.

Jalap—a drastic cathartic obtained from the Mexican vine *Exogonium jalapa*. Among the ingredients of Dr. Rush's "Thunderclapper" pills.

Laudanum—tincture of opium, about a 10 percent opium solution. First concocted in 1510.

Magnesia—a cathartic magnesium salt.

Mercury ointment—the mainstay of syphilis treatment. Applied directly to the lesion and other areas. Patients were often treated until they showed signs of mercury poisoning such as excessive salivation or sore gums. Potentially curative, but highly toxic and unreliable.

Nutmeg, cloves, and cinnamon—used to flavor foul-tasting medicines as well as lessen the cramping action of cathartics.

Peruvian bark—The Corps took more of this than any other medicine, fifteen pounds in the powdered form. Obtained from the genus *Cinchona*, a tree of Peru; used as a tonic and in many concoctions for fever, snakebites, abdominal pain, and just about anything else. Contains quinine, which was effective against "ague" or malaria.

Rhubarb—a purgative, cathartic (powdered).

Sugar of lead—Lead acetate, used in eye washes. On the return trip, the captains traded medical services, especially this treatment, with Indians of the Columbia River drainage.

Tartar emetic—an antimony-potassium compound, with a sweet, metallic taste, which produces vomiting.

Tragacanth—a gummy exudate from the plant *Astragalum gummifor*, a non-greasy lubricant used in lotions, emollients.

Turkish opium—obtained from immature capsules of the opium poppy, *Papaver somniferum*, used to relieve pain, and as a sedative to lessen nervous excitability. Mixed with alcohol to make laudanum.

White vitriol—zinc sulfate, used with lead acetate in the captains' eye wash. The Corps carried only 4 ounces.

Wine (30 gallons) and whiskey—Medicinal (of course!), following Dr. Rush's Rx. They ran out of whiskey on the Fourth of July 1805.

Instruments and Other Supplies

Best lancets (3)—used to cut open a vein and get rid of that irritating blood!

Clyster syringe (1)—a large syringe used to administer enemas.

"Emplast. Diach. S."—Lead oleate, a plaster of lead probably used as a casting material, or to apply to the skin after it was spread with medication on muslin or leather.

Penis syringes (4)—Likely to adminster penile lavages of balsam of copaiba to treat gonorrhea. The journals do not mention the use of these items.

Pocket instruments—Likely small surgical instruments.

Teeth instruments—Dental instruments.

Tourniquet (1)

Patent lint—used to pack wounds, especially Capt. Lewis's gunshot in the buttocks.

Various canisters, tincture bottles, all stored in a walnut chest and a pine chest.

Notes

The primary source for quotations from expedition journals is Gary E. Moulton, ed., *Journals of the Lewis and Clark Expedition*, Volumes 2 through 11, published by University of Nebraska Press, Lincoln, from 1986 through 1997. Where the current text quotes from either Lewis or Clark and states the date of the quotation, the Moulton volumes are not footnoted, for the sake of simplicity.

Chapter 1: Politics and Passion

1. Stephen E. Ambrose, *Undaunted Courage: Meriwether Lewis, Thomas Jefferson, and the Opening of the American West* (New York: Simon & Schuster, 1996), p. 3.

2. Frederick Jackson Turner, *The Frontier in American History* (New York: Dover, 1996), p. 5.

3. Robert Leckie, *George Washington's War* (New York: Harper Collins, 1992), p. 14.

4. Michael B.A. Oldstone, *Viruses, Plagues, & History* (New York: Oxford University Press, 1998), p. 50.

5. Gary E. Moulton, ed., *The Journals of the Lewis & Clark Expedition* (Lincoln: University of Nebraska Press, Vols. 2-11, 1986-1997), vol. 10 (1996), p. 1.

Chapter 2: Meriwether Lewis and William Clark

1. Donald Jackson, ed., *Letters of the Lewis and Clark Expedition, with Related Documents*: 1783-1854, 2nd ed. (Urbana: University of Illinois Press, 1978), vol. 1, p. 17.

2. Stephen E. Ambrose, *Undaunted Courage: Meriwether Lewis, Thomas Jefferson, and the Opening of the American West* (New York: Simon & Schuster, 1996), p. 25.

3. Roy Appleman, *Lewis and Clark: Historic Places Associated with Their Transcontinental Exploration (1804-06)* (Washington: United States Department of the Interior, National Park Service, 1975), p. 52.

4. Ibid., p. 54.

5. John Alden, *A History of the American Revolution* (New York: DaCapo, 1969), pp. 438-441.

6. Ibid.

7. Ambrose, *Undaunted Courage*, p. 45.

8. Jackson, *Letters*, vol. 1, p. 2.

Chapter 3: Just Doing the Best We Can

1. Daniel J. Boorstin, *The Americans: The Colonial Experience* (New York: Oxford Univ. Press, 1997), p. 218.

2. Ibid., pp. 233-234.

3. Ibid., p. 237.

4. Ibid., p. 212.

5. One of the great scourges of mankind has been smallpox. This tiny virus, a bit of DNA wrapped inside a protein coat, exists in three forms that can produce disease of varying severity. A form present chiefly in cattle, called cowpox, is termed Variola vaccinae, and is usually very mild in humans. Another mild form termed *Variola minor* or *alastrim*, affects humans but is usually a minor childhood illness. The full-blown and virulent form is called *Variola major*.

6. As medicine advanced, new forms of the weakened smallpox virus were used in immunizing patients. Due to extensive immunization of the world's population, this once dreaded disease had its last reported case in the mid-1970s in Bangladesh and, in 1979, was declared "eradicated from nature" by the World Health Organization. Governments continue to keep the virus in labs, and it was reported in September 2000 that the former Soviet Union had developed an extensive program of biological warfare using the smallpox virus.

7. http://www.colonialhall.com/rush/rush.asp/

8. Both Drs. Shippen and Morgan would go on to serve as a Director-General of the Continental Army during the American Revolution. Morgan was ousted from that position by the Continental Congress due to his zealous and unappreciated attempts to improve the health of the troops. Shippen's military career was stained by charges of dishonesty, which included a court-martial for "Scandalous and infamous practices such are unbecoming the Character of an Officer and Gentleman." He was acquitted by one vote. C. Keith Wilbur, *Revolutionary Medicine 1700-1800* (Philadelphia: Chelsea House, 1980), p. 7.

9. Fermentation is defined according to *Stedman's Medical Dictionary*, 25th ed., as "A chemical change induced in a complex organic compound by the action of an enzyme, whereby the substance is split into simpler compounds," or, "In bacteriology, the anaerobic dissimilation of substrates with the production of energy and reduced compounds; the mechanism of fermentation does not involve a respiratory chain or cytochrome, hence oxygen is not the final electron acceptor as it is in oxidation."

10. E.G. Chuinard, *Only One Man Died: The Medical Aspects of the Lewis and Clark Expedition* (Washington: Ye Galleon Press, 1974), p. 130.

11. http://members.aol.com/Fever1793/ch1.html

12. http://www.colonialhall.com/rush/rush.asp

13. Benjamin Rush, letter of Sept. 10, 1793. http://www.members.aol.com/Fever1793/Kuhn.html

14. A.S. Blumgarten, M.D. *Textbook of Materia Medica*, 4th ed. (New York: Macmillan Co. 1927), p. 178-79. By the time of the expedition, Rush had combined his calomel and jalap and produce his "Bilious Pills of Dr. Rush" that were thought to be efficacious for nearly every known and unknown disease.

15. Chuinard, *Only One Man Died*, p. 137.

16. http://www.godstruthfortoday.org/ElhananWinchester/Winchester.019.html

17. Chuinard, *Only One Man Died*, p. 138.

Chapter 4: Into the Starting Blocks

1. Donald Jackson, ed., *Letters of the Lewis and Clark Expedition, with Related Documents: 1783-1854*, 2nd ed. (Urbana: University of Illinois Press, 1978), vol. 1, p. 54.

2. E.G. Chuinard, *Only One Man Died: The Medical Aspects of the Lewis and Clark Expedition* (Washington: Ye Galleon Press, 1979), p. 102.

3. DEET is the active ingredient in modern insect repellents. Its organic chemical name is N,N-diethyl-meta-toluamide.

4. Jackson, *Letters*, p. 55.

5. Ibid., p. 57.

6. Ibid., p. 103.

7. Ibid., p. 110.

8. Ibid., p. 112.

9. Paul Cutright, *Lewis and Clark: Pioneering Naturalists* (Lincoln: University of Nebraska Press, 1969), p. 26.

Chapter 5: "Misqutrs" on the Ohio

1. Robert B. Betts, *In Search of York: The Slave Who Went to the Pacific with Lewis and Clark* (Boulder: Colorado Associated University Press, 1985), p. 92.

2. George H. Yater and Carolyn Denton, "Nine Young Men from Kentucky," *We Proceeded On*, Publication No. 11 (May 1992), p. 4.

3. Ibid., p. 6.

4. Donald Jackson, ed., *Letters of the Lewis and Clark Expedition, with Related Documents: 1783-1854*, 2nd ed. (Urbana: University of Illinois Press, 1978), vol. 1, p. 367.

5. Yater and Denton, "Nine Young Men from Kentucky," pp. 7-8.

6. Ibid., p. 9.

7. Ibid., pp. 10-11.

8. Ibid., pp. 11-12.

9. Gary E. Moulton, ed., *The Journals of the Lewis & Clark Expedition* (Lincoln: University of Nebraska Press, Vols. 2-11, 1986-1997), vol. 2 (1986), pp. 513-515.

10. Ibid., p. 516.

11. Ibid., pp. 517-524.

12. E.G. Chuinard, *Only One Man Died: The Medical Aspects of the Lewis and Clark Expedition* (Washington: Ye Galleon Press, 1979), p. 173.

13. Malaria and ague are derivations from the Italian words "mal" and "aria," referring to bad air being the source of the disease. "Ague" reportedly is a corruption of the French term "aigu," meaning "sharp," a term that describes the rapid elevation in temperature that is characteristic of this disease.

14. Donald J. Krogstad, Chapter 264 "Plasmodium Species (Malaria)," in *Principles and Practice of Infectious Diseases*, Mandel et al., eds.; 5th ed (New York: Churchill Livingstone, 2000), vol. 2, p. 2819.

15. Ibid., p. 2818.

16. Carl Schreck, "Protection from Blood-Feeding Arthropods," in Paul S. Auerbach, ed., *Wilderness Medicine: Management of Wilderness and Environmental Emergencies*, 3rd ed. (St. Louis: Mosby, 1995), p. 823.

17. Jackson, *Letters*, vol. 1, p. 130.

18. W.H. Lewis and Memory P.F. Elvin-Lewis, *Medical Botany: Plants Affecting Man's Health* (New York: John Wiley & Sons, 1977), p. 363.

19. Chuinard, *Only One Man Died*, p. 190.

Chapter 6: Snakes in the Grass and Bugs in the River

1. P. Erik Gundersen, *The Handy Physics Answer Book* (Farmington Hills, MI: Visible Ink Press, 1999), pp. 332-334.

2. Robert R. Hunt, "Tents Shreds & Pieces," *We Proceeded On*, Vol. 22, No. 1 (February 1996), p. 4.

3. Gary E. Moulton, ed., *The Journals of the Lewis & Clark Expedition* (Lincoln: University of Nebraska Press, Vols. 2-11, 1986-1997), vol. 2 (1986), p. 299 note.

4. H. Dupont and H. Backer, Chapter 42 "Infectious Diarrhea from Wilderness and Foreign Travel," in Paul S. Auerbach, ed., *Wilderness Medicine: Management of Wilderness and Environmental Emergencies*, 3rd ed. (St. Louis: Mosby, 1995), pp. 1048-1049.

5. Ibid.

6. Ibid.

7. Ibid., p. 1051.

8. Ibid., pp. 1051-1053.

9. Ibid., p. 1053.

10. Moulton, ed., *Journals of the Lewis & Clark Expedition*, vol. 2, p. 325 note.

11. J.B. Sullivan, Jr., et al., Chapter 28 "North American Venomous Reptile Bites," in P.S. Auerbach, ed., *Wilderness Medicine*, 3rd ed. (St. Louis: Mosby, 1995), p. 681.

12. Ibid., p. 688. Venom potency is measured in the amount it takes to kill 50 percent of experimental animals it is injected into, in milligrams of venom per kilograms of victim's weight.

13. Ibid., pp. 685-687.

14. Ibid., p. 685.

15. The antivenin antibodies are produced by horses that have been injected with small amounts of crotalid venom. The horse's immune system recognizes the rattlesnake venom as a foreign invader and starts producing antibodies to combat it. After several weeks, the horse blood is collected and the horse serum is purified and manufactured into commercial antivenin.

Chapter 7: The Sun and Dying Young

1. R. Hubbard, et al., "Heat-Related Illness," in Paul S. Auerbach, ed., *Wilderness Medicine: Management of Wilderness and Environmental Emergencies*, 3rd ed. (St. Louis: Mosby, 1995), pp. 168-169.

2. Ibid., p. 173.

3. Ibid.

4. Ibid., p. 169.

5. James P. Ronda, *Lewis & Clark Among the Indians* (Lincoln: University of Nebraska Press, 1984), p. 16.

6. Donald Jackson, ed., *Letters of the Lewis and Clark Expedition, with Related Documents: 1783-1854*, 2nd ed. (Urbana: University of Illinois Press, 1978), vol. 1, p. 50.

7. Ronda, *Lewis & Clark Among the Indians*, pp. 30-31.

8. B. Tuckman, "Developmental Sequence in Small Groups," *Psychological Bulletin*, vol. 63, no. 6 (1965), pp. 384-399.

9. W. Silen, "Acute Appendicitis," in Petersdorf, et al., eds., *Harrison's Principles of Internal Medicine*; 10th ed. (New York: McGraw-Hill, 1983), p. 1768.

10. M.L. Callahan, "Bites and Injuries Inflicted by Mammals," in Auerbach, ed., *Wilderness Medicine*, 3rd ed., p. 955.

11. J. Cross, Jr., R. Penn, Chapter 216 "Francisella tularensis (Tularemia), in Mandel, et al., eds., *Principles and Practice of Infectious Diseases*; 5th ed. (New York: Churchill Livingstone, 2000), vol. 2, pp. 2395-2397.

12. Ibid., p. 2401.

13. Ibid., p. 2399.

14. Ronda, *Lewis & Clark Among the Indians*, pp. 23-26.

15. Moulton, ed., *Journals of the Lewis & Clark Expedition*, vol.11 (1997), p. 72.

16. Ibid., vol. 9 (1995), p. 68

17. Ibid., vol. 11 (1997), p. 85.

18. Ronda, *Lewis & Clark Among the Indians*, pp. 44-51.

19. Ibid., p. 52.

Chapter 8: They Should Have Danced All Night

1. F. Cartwright, and M. Biddiss, *Diseases & History*, 2nd ed. (Great Britain: Sutton Publishing Company, 2000), p. 44.

2. Ibid.

3. E.C. Tramont, Chapter 27 "Treponema pallidum (Syphilis)," in Mandel, et al., eds., *Principles and Practice of Infectious Diseases*; 5th ed. (New York: Churchill Livingstone, 2000), vol. 2, pp. 2476-2477.

4. Ibid., pp. 2477-2482.

5. Ibid.

6. Ibid.

7. John S. Haller and Robin M. Haller, *The Physician and Sexuality in Victorian America* (Urbana: University of Illinois Press, 1974), p. 262.

8. Ibid., p. 267.

9. C. Klaasen, "Heavy Metals and Heavy-Metal Antagonist," in Goodman & Gilman, *The Pharmacological Basis of Therapeutics*; 10th ed. (New York: McGraw Hill, 2001), p. 1858.

10. Ibid., p. 1860.

11. P. Sparling and H. Hansfield, Chapter 200 "Neisseria gonorrhea," in Mandel, et al., eds., *Principles and Practice of Infectious Diseases*; 5th ed. (New

York: Churchill Livingstone, 2000), vol. 2, pp. 2242-2255.

Chapter 9: Cold Toes and a Baby Boy

1. James P. Ronda, *Lewis & Clark Among the Indians* (Lincoln: Univ. of Nebraska Press, 1984), p. 73.

2. Ibid., p. 75.

3. Gary E. Moulton, ed., *The Journals of the Lewis & Clark Expedition* (Lincoln: University of Nebraska Press, Vols. 2-11, 1986-1997), Vol. 3 (1987), map p. 202.

4. S. McCauley, et al., Chapter 7 "Frostbite," in Auerbach, ed., *Wilderness Medicine*, 4th ed. (St. Louis: Mosby, 2001), pp. 178-194.

5. Ibid., p. 186.

6. Stephen E. Ambrose, *Undaunted Courage: Meriwether Lewis, Thomas Jefferson, and the Opening of the American West* (New York: Simon & Schuster, 1996), p. 195.

Chapter 10: Wild Times in Old Montana: Act One

1. F.M. Seesee, D.E. Worley, "Taenia ovis krabbei" from "Grizzly Bears, Ursus artos, in Montana and Adjacent Areas," *Proceedings of Helminthological Society*, Washington Vol. 53, No. 2 (1986), pp. 298-300.

2. Keith Aune, Ph.D., Montana Fish, Wildlife & Parks, Wildlife Research Lab, Montana State University, Bozeman, MT, conversation with author, September 2000.

3. E.G. Chuinard, *Only One Man Died: The Medical Aspects of the Lewis and Clark Expedition* (Washington: Ye Galleon Press, 1979), p. 159.

4. Petersdorf, et al., eds., *Harrison's Principles of Internal Medicine*; 10th ed. (New York: McGraw-Hill, 1983), p. 466-467.

5. Ibid.

6. Gary E. Moulton, ed., *The Journals of the Lewis & Clark Expedition* (Lincoln: University of Nebraska Press, Vols. 2-11, 1986-1997), vol. 4 (1987), p. 156, note.

Chapter 11: Wild Times in Old Montana: Act Two

1. Gary E. Moulton, ed., *The Journals of the Lewis & Clark Expedition* (Lincoln: University of Nebraska Press, Vols. 2-11, 1986-1997), vol. 4 (1987), p. 269, note.

2. Paul M. Dewick, *Medicinal Natural Products: A Biosynthetic Approach*

(New York: John Wiley & Sons, 1997), pp. 418-419.

3. Moulton, ed., *Journals*, vol. 11 (1997), p. 214

Chapter 12: From a Torrent to a Trickle

1. A.D. Nell and J. E. Taylor, *Lewis and Clark in the Three Rivers Valleys* (Tucson: The Patrice Press, 1996), p. 274.

2. WD. Gentile, "A Tick Borne Disease," in Paul S. Auerbach, ed., *Wilderness Medicine: Management of Wilderness and Environmental Emergencies*, 3rd ed. (St. Louis: Mosby, 1995), p. 804.

3. Ronald V. Loge, "Two Dozes of Bark's and Opium: Lewis and Clark as Physicians," *We Proceeded On,* Feb. 1997, p. 15.

4. Ibid.

5. Ronald V. Loge, "Acute Hepatitis Associated with Colorado Tick Fever, *Western Journal of Medicine*, Vol. 142 (1985), p. 91, as cited in Mandel, et al., eds., *Principles and Practice of Infectious Diseases*; 5th ed. (New York: Churchill Livingstone, 2000), vol. 2, pp. 1695-1696.

6. Tom Schwan, Ph.D., Rocky Mountain Labs: Hamilton, Montana, conversation with author, September 2000.

7. Moulton, ed., *Journals*, vol. 11 (1997), p. 257.

8. Ambrose, *Undaunted Courage*, p. 275.

9. Biddle, Nicholas, ed. *The Journals of the Expedition Under the Command of Capts. Lewis and Clark*; 2 vols. (New York: The Heritage Press, 1962), vol. 2, p. 233.

Chapter 13: No Place for Mockersins

1. W.H. Lewis and Memory P.F. Elvin-Lewis, *Medical Botany: Plants Affecting Man's Health* (New York: John Wiley & Sons, 1977), p. 193.

2. Paul M. Dewick, *Medicinal Natural Products: A Biosynthetic Approach* (New York: John Wiley & Sons, 1997), pp. 160-161, 165.

3. Gary E. Moulton, ed., *The Journals of the Lewis & Clark Expedition* (Lincoln: University of Nebraska Press, Vols. 2-11, 1986-1997), vol. 11 (1997), p. 216.

4. Ibid., vol. 10 (1996), p. 135.

5. Ibid., vol. 11, p. 295; vol. 9 (1995), p. 216.

6. Ibid., vol. 9, p. 216.

7. Ibid., p. 218.

8. Ibid., vol. 11, p. 300.

9. Ibid., p. 301.

10. Ibid., p. 306.

11. Ibid., vol. 10, p. 139.

12. Ibid., p. 141.

13. Ibid., p. 142.

14. Ibid., p. 143.

15. Biddle, Nicholas. *The Journals of the Expedition Under the Command of Capts. Lewis and Clark*; 2 vols. (New York: The Heritage Press, 1962), Vol. 2, p. 272.

16. Moulton, ed., *Journals*, vol. 10, p. 143

17. Moulton, ed., *Journals*, vol. 5 (1988), p. 214, note.

18. E.G. Chuinard, *Only One Man Died: The Medical Aspects of the Lewis and Clark Expedition* (Washington: Ye Galleon Press, 1979), pp. 160-161.

19. Aune, Keith, Ph.D., Wildlife Research Lab, Bozeman, Montana. Conversation with author, September 2000.

20. C.H. King, Chapter 250 "Cestodes (Tapeworms)," in Mandel et al., eds., *Principles and Practice of Infectious Diseases*; 5th ed (New York: Churchill Livingstone, 2000), vol. 2, p. 2957.

21. Ibid., p. 2963.

22. Ibid., pp. 2958-2959.

23. B.J. Bogitsch and T.C. Cheng, *Human Parasitology*; 2nd ed. (San Diego: Academic Press, 1998), pp. 373-374.

24. Moulton, ed., *Journals*, vol. 11, p. 369

25. Moulton, ed., *Journals*, vol. 5 (1998), p. 291, note.

Chapter 14: A Winter of Pore Elk and Flees

1. Gary E. Moulton, ed., *The Journals of the Lewis & Clark Expedition* (Lincoln: University of Nebraska Press, Vols. 2-11, 1986-1997), vol. 6 (1997), p. 74.

2. Moulton, ed., *Journals*, vol. 11 (1997), p. 405.

3. T. Butler, Chapter 218 "Yersina Species," in G. Mandel, et al., eds., *Principles and Practice of Infectious Diseases*; 5th ed. (New York: Churchill Livingstone, 2000), vol. 2, pp. 2406-2409.

4. Ibid., pp. 2050-2055.

5. Moulton, ed., *Journals*, vol. 11, p. 407.

6. Ibid., vol. 6, p. 416.

7. Ibid., p. 75.

8. Ibid., p. 239

9. Ibid., p. 356.

10. Ibid., p. 416.

11. Ibid., p. 240.

12. Ibid.

13. Ibid., p. 65.

14. Ibid., p. 74.

15. Ibid., p. 142.

16. Ibid., p. 429-430.

17. Ibid., pp. 447, 459.

Chapter 15: A Clash of Cultures

1. Stephen E. Ambrose, *Undaunted Courage: Meriwether Lewis, Thomas Jefferson, and the Opening of the American West* (New York: Simon & Schuster, 1996), p. 357.

2. This may have been Haystack Butte, Klickitat County, Washington, directly opposite the Deschutes River. Gary E. Moulton, ed., *The Journals of the Lewis & Clark Expedition* (Lincoln: University of Nebraska Press, Vols. 2-11, 1986-1997), vol. 7 (1991), p. 159, note.

Chapter 16: Frontier Doctor and Medical Diplomats

1. James P. Ronda, *Lewis & Clark Among the Indians* (Lincoln: Univ. of Nebraska Press, 1984), p. 105.

2. Gary E. Moulton, ed., *The Journals of the Lewis & Clark Expedition* (Lincoln: University of Nebraska Press, Vols. 2-11, 1986-1997), vol. 9 (1995), p. 299.

3. Paul Cutright, *Lewis and Clark: Pioneering Naturalists* (Lincoln: University of Nebraska Press, 1969), p. 285.

4. C. Keith Wilbur, *Revolutionary Medicine 1700-1800* (Philadelphia: Chelsea House, 1980), p. 25.

5. A.S. Blumgarten, M.D., *Textbook of Materia Medica*, 4th ed. (New York: The Macmillan Co., 1927), p. 166.

6. W.H. Lewis and Memory P.F. Elvin-Lewis, *Medical Botany: Plants Affecting Man's Health* (New York: John Wiley & Sons, 1977), pp. 316, 333, 348, 353.

7. Moulton, ed., Journals, vol. 7, p. 285, note.

8. Petersdorf, et al., eds., *Harrison's Principles of Internal Medicine*; 10th ed. (New York: McGraw-Hill, 1983), p. 2159.

9. Harold Cook, Chapter 6 "From the Scientific Revolution to the Germ

Theory," in Irving Loudin, ed., *Western Medicine* (New York: Oxford University Press, 1997), p. 88.

Chapter 17: Wild Times in Old Montana: Act Three

1. W.H. Lewis and Memory P.F. Elvin-Lewis, *Medical Botany: Plants Affecting Man's Health* (New York: John Wiley & Sons, 1977), p. 374.

2. Gary E. Moulton, ed., *The Journals of the Lewis & Clark Expedition* (Lincoln: University of Nebraska Press, Vols. 2-11, 1986-1997), vol. 8 (1993), pp. 87-88, 235 note.

3. I sometimes sit on my property near Stonewall Creek, outside Lincoln, Montana, by an immense ponderosa pine with a diameter of more than three feet, which was clearly growing for centuries prior to the time that Lewis walked through the Blackfoot Valley. Given where he camped near Beaver Creek, which is less than a mile away, Lewis could have walked by my tree, now unofficially designated "The Meriwether Lewis Memorial Ponderosa Pine."

4. Moulton, ed., *Journals*, vol. 8, p. 133, note.

5. Ibid., vol. 9, p. 342.

6. Ibid., vol. 8, p. 137, note.

Chapter 18: Near Disaster and Then...

1. E.G. Chuinard, *Only One Man Died* (Washington: Ye Galleon Press, 1979), p. 395

2. Ann Rogers, "Was it the Pawpaws?" *We Proceeded On*, vol. 13, pp. 17-18.

3. Gary E. Moulton, ed., *The Journals of the Lewis & Clark Expedition* (Lincoln: University of Nebraska Press, Vols. 2-11, 1986-1997), vol. 9 (1995), p. 365.

4. Donald Jackson, ed., *Letters of the Lewis and Clark Expedition, with Related Documents: 1783-1854*, 2nd ed. (Urbana: University of Illinois Press, 1978), vol. 1, pp. 319-20.

5. Moulton, *Journals*, vol. 9, p. 366.

Chapter 19: Ghosts of Explorations Past

1. Gary E. Moulton, ed., *The Journals of the Lewis & Clark Expedition* (Lincoln: University of Nebraska Press, Vols. 2-11, 1986-1997), vol. 2 (1986), p. 516.

2. George H. Yater and Carolyn Denton, "Nine Young Men From Kentucky," *We Proceeded On*, May 1992, p. 3.

3. Ibid., p. 4.

4. Ibid., p. 7.

5. Ibid., p. 8.

6. Moulton, ed., *Journals*, vol. 2, p. 513.

7. Ibid., p. 515.

8. Merrill G. Burlingame, *The Montana Frontier* (Helena: State Publishing Company, 1942), pp. 9-12.

9. Yater and Denton, "Nine Young Men From Kentucky," p. 10.

10. Burlingame, *The Montana Frontier*, p. 10.

11. Robert E. Lange, "William Bratton: One of Lewis and Clark's Men," *We Proceeded On*, Vol. 7 No. 1 (February 1981), p. 8.

12. Moulton, ed., *Journals*, vol. 2, p. 515.

13. Ibid., p. 518.

14. Ibid., p. 519.

15. Ibid.

16. Ibid.

17. Ibid., pp. 521-522; Carolyn Denton, "George Shannon of the Lewis and Clark Expedition: His Kentucky Years," *We Proceeded On*, Vol. 18, No. 2 (May 1992), p. 21.

18. Moulton, ed., *Journals*, vol. 2, p. 525.

19. Ibid., p. 524.

20. Roy Appleman, *Lewis and Clark: Historic Places Associated with Their Transcontinental Exploration (1804-06)* (Washington: United States Department of the Interior, National Park Service, 1975), p. 252.

21. Ibid.

22. Moulton, ed., *Journals*, vol. 2, p. 513; Appleman, p. 249.

23. Stephen E. Ambrose, *Undaunted Courage: Meriwether Lewis, Thomas Jefferson, and the Opening of the American West* (New York: Simon & Schuster, 1996), p. 460.

24. Chuinard, E.G., "How Did Meriwether Lewis Die? It Was Murder," *We Proceeded On*, Vol. 17 No. 3 (August 1991), pp. 4-11; Vol. 17 No. 4 (November 1991); Vol. 18 No. 1 (January 1992), pp. 4-7.

25. Chuinard, "It Was Murder," Vol. 17 No. 4, p. 7.

26. Ibid., p. 8.

27. S. Oake, et al., eds., *Malaria: Obstacles and Opportunities* (Washington, DC: National Academy Press, 1991), p. 38

28. Donald J. Krogstad, Chapter 264 "Plasmodium Species (Malaria)" in Mandel, et al., eds., *Principles and Practice of Infectious Diseases*; 5th ed. (New

York: Churchill Livingstone, 2000), vol. 2, pp. 2819, 2821-2823.

29. Ibid., p. 2822.

30. Ibid., p. 2819.

31. Ibid., p. 2824.

32. Reimert Thorolf Ravenholt, "Self Destruction on the Natchez Trace: Meriwether Lewis's Act of Ultimate Courage," *Columbia: The Magazine of Northwest History*, Vol. 13, No. 2 (Summer 1999), pp. 3-6.

33. Lewis P. Rowland, *Merritt's Textbook of Neurology*; 8th ed. (Philadelphia: Lea & Febiger 1989), p. 152.

34. E. Tramont, Chapter 227 "Treponema pallidum (Syphilis)," in Mandel, et al., eds., *Principles and Practice of Infectious Diseases*; 5th ed. (New York: Churchill Livingstone, 2000), vol. 2, pp. 2474-2482.

35. E.G. Clark and N. Danbolt, "The Oslo Study of the Natural Course of Untreated Syphilis," cited in Mandel, et al., eds., *Principles and Practice of Infectious Diseases*; 5th ed., vol. 2, p. 2477.

36. D.H. Rockwell, A.R. Yobs, M.B. Moore, "The Tuskeegee Study of Untreated Syphilis: The 30th Year of Observation," *Archives of Internal Medicine*, Vol. 114 (1964), p. 792, cited in Mandel, et al., eds., *Principles and Practice of Infectious Diseases*; 5th ed., vol. 2, pp. 2477-2478.

37. Ravenholt, "Self Destruction on the Natchez Trace," p. 6.

38. *Diagnostic and Statistical Manual of Mental Disorders*, 4th ed. (Washington, DC: American Psychiatric Association, 1994), p. 340.

Chapter 20: Fiddles and Friendships

1. Gary E. Moulton, ed., *The Journals of the Lewis & Clark Expedition* (Lincoln: University of Nebraska Press, Vols. 2-11, 1986-1997), vol. 11 (1997), p. 7.

2. Joseph A. Mussulman, "Men in High Spirits: Humor on the Lewis and Clark Trail," *We Proceeded On*, Vol. 22, No. 2 (May 1996), pp. 10-16.

3. *Outside Magazine*, Vol. XXV, No. 12 (December 2000).

Appendix One: Riddles of Nature

1. Erwin Ackerknecht, *A Short History of Medicine* (Baltimore: Johns Hopkins Univ. Press, 1982), p. 12.

2. Ibid., p. 47.

3. Ibid., p. 52.

4. Ibid., p. 54.

5. Roy Porter, ed., *Medicine: A History of Healing* (New York: Marlowe &

Company, 1997), pp. 20, 21, 122, 173, 196.

6. Ackerknecht, *A Short History of Medicine*, p. 61.

7. Irvin Loudin, ed., *Western Medicine: An Illustrated History* (Oxford: Oxford Univ. Press, 1997), pp. 35-36.

8. Ibid., pp. 40, 48, 55, 75.

9. Ackerknecht, *A Short History of Medicine*, pp. 73-79.

10. Ibid., pp. 73-77.

11. Ibid.

12. Ibid.

13. Ibid., p. 90.

14. T. Butler, Chapter 218 "Yersinia Species, Including Plague," in Mandel, et al., eds., *Principles and Practice of Infectious Diseases*, 5th ed. (New York: Churchill Livingstone, 2000), vol. 2, p. 2406.

15. Cartwright & Biddiss, *Disease and History* (New York: Sutton Publishing, 1972), p. 22.

16. Ackerknecht, *A Short History of Medicine*, pp. 94-104.

17. Ibid., pp. 103-105.

18. Ibid., pp. 105-108.

19. Roberto Margotta, *The History of Medicine* (New York: Smithmark Publishers, 1996), pp. 82, 86.

20. F.E. Udwadia, *Man and Medicine: A History* (New York: Oxford University Press, 2001), p. 222.

21. Ackerknecht, *A Short History of Medicine*, p. 129.

22. Loudin, ed., *Western Medicine*, p. 88.

23. Lester S. King, *The Medical World of the Eighteenth Century* (Chicago: The University of Chicago Press, 1958), Chapters 3 & 4.

24. Fielding Garrison, *An Introduction to the History of Medicine*, 3rd ed. (Philadelphia: W.B. Saunders, 1924), pp. 319, 320; Johannes Hermann, translated by H.E. Handerson, *The History of Medicine and the Medical Profession* (New York: J.H. Vail & Co., 1889), pp. 634, 637.

Bibliography

Ackerknecht, Erwin H. *A Short History of Medicine*; rev. ed. Baltimore: The Johns Hopkins University Press, 1982.

Alden, John. *A History of the American Revolution*. New York: DaCapo, 1969.

Ambrose, Stephen E. *Undaunted Courage: Meriwether Lewis, Thomas Jefferson, and the Opening of the American West*. New York: Simon & Schuster, 1996.

Appleman, Roy E. *Lewis & Clark Historic Places Associated with Their Transcontinental Exploration 1804-1806*. Washington, D.C.: National Park Service, 2000.

Auerbach, Paul S. *Wilderness Medicine: Management of Wilderness and Environmental Emergencies*; 3rd ed. St. Louis: Mosby, 1995.

Auerbach, Paul S., ed. *Wilderness Medicine*; 4th ed. St. Louis: Mosby, 2001.

Betts, Robert B. *In Search of York: The Slave Who Went to the Pacific with Lewis and Clark*. Boulder, CO: Associated University Press, 1985.

Biddle, Nicholas, ed. *The Journals of the Expedition Under the Command of Capts. Lewis and Clark*; volumes 1 & 2. New York: The Heritage Press. 1962.

Blumgarten, A.S. *Textbook of Materia Medica*, 4th ed. New York: The Macmillan Company, 1927.

Bogitsch, B.J., and T.C. Cheng. *Human Parasitology*; 2nd ed. San Diego: Academic Press, 1998.

Boorstin, Daniel J. *The Americans: The Colonial Experience*. New York: Vintage Books, 1958.

Brinkley, Douglas. *History of the United States: American Heritage*. New York: Viking, 1998.

Brown, Harold W. *Basic Clinical Parasitology*; 4th ed. New York: Appleton-Century-Crofts, 1975.

Burlingame, M.G. *The Montana Frontier*. Helena: State Publishing Company, 1942.

Cartwright, Frederick F. & Michael Biddiss. *Disease & History*, 2nd ed. New York: Sutton Publishing, 1972.

Chuinard, E.G. *Only One Man Died: The Medical Aspects of the Lewis and Clark Expedition*. Washington: Ye Galleon Press, 1979.

Cook, Harold, ed. *Western Medicine* (New York: Oxford University Press, 1997.

Cunningham, Noble E., Jr. *In Pursuit of Reason: The Life of Thomas Jefferson*. New York: Ballantine Books, 1987.

Cutright, Paul R. *Lewis & Clark: Pioneering Naturalists*. Lincoln and London: University of Nebraska Press, 1969.

Davison, Forrest R. *Handbook of Materia Medica, Toxicology, and Pharmacology*; 4th ed. St. Louis: The C.V. Mosby Company, 1949.

Dewick, Paul M. *Medicinal Natural Products: A Biosynthetic Approach*. Chichester: John Wiley & Sons, 1997.

Diagnostic and Statistical Manual of Mental Disorders; 4th ed. Washington, DC: American Psychiatric Association, 1994.

Drake, Daniel, ed. by Norman D. Levine. *Malaria in the Interior Valley of North America*. Urbana: Univ. of Illinois Press, 1964.

Garrison, F. *An Introduction to the History of Medicine*; 3rd ed. Philadelphia: W.B. Saunders, 1924.

Goodman and Gilman. *The Pharmacological Basis of Therapeutics*; 10th ed. New York: McGraw-Hill, 2001.

Gordon, Maurice. *Aesculapius Come to the Colonies*. New Jersey: Ventnor Publishers, 1949.

Gundersen, P. Erik. *The Handy Physics Answer Book*. Farmington Hills, MI: Visible Ink Press, 1999.

Haller, John S., Jr., and Robin M. Haller. *The Physician and Sexuality in Victorian America*. Urbana: Univ. of Illinois Press, 1974.

Hermann, J., translated by H.E. Handerson. *The History of Medicine and the Medical Profession*. New York: J.H. Vail & Co., 1889.

Jackson, Donald, ed. *Letters of the Lewis and Clark Expedition with Related Documents, 1783-1854*. 2 volumes. Urbana: Univ. of Illinois Press, 1978.

King, Lester S. *The Medical World of the Eighteenth Century*. Univ. of Chicago Press, 1958.

Leckie, Robert. *George Washington's War: The Saga of the American Revolution*. New York: HarperCollins Publishers, 1992.

Lewis, Walter H., and Memory P.F. Elvin-Lewis. *Medical Botany: Plants Affecting Man's Health*. New York: John Wiley & Sons, 1977.

Loudin, Irvine, ed. *Western Medicine: An Illustrated History*. Oxford Univ. Press, 1997.

Mandel, Douglas, and Bennett, eds. *Principles and Practice of Infectious Diseases*; 5th ed. 2 volumes. New York: Churchill Livingstone, 2000.

Margotta, Roberto. *The History of Medicine*. New York: Smithmark Publishing, 1996.

Moulton, Gary E., ed. *The Journals of the Lewis & Clark Expedition*. 13 volumes. Lincoln: Univ. of Nebraska Press, 1986-2000.

Nell, Donald F., and John E. Taylor. *Lewis and Clark in the Three Rivers Valleys*. Tucson: The Patrice Press, 1996.

Oldstone, Mechael B.A. *Viruses, Plagues, & History*. Oxford Univ. Press, 1998.

Petersdorf, et al., eds. *Harrison's Principles of Internal Medicine*; 10th ed. New York: McGraw-Hill, 1983.

Porter, Roy, ed. *Medicine: A History of Healing, Ancient Traditions to Modern Practices*. New York: Marlowe & Company, 1997.

Ronda, James P. *Lewis and Clark Among the Indians*. Lincoln: Univ. of Nebraska Press, 1984.

Rowland, L.P., ed. *Merritt's Textbook of Neurology*; 8th ed. Philadelphia: Lea & Febiger, 1989.

Smith, A.W., and J.N. Cooper. *Elements of Physics*; 9th ed. New York: McGraw-Hill Book Company, 1979.

Turner, F.J. *The Frontier in American History*. New York: Dover, 1996.

We Proceeded On. Journal of The Lewis and Clark Trail Heritage Foundation. Great Falls, Montana.

Wilbur, C. Keith. *Revolutionary Medicine 1700-1800*. Philadelphia: Chelsea House, 1980.

Udwadia, F.E.. *Man and Medicine: A History*. New York: Oxford University Press, 2000.

Voyles, Bruce A. *The Biology of Viruses*. St. Louis: Mosby, 1993.

Index

action of 65; ineffective uses 89, 92, 160, 161, 227, 304

Philadelphia 31, 49; Benjamin Rush in 40, 41-45; Lewis in 46-47, 48-52

Philanthropy River: See Ruby River

Pierre, SD 110

Pioneer Mountains 262

Pirogues 137, 155, 166; cached 159, 272; destroyed 272; purchased 57, 60-61

Pittsburgh 52, 54

Plague 314; bilious 44-45; bubonic 220

Plasmodium 62, 63-64, 65, 294-295; *P. falciparum* 63-64, 294; *P. malariae* 63; *P. ovale* 63-64, 294-295; *P. vivax* 63-64, 294-295

Platte River 96-97, 287

Pleurisy 129-130

Plums 81, 99

Pneumonia 26, 74, 229, 237, 273, 289, 290, 304

Pneumothorax 269-270

Point William 233

Pompey: See Charbonneau, Jean Baptiste

Potassium 49, 94-95, 161, 208, 315-316, 323

Potassium bitartrate 245

Potassium nitrate 96, 166, 226

Potlatch River 245

Potts, John 73, 78, 173, 263, 287; injured 256, 257, 261-262, 280-281

Poultices 89, 129-130, 252-253; defined 148

Prickly Pear Creek 174

Prickly Pear Valley 173-174

Primaquine 65

Pronghorn 138, 142, 143-144, 175

Pryor Mountains 287

Pryor, MT 287

Pryor, Nathaniel 58, 109, 173, 227; after expedition 286-287; dislocated shoulder 124-125, 179, 218; leads horse party 258; out alone 69-70

Pryor, OK 287

Psychiatry 46, 251, 252

Pythagoras 310

Quinine 65, 66, 92, 227, 318

Rabbits 72, 110; as disease source 106, 144-145

Rainbow Falls 266-267

Raspberries 88, 99

Rattlesnakes 153-154, 165-166, 170, 173, 241; action of venom 89-92; rattles of 90, 134

Red osier dogwood 233

Redman, John 40

Reed, Moses 59, 100-101, 135

Return party 73, 135, 137

Rhubarb 49, 323

Rickettsia 178-179, 221

Rifles: See Arms and ammunition

Ritalin 277

RNA 178

Robertson, John 59, 74-75

Rocky Mountain spotted fever 178-179, 221

Rocky Mountains 22, 131, 135, 155-156, 159, 171, 195; eastward crossing 253, 255-258; Lewis "sees" for first time 155-156; westward crossing 197-208

Rogers, Ann 281

Ronda, James 99-100, 242-243

Ross's Hole 262

Ruby River 181

Rush, Benjamin 97; biography 38-46; bloodletting theory 42-43, 45-46, 95-96, 97; formula of Dr. Rush's Pills 51; trains Lewis 47, 48-49

Russell, Gilbert 292

Ryan Dam 266-267

Sacagawea 138, 142, 154, 190, 201-202, 221, 258; after expedition 278, 290; early life 131-132; at Fort Clatsop 223, 229; gives birth 133-134; ill 159-162, 166-167; information of 147-148, 175, 176-177, 179, 182, 263; and Shoshones 186

Saccacommis 233

Sacramento, CA 289-290

Sage tea 130

St. Charles, MO 282

St. Louis 69, 258-259, 282-283; Lewis in 71, 73, 75

St. Peters River 98

Salish Indians 195

Salmon; as disease source 208-209; dried 184, 205, 206, 211, 213, 218, 228; purchased 193; scarcity 234; seasonal runs 206

Salmon River 188-189

Salmon, ID 184

Salmonella 86

Salt 223, 229, 315-316

Salt Camp 222

Saltpeter: See Potassium nitrate

Santa Barbara, CA 140

Sapphire Mountains 262

Sarsaparilla 116

Saskatchewan River 268

Sassafras 116

Sauk Indians 82-83

Scannon: See Seaman

Sciatic nerve 276, 277

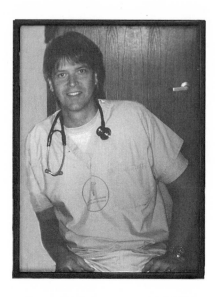

David J. Peck is a board certified physician in Family Practice who currently practices in the Urgent Care Department of the Sharp Rees-Stealy Medical Group in San Diego, California. He also holds Bachelor's and Master's degrees in Biology/Secondary Education from Arizona State University and taught high school biology prior to obtaining his medical degree at Western University of Health Sciences.

Dr. Peck is an avid outdoorsman and has family roots in the Helena, Montana, area, where he frequently explores the Lewis and Clark trail. He is a popular speaker on the medical aspects of the Lewis and Clark Expedition. His audiences have included the University of California at San Diego/Wilderness Medicine Society annual conference in Colorado, medical groups, chapter meetings of the Lewis and Clark Trail Heritage Foundation, and visitors to the Lewis and Clark National Historic Trail Interpretive Center in Great Falls, Montana. He lives with his wife, Marti, a clinical psychologist, in San Diego.